Sports Nutrition

Vitamins and Trace Elements

NUTRITION in EXERCISE and SPORT

Editors, Ira Wolinsky and James F. Hickson, Jr.

Published Titles

Nutrients as Ergogenic Aids for Sports and Exercise
Luke Bucci

Nutrition in Exercise and Sport, 2nd Edition
Ira Wolinsky and James F. Hickson, Jr.

Exercise and Disease
Ronald R. Watson and Marianne Eisinger

Nutrition Applied to Injury Rehabilitation and Sports Medicine
Luke Bucci

Nutrition for the Recreational Athlete
Catherine G.R. Jackson

NUTRITION in EXERCISE and SPORT

Editor, Ira Wolinsky

Published Titles

Nutrition, Physical Activity, and Health in Early Life
Jana Pařízková

Exercise and Immune Function
Laurie Hoffman-Goetz

Sports Nutrition: Minerals and Electrolytes
Constance Kies and Judy Driskell

Nutrition and the Female Athlete
Jaime S. Ruud

Body Fluid Balance: Exercise and Sport
E.R. Buskirk and S. Puhl

Sports Nutrition: Vitamins and Trace Elements
Ira Wolinsky and Judy A. Driskell

Forthcoming Titles

Biochemical Methods for Exercise Assessment
Jon Karl Linderman

Amino Acids and Proteins for the Athlete — The Anabolic Edge
Mauro G. Di Pasquale

Sports Nutrition
Vitamins and Trace Elements

Edited by

Ira Wolinsky, Ph.D.
University of Houston
Houston, Texas

Judy A. Driskell, Ph.D.
University of Nebraska
Lincoln, Nebraska

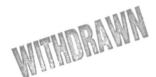

CRC Press
Boca Raton   New York   London   Tokyo

Publisher:	Robert B. Stern
Project Editor:	Renee Taub
Marketing Manager:	Susie Carlisle
Direct Marketing Manager:	Becky McEldowney
Cover design:	Jason Toemmes
PrePress:	Kevin Luong
Manufacturing:	Sheri Schwartz

Library of Congress Cataloging-in-Publication Data

Sports nutrition : vitamins and trace elements / edited by Ira
    Wolinsky, Judy A. Driskell.
        p. cm. — (Nutrition in exercise and sport)
      Includes bibliographical references and index.
      ISBN 0-8493-8192-4 (alk. paper)
      1. Vitamins in human nutrition. 2. Trace elements in nutrition.
    3. Athletes—Nutrition. I. Wolinsky, Ira. II. Driskell, Judy A.
    (Judy Anne) III. Series.
    QP771.S68   1996
    613.2'8—dc20

                                        96-27158
                                           CIP

No claim to original U.S. Government works
International Standard Book Number 0-8493-8192-4
Library of Congress Card Number 96-27158
Printed in the United States of America 1 2 3 4 5 6 7 8 9 0
Printed on acid-free paper

DEDICATION

This book is dedicated to all the athletes and others who, by their questions, have encouraged researchers to expand knowledge of the relationships between nutrition and exercise. Those who have approached the co-editors have helped us to realize the need for a book relating vitamin and trace element nutrition to athletic performance. We thank them for their encouragement. We also thank the authors for contributing the excellent chapters found in this book.

The CRC Series on Nutrition in Exercise and Sport provides a setting for in-depth exploration of the many and varied aspects of nutrition and exercise, including sports. The topic of exercise and sports nutrition has been a focus of research among scientists since the 1960s, and the healthful benefits of good nutrition and exercise have been appreciated. As our knowledge expands, it will be necessary to remember that there must be a range of diets and exercise regimes that will support excellent physical condition and performance. There is not a single diet-exercise treatment that can be the common denominator, or the single formula for health, or panacea for performance.

This Series is dedicated to providing a stage upon which to explore these issues. Each volume provides a detailed and scholarly examination of some aspects of the topic, and, as such, will be of interest to professionals as well as educated laymen.

Contributors from any bona fide area of nutrition and physical activity, including sports and the controversial, are welcome.

I and Dr. Judy Driskell are pleased to add our contribution to the Series. We trust you will find it timely and useful.

Ira Wolinsky, Ph.D.
Series Editor

This book addresses the relationships of vitamin and trace element needs and interactions to sports and exercise. A body of research indicates that work capacity, oxygen consumption, and other measures of physical performance of individuals including athletes are affected by deficiency or borderline deficiency of specific vitamins or essential trace elements. Athletes as well as the public in general often have low dietary intakes of many of the vitamins and essential trace elements. The findings of some researchers indicate that large doses of certain vitamins and trace elements given to individuals who had adequate status of that vitamin or trace element improved various measures of physical performance. Other researchers have reported conflicting findings. A critical review of these reports is included in this book.

This volume includes a collection of chapters written by scientists from several academic disciplines who have expertise in an area of vitamin or trace element nutrition as it relates to sports and exercise. The book reviews the convincing evidence that exists that exercise and sport activities do affect the vitamin and trace element status of individuals and vice versa. Following an Introduction, are reviews of exercise and sports as they relate to Ascorbic Acid, Thiamin, Riboflavin and Niacin, Vitamin B_6, Folate and Vitamin B_{12}, Pantothenic Acid and Biotin, Vitamin A and Carotenoids, Vitamins D and K, Vitamin E, Iron, Zinc, Copper, Chromium, Selenium, as well as Other Substances in Foods, and ending with a Summary. Researchers, practitioners, and students will benefit from reading the book.

Editors
Ira Wolinsky, Ph.D.
Judy A. Driskell, Ph.D.

Ira Wolinsky, Ph.D. is a Professor of Nutrition at the University of Houston. He received his B.S. degree in Chemistry from the City College of New York in 1960 and his M.S. (1965) and Ph.D. (1968) degrees in Biochemistry from Kansas University. He has served in research and teaching positions at the Hebrew University (Medical School and Faculty of Agriculture), the University of Missouri, and Pennsylvania State University, as well as conducting basic research in NASA life sciences facilities.

Dr. Wolinsky is a member of the American Institute of Nutrition and the American Society for Clinical Nutrition, among other honorary and scientific organizations.

Dr. Wolinsky has contributed numerous nutrition research papers in the open literature. His current major research interests relate to the nutrition of bone and calcium and to sports nutrition. He has been the recipient of research grants from both public and private sources.

Dr. Wolinsky has co-authored a book on the history of the science of nutrition, *Nutrition and Nutritional Diseases. The Evolution of Concepts,* and co-edited the CRC Press volume *Nutrition in Exercise and Sport* and the volume *Nutritional Concerns of Women.* He is also editor of the *CRC Series* on *Modern Nutrition* and the *CRC Series on Nutrition in Exercise and Sport* and co-editor of the *CRC Series on Methods in Nutrition Research.*

Judy Anne Driskell, Ph.D., R.D., is Professor of Nutritional Science and Dietetics at the University of Nebraska.

Dr. Driskell received her B.S. degree in Biology in 1965 from the University of Southern Mississippi in Hattiesburg. Her M.S. and Ph.D. degrees were obtained from Purdue University in Indiana in 1967 and 1970, respectively. She served as an Assistant Professor of Nutrition and Foods at Auburn University in Alabama from 1970 to 1972, an Assistant Professor of Foods and Nutrition at Florida State University in Tallahassee from 1972 to 1974, an Associate Professor and Professor of Human Nutrition and Foods at Virginia Polytechnic Institute and State University in Virginia from 1974 to 1989, and Professor of Nutritional Science at the University of Nebraska in Lincoln from 1989 to present. She was the Nutrition Scientist for the U.S. Department of Agriculture/Cooperative State Research Service in Washington, D.C. in 1981 to 1982, and part-time in 1985.

Dr. Driskell is a member of numerous professional organizations including the American Institute of Nutrition, the American Society for Clinical Nutrition, the Institute of Food Technologists, and the American Dietetic Association. In 1993 she received the Professional Scientist Award of the Food Science and Human Nutrition Section of the Southern Association of Agricultural Scientists. In addition, she was the 1987 recipient of the Borden Award for Research in Applied Fundamental Knowledge of Human Nutrition. She served as a member and chair of the Subcommittee for Human Nutrition of the Experiment Station Committee on Policy and Organization from 1981 to 1987. She is listed as an expert in B-complex vitamins by the Vitamin Nutrition Information Service.

Dr. Driskell recently co-edited the CRC book *Sports Nutrition: Minerals and Electrolytes* with Constance V. Kies (deceased). She has published about 100 refereed research articles and 10 book chapters as well as several publications intended for lay audiences and has given numerous professional and lay presentations. Her current research interests center around vitamin metabolism and requirements, including the interrelationships between exercise and water-soluble vitamin requirements.

CONTRIBUTORS

Jenna Anding, Ph.D., R.D.
Department of Human Development
University of Houston
Houston, Texas

John Beard, Ph.D.
Department of Nutrition
Pennsylvania State University
University Park, Pennsylvania

Mallory L. Boylan, Ph.D., R.D.
Department of Education, Nutrition,
  Restaurant Hotel Management
Texas Tech University
Lubbock, Texas

Luke R. Bucci, Ph.D., R.D., C.C.N.
Weider Nutrition Group
Salt Lake City, Utah

Barbara Mc. Chrisley, Ph.D., R.D.
Department of Health Services
Radford University
Radford, Virginia

Judy A. Driskell, Ph.D., R.D.
Department of Nutritional Science and
  Dietetics
University of Nebraska
Lincoln, Nebraska

Roger Fielding, Ph.D.
Department of Health and Science
Boston University
Boston, Massachussets

Nader Fotouhi. Ph.D.
USDA — Human Nutrition Research
Center on Aging
Tufts University
Boston, Massachussets

Andrea M. Frederick, M.S.
Department of Nutritional Science and
  Dietetics
University of Nebraska
Lincoln, Nebraska

Robert E. Keith, Ph.D., R.D., F.A.C.S.M.
Department of Nutrition and Food
  Science
Auburn University
Auburn, Alabama

Dorothy Klimis-Tavantzis, Ph.D., R.D.
Department of Food Science and Human
  Nutrition
University of Maine
Orono, Maine

Nancy M. Lewis, Ph.D., R.D., F.A.D.A.
Department of Nutritional Science and
  Dietetics
University of Nebraska
Lincoln, Nebraska

Richard D. Lewis, Ph.D., R.D.
Department of Foods and Nutrition
The University of Georgia
Athens, Georgia

Henry C. Lukaski, Ph.D.
Grand Forks Human Nutrition Research
  Center
Agricultural Research Service
U.S. Department of Agriculture
Grand Forks, North Dakota

Kenneth McMartin, Ph.D.
Department of Pharmacology and
  Therapeutics
Louisiana State University Medical
  Center
Shreveport, Louisiana

Mohsen Meydani, D.V.M., Ph.D.
USDA — Human Nutrition Research
Center on Aging
Tufts University
Boston, Massachussets

James J. Peifer, Ph.D.
Department of Foods and Nutrition
The University of Georgia
Athens, Georgia

Philip G. Reeves, Ph.D.
*Grand Forks Human Nutrition Research
  Center
Agricultural Research Service
U.S. Department of Agriculture
Grand Forks, North Dakota*

David A. Sampson, Ph.D.
*Department of Food Science and
  Nutrition
Colorado State University
Ft. Collins, Colorado*

Julian F. Spallholz, Ph.D.
*Department of Education, Nutrition,
  Restaurant Hotel Management
Texas Technical University
Lubbock, Texas*

Maria Stacewicz-Sapuntzakis, Ph.D.
*Human Nutrition and Dietetics
University of Illinois at Chicago
Chicago, Illinois*

Elizabeth A. Thomas, Ph.D., R.D.
*Department of Human Nutrition, Foods, and
  Exercise
Virginia Polytechnic Institute and State
  University
Blacksburg, Virginia*

Brian W. Tobin, Ph.D.
*Division of Basic Medical Sciences
Mercer University School of Medicine
Macon, Georgia*

Ira Wolinsky, Ph.D.
*Department of Human Devleopment
University of Houston
Houston, Texas*

TABLE OF CONTENTS

Chapter 1

INTRODUCTION

Luke R. Bucci

CONTENTS

I. INTRODUCTION

Pursuit of excellence in sports and exercise demands sustained and/or peak outputs of bioenergetic functions of muscles and integration of the musculoskeletal, bioenergetic, neuroendocrine, psychological, and immune systems. Fuel (carbohydrates, fats, amino acids, and their metabolic byproducts), water, and electrolytes (sodium, potassium, calcium, magnesium, chloride, and phosphate) are required for all systems to operate efficiently. The effects of these macronutrients on exercise have been extensively studied, and clear guidelines for maintenance of optimum performance by macronutrient manipulation or supplementation have been consistently observed, reported, and recommended.[1-6]

0-8493-8192-4/97/$0.00+$.50
© 1997 by CRC Press, Inc.

All cells of the human body require relatively small amounts (intakes from micrograms to milligrams per day) of certain biochemical compounds (classified as vitamins) and a few atomic elements (classified as essential trace minerals) to enable all body systems to utilize fuel, water, and electrolytes for everyday survival, including exercise.

This introductory chapter will briefly familiarize the reader with the vitamins and minerals discussed in successive chapters. Any redundancy with other chapters was deemed useful by the editors to provide convenience and reinforcement. Emphasis here will be placed on results of multiple vitamin/mineral supplementation trials on nutrient status and exercise performance, since other chapters are devoted to single nutrients. The variables affecting research on exercise and nutrients will be explored, with consideration of biological variability and statistical power. This knowledge is extremely important to generate accurate conclusions from the available data. Furthermore, indirect relationships of vitamins and trace minerals with other body systems that influence exercise performance will be mentioned. One example is maintenance of immune functions, which may prevent minor illnesses or infections from delaying the effects of training or competitions.

Some of the conclusions of this chapter may seem at variance with other reviews. Unlike other reviews, this chapter has analyzed more published journal papers on the effects of multiple vitamin/mineral supplements, utilized statistical power analysis retrospectively (also unique), rated studies according to their scientific merit by a scale designed for human drug trials (also unique), and considered other measurements of performance. When more data and analyses are available, a more accurate assessment of results becomes obvious. Before discovery of the microscope, there was no direct proof for the existence of germs. Of course germs were always there, awaiting more focused attention. This chapter has simply focused more attention on the effects of multiple vitamin/mineral supplements on exercise than previous attempts. Naturally, new conclusions are a direct outgrowth of new data.

II. IDENTITY AND ROLES OF VITAMINS AND TRACE MINERALS

Vitamins are an extremely diverse range of biochemical compounds which have been classified by legislative definitions rather than biochemical functions. For example, vitamins were originally supposed to be coenzyme factors for essential enzyme functions. However, vitamins A, C, D, and E function via noncoenzymatic or hormonal mechanisms for their major roles. These disparate functions mean that some vitamins and trace minerals remain untested for specific effects on exercise performance because they do not participate directly in intermediary metabolism.

Table 1 lists each vitamin with brief descriptions of its roles, functions, dietary needs, deficiency symptoms, populations at risk for deficiency symptoms, and major dietary sources. For further information on each vitamin, the reader is referred to several reviews that have been published recently.[3,7-13] Generally speaking, the B vitamins function as enzyme activators, while the fat-soluble vitamins function without enzymes. Vitamins A and C function with and without enzymes.

Table 2 lists the trace minerals known to be essential, and a few that await confirmation of essentiality in humans. Again, the reader is referred to several recent reviews on trace minerals for further information.[3,12-19] Daily trace mineral needs are in the microgram to milligram range, as opposed to hundreds of milligrams to grams for other essential minerals. Like B vitamins, most trace minerals are involved with enzyme activation or function, forming metalloenzymes.

TABLE 1 Roles, Functions, Deficiency Symptoms, and Dietary Sources of Vitamins

Vitamin A (Retinol Equivalents, Carotenoid Precursors)

Roles:	Vision, differentiation and maintenance of epithelial tissues (skin, bone, cartilage, loose connective tissues, linings), immune responses, growth, reproduction, anticarcinogens
Functions:	Retinols: visual purple formation and operation, hormone-like activation of genes, cofactor for sugar transport in glycosylation reactions; electron transfer coenzyme for membrane stability Carotenoids: antioxidants, precursor for retinol
Dietary Needs:	The 1995 RDI for vitamin A is 5000 International Units (IU) = 1000 Retinol Equivalents (RE) (1 RE = 1 μg all-*trans* retinol or 6 μg all-*trans* beta-carotene) for adults
Deficiency Symptoms:	Night blindness, xerophthalmia, Bitot's spots, keratomalacia, follicular hyperkeratosis of skin, phrynoderma, impaired immune functions, decreased resistance to infections, impaired wound healing, bone loss, decreased cytokine response
Deficiency Risk:	Malnourished, severe injuries (trauma, burns, fractures), liver damage, long-term TPN, chronic fat malabsorption syndromes, alcoholics, elderly, anorexics, dieters, zinc and vitamin E deficiencies
Dietary Sources:	Retinol: nutritional supplements, fish liver oils, liver, organ meats, whole eggs, fortified dairy products, small whole fish Carotenoids: nutritional supplements, *Dunaliella* algae, red palm oil, carrots, green leafy vegetables, yams, sweet potatoes, papayas, mangoes, peaches, oranges

Vitamin B$_1$ (Thiamin)

Roles:	Energy production from foodstuffs, especially carbohydrates
Functions:	Coenzyme for transketolase (pentose phosphate pathway), pyruvate dehydrogenase and α-ketoglutarate dehydrogenases (entry of acetyl groups and α-ketoglutarate into tricarboxylic acid cycle)
Dietary Needs:	The 1995 RDI for thiamin is 1.5 mg for adults (0.5 mg/1000 kcal)
Deficiency Symptoms:	Early: fatigue, loss of appetite, nausea, constipation, irritability, mental depression, peripheral neuropathy Moderate = Wernicke-Korsakoff Syndrome: ataxia, loss of fine motor control, mental confusion, loss of eye coordination, sonophobia Severe = beriberi: muscular weakness, muscular atrophy, edema, heart failure
Deficiency Risk:	Malnutrition or starvation, malabsorption syndromes, alcoholism, elderly, restricted diets, increased metabolic rate (pregnancy, lactation, fever, infection, trauma), prolonged hemodialysis, gastric partitioning surgery, and inherited thiamin-responsive metabolic disorders
Dietary Sources:	Nutritional supplements; nutritional yeasts, *Spirulina* algae, rice bran, rice polish, wheat germ, pork, enriched grains and grain products (cereals), legumes (beans, peas, soybeans, lentils) Other meats, milk and milk products, fruits, and vegetables have lower amounts of thiamin but can be a significant source if consumed in large quantities Excessive ingestion of certain raw freshwater fish and shellfish, tea, coffee, blueberries, and red cabbage should be avoided, as these foods may contain antithiamin factors

Vitamin B$_2$ (Riboflavin)

Roles:	Energy production and cellular respiration
Functions:	Unique component of coenzymes flavin adenine dinucleotide (FAD) and flavin mononucleotide (FMN), essential for large number of redox reactions, releasing energy from carbohydrates, fats, and amino acids (proteins)

TABLE 1   Roles, Functions, Deficiency Symptoms, and Dietary Sources of Vitamins (continued)

Dietary Needs:	The 1995 RDI for riboflavin is 1.7 mg for adults (0.6 mg/1000 kcal)
Deficiency Symptoms:	Scaly dermatitis, glossitis, angular cheilitis (fissures at corner of mouth), alopecia, cataracts, depression, photophobia
Deficiency Risk:	Malnourished; malabsorption syndromes, elderly, hypothyroidism, increased metabolic rate (trauma, fever, infection, pregnancy, lactation)
Dietary Sources:	Nutritional supplements, nutritional yeasts, meats and dairy products, green leafy vegetables, enriched grains and grain products

Niacin, Niacinamide (Nicotinic Acid, Nicotinamide)

Roles:	Energy production, cellular respiration, fat synthesis
Functions:	Unique component of coenzymes nicotinamide adenine dinucleotide (NAD) and nicotinamide adenine dinucleotide phosphate (NADP), essential for many redox reactions, releasing energy from breakdown of carbohydrates, fats, and amino acids (proteins); glycogen synthesis
Dietary Needs:	The 1995 RDI for niacin is 20 mg for adults [6.6 Niacin Equivalents (NE) per 1000 kcal (1 NE = 1 mg niacin)]
Deficiency Symptoms:	Early: fatigue, muscular weakness, anorexia, indigestion, skin eruptions, depression, headaches, irritability, limb pains
	Severe = pellagra: glossitis, tremors, diarrhea, dementia, dermatitis with dark pigmentation (3 D's), confusion, memory impairment
Deficiency Risk:	Alcoholics; malnourished, malabsorption, elderly, low food intake, high consumption of corn with little protein, high consumption of sorghum or millet, increased metabolic rate (trauma, fever, infection, pregnancy, lactation)
Dietary Sources:	Dietary sources of niacinamide are expressed as niacin equivalents, taking into account tryptophan's contribution
	Richest sources (per serving) include nutritional supplements, nutritional yeasts, meats; legumes including peanuts, enriched cereals; potatoes

Vitamin B_6 (Pyridoxine, Pyridoxal, Pyridoxamine)

Roles:	Amino acid metabolism and energy production
Functions:	Unique component of coenzyme pyridoxal phosphate, essential for numerous reactions involving transamination (transfer of amino groups), deamination (removal of amino groups), desulfuration (transfer of sulfhydryl groups), decarboxylation (removal of organic acid group), cofactor for lysyl oxidase (collagen and elastin maturation), heme formation, conversion of tryptophan to niacin, glycogen breakdown, eicosanoid synthesis, one-carbon metabolism, hormone modulation, gluconeogenesis, neurotransmitter synthesis
Dietary Needs:	The 1995 RDI for vitamin B_6 is 2.0 mg for adults
Deficiency Symptoms:	Early: irritability, nervousness, depression, peripheral neuropathy, sideroblastic anemia, acne, fatigue, irritability, nervousness
	Severe: peripheral neuritis, convulsions, nausea, vomiting, dermatitis, mucous membrane lesions, alopecia, sideroblastic anemia, arthritis, cheilosis, conjunctivitis, numbness, paresthiasis, seizures
Deficiency Risk:	Pregnancy, lactation, oral contraceptive users, alcoholism, inherited metabolic disorders, malabsorption, malnourished, isoniazid therapy for tuberculosis, penicillamine therapy
Dietary Sources:	Nutritional supplements, nutritional yeasts, potatoes, meats, wheat germ, bananas, legumes, fortified cereal products

Vitamin B_{12} (Cobalamins, Cyanocobalamin, Hydroxocobalamin, Cobamamide)

Roles:	Prevention of anemia and neuropathy, cell division (DNA synthesis)
Functions:	Essential for one-carbon metabolism and recycling of folate, breakdown of odd-chain fatty acids and branched-chain amino acids
Dietary Needs:	The 1995 RDI for vitamin B_{12} is 6.0 µg for adults

TABLE 1   Roles, Functions, Deficiency Symptoms, and Dietary Sources of Vitamins (continued)

Deficiency Symptoms:	Mental depression, pernicious anemia (macrocytic anemia), fatigue, shortness of breath, weakness, peripheral neuropathy followed by irreversible neurological damage, constipation, gastrointestinal disturbances, glossitis, headaches, irritability, numbness, palpitations, spinal cord degeneration
Deficiency Risk:	Malabsorption disorders, loss of gastric acidity, loss of ileum surface, long-term, strict vegetarians
Dietary Sources:	Dietary sources for cobalamins are strictly from animal foodstuffs. Vitamin B_{12} is not found in plant foodstuffs. Dietary supplements can also contain vitamin B_{12}.

Folic Acid (Folate, Folacin, Folinic Acid, Pteroylglutamates)

Roles:	Blood cell formation and cell division (DNA synthesis)
Functions:	Primary carrier of one-carbon units used for numerous biosynthetic events
Dietary Needs:	The 1995 RDI for folate is 400 µg for adults
Deficiency Symptoms:	Macrocytic anemia (fatigue, weakness, shortness of breath), gastrointestinal symptoms, glossitis, depressed ankle jerks, anorexia, apathy, constipation, growth impairment, headaches, insomnia, memory impairment, restless legs, loss of vibratory sensation in legs
Deficiency Risk:	vitamin B_{12} deficiency, malnourished, malabsorption, pregnant and lactating women, increased rate of cellular division (burns, trauma, malignancies, hemolytic anemias), alcoholics, anticonvulsant therapy (phenytoin, barbiturates, primidone), folate antagonist therapy (methotrexate, 5-fluorouracil, pyrimethamine), tuberculosis therapy (isoniazid plus cycloserine), oral contraceptive users; sulfasalazine therapy, elderly, infants, inherited folate disorders
Dietary Sources:	Nutritional supplements, legumes, vitamin-fortified cereals, green leafy vegetables, wheat germ, seeds, nuts, liver

Pantothenic Acid (Pantothenate)

Roles:	Energy production from carbohydrates, fats, amino acids (proteins)
Functions:	Unique component of coenzyme A, essential for entry of carbohydrates, fats and amino acids (proteins) into tricarboxylic acid cycle; coenzyme A used in many biosynthetic pathways
Dietary Needs:	The 1995 RDI for pantothenate is 10 mg for adults
Deficiency Symptoms:	Anorexia, burning feet, impaired coordination, depression, eczema, fatigue, hypotension, infections, insomnia, irritability, muscle spasms, nausea, nervousness
Deficiency Risk:	Malnourished, malabsorption, greatly increased metabolic rate (trauma).
Dietary Sources:	Nutritional supplements, nutritional yeast, meats, legumes, whole grain products, wheat germ, vegetables, nuts, seeds

Biotin

Roles:	Energy production and fat metabolism
Functions:	Biosynthesis of fatty acids, replenishment of tricarboxylic acid cycle, gluconeogenesis
Dietary Needs:	The 1995 RDI for biotin is 300 µg for adults
Deficiency Symptoms:	Fatigue, muscle weakness and pain, dermatitis (especially nose and mouth), depression, hair loss, anemia, anorexia, nausea, hypercholesterolemia, hyperglycemia, insomnia, gray skin, pale smooth tongue
Deficiency Risk:	Persons consuming excessive amounts of raw egg whites, inherited disorders of biotin metabolism, extended total parenteral nutrition (biotin-free), loss of enteric gut microflora from antibiotic therapy or altered gut motility, pregnant and lactating women, antiepileptic drug therapy, alcoholics, trauma (burns and surgery), elderly, malabsorption (especially achlorhydria)
Dietary Sources:	Nutritional supplements, liver, egg yolk, nutritional yeast, royal jelly, legumes, rice bran, whole grains, fish

TABLE 1   Roles, Functions, Deficiency Symptoms, and Dietary Sources of Vitamins (continued)

Vitamin C (Ascorbic acid)

Roles:	Enzyme cofactor, water-soluble antioxidant, reducing agent
Functions:	Xenobiotic detoxification; collagen modifications; hydroxylations; synthesis of carnitine, catecholamines, neurotransmitters, and vasoactive amines; folate metabolism; tyrosine metabolism; interaction with tocopherol and glutathione; sulfating agent; cyclic nucleotide metabolism; eicosanoid metabolism
Dietary Needs:	The 1995 RDI for vitamin C is 60 mg for adults
Deficiency Symptoms:	Early: fatigue, decreased immune functions, muscle weakness, increased lipid peroxidation, elevated plasma histamine, altered eicosanoid and catecholamine metabolism, mineral imbalances, hypercholesterolemia, depression
	Severe = scurvy: tiredness, malaise, joint and bone pains, loose teeth, impaired wound healing, bleeding gums, easy bruising, irritability, depression, anemia, edema
Deficiency Risk:	Malnourished, elderly, pregnancy, lactation, dietary lack of fruits or vegetables, smokers, acute emotional or environmental stresses, high-dose aspirin, oral contraceptive users
Dietary Sources:	Nutritional supplements, willow leaves, acerola fruit, rose hips, peppers, citrus fruits, cruciferous vegetables, green leafy vegetables, berries, potatoes, tomatoes

Vitamin D (Calciferols)

Roles:	Precursor for 1,25-dihydroxycholecalciferol, bone mass formation and maintenance, calcium absorption, immune response
Functions:	Enhances intestinal absorption of calcium, phosphorus, magnesium; maintain calcium homeostasis, aiding in bone mass maintenance; activation of immune system cells; differentiation of bone marrow cells
Dietary Needs:	The 1995 RDI for vitamin D is 400 IU (10 µg cholecalciferol) for adults
Deficiency Symptoms:	Bone loss, increased fracture risk, secondary hyperparathyroidism, depressed immune responses severe = rickets, osteomalacia
Deficiency Risk:	Malnourished, elderly, pregnancy, lactation, fat malabsorption syndromes
Dietary Sources:	Sunlight, nutritional supplements, fish liver oil, fortified dairy products

Vitamin E (Tocopherols)

Roles:	Lipid antioxidant
Functions:	Removes oxidative species before cell structures are damaged (anticarcinogen, immune function, neurological function)
Dietary Needs:	The 1995 RDI for vitamin E is 30 IU tocopherol equivalents (TEs) (1 mg RRR-d-alpha tocopherol = 1 TE = 1.49 IU) for adults
Deficiency Symptoms:	Neurological degeneration, hemolysis, immune impairment, lipofuscin accumulation, increased risk of cancer, increased risk of cardiovascular disease, retinopathy, neuromuscular defects
Deficiency Risk:	Malnourished, elderly, pregnancy, lactation, fat malabsorption syndromes, preterm infants, abetalipoproteinemia, cirrhosis, zinc deficiency
Dietary Sources:	Nutritional supplements, fish liver oil, wheat germ oil, rice bran oil, nuts, seeds, vegetable oils, whole grains, green leafy vegetables, margarine

Vitamin K (Phylloquinones)

Roles:	Cofactor for gamma-carboxyglutamyl synthetases, redox reactions
Functions:	Gamma-carboxylated proteins necessary for blood clotting, bone formation, calcium binding
Dietary Needs:	The 1995 RDI for vitamin K is 80 µg for adults
Deficiency Symptoms:	Impaired blood clotting, bone loss (osteoporosis)

TABLE 1   Roles, Functions, Deficiency Symptoms, and Dietary Sources of Vitamins (continued)

Deficiency Risk:	Malnourished, elderly, fat malabsorption syndromes, neonates, coumarin administration, antibiotic sterilization of gut, long-term TPN, salicylate therapy
Dietary Sources:	Nutritional supplements; green leafy vegetables

III. ASSESSMENT TECHNOLOGIES OF VITAMIN AND TRACE MINERAL STATUS

Determining the status of vitamins and trace minerals in individual humans is a daunting task. Table 3 lists some of the current methodologies that are being used to assess vitamin and trace mineral status.[20-25] Each method leaves much to be desired as a reliable measure of status. Vitamins and trace minerals function *intracellularly*, but their usual analysis is performed on extracellular fluids because of ease of collection. While low levels of vitamins or trace minerals in extracellular fluids usually signify a deficient status throughout the body, it is not a guarantee of deficient status since some tissues may avidly retain enough vitamins or minerals to function adequately.[12,13] Ideally, an assay would reflect *intracellular function* of a nutrient for each individual. Validation of such assays are difficult, since other comparative methods of assessment may be inferior.

An analogy of Galileo with the first telescope comes to mind. With his new and more sensitive assessment tool, Galileo saw rings around Saturn. Of course, the rings could not be verified without a telescope, so it remained easy for disbelievers to attribute the observed rings to the telescope or Galileo's imagination, and not to Saturn. Ultimately, the best method of assessment of status for many nutrients remains a clinical trial of supplementation.[13,24] As long as delivery of nutrient to cells can be verified, any resulting changes in functions (cell, tissue, organ, or whole-body system) can be assumed to have repleted a deficient functional status or perhaps augmented adequate status.

Another difficulty with assessment of vitamin and trace mineral status in populations is the large degree of normal biological variation. Often, the variation requires large numbers of subjects in order to reach statistical power — an event which has seldom been attained and which will be discussed in more detail in this chapter.

IV. EFFECTS OF MICRONUTRIENT DEFICIENCIES ON EXERCISE PERFORMANCE

Effects of micronutrient deficiencies on exercise performance have been studied for many years, and will be discussed in detail in subsequent chapters. Usually, decreases in physical performance are found when one or more vitamins and/or trace minerals are known to be deficient, based on an extended lack of dietary intakes or reduced serum levels.[26-38] These findings were first demonstrated in the 1940s, before fortification of refined foods with iron and a few B vitamins was widespread. It is also unknown if deficiencies of essential vitamins or trace minerals not yet characterized affected results. Decrements in physical performance due to a deficient status in one or more vitamins or trace minerals continue to be documented in recent times by experimental design or by examination of subjects in countries without food fortification.[30-38] Iron-deficiency anemia in endurance athletes is still encountered, and is well known to reduce performance.[29,35,36,39,40] At this time, it is generally agreed that measurable deficiencies of vitamins thiamin, riboflavin, B$_6$, C, E, or iron (singly or in combination) are detrimental to human physical performance. There are insufficient data or

TABLE 2   Roles, Functions, Deficiency Symptoms, and Dietary Sources Of Trace Minerals

Iron

Roles:	Oxidation-reduction reactions, oxygen and carbon dioxide transport, metalloenzyme component
Functions:	Oxygen transport (hemoglobin), myoglobin activity, cytochromes (energy production), catalase activity (antioxidant activity), iron-sulfur oxidoreductases (transfer of electrons), cytochrome P-450 (detoxication of xenobiotics), collagen and elastin modification (lysyl and prolyl hydroxylases), α-glycerophosphate dehydrogenase activity (aerobic metabolism), myeloperoxidase (immune function), aconitase (cell energy metabolism), ribonucleotide reductase (DNA, RNA synthesis), phosphoenolpyruvate carboxykinase (gluconeogenesis)
Dietary Needs:	The 1995 RDI for iron is 18 mg for adults
Deficiency Symptoms:	Microcytic anemia, fatigue, tiredness, weakness, impaired work tolerance, decreased cold tolerance, secondary thyroid hormone deficiency, pallor, shortness of breath, depression, gastrointestinal complaints, pica, spoon-shaped nails (koilonychia), edema, immune depression, increased rate of infections, growth retardation, behavioral disturbances, impaired cognitive function, electrocardiogram abnormalities, glossitis, angular stomatitis, dysphagia
Deficiency Risk:	Pregnancy, malnourished (anorexics, dieters, adolescents, infants), elderly, blood loss (menorrhagia, gastrointestinal ulcers, hookworm infestation, hemorrhoids, salicylates, NSAIDs, colorectal tumors, iatrogenic phlebotomy, excess blood donations, runner's hemolysis?), thalassemias, female endurance athletes, gastrectomy, malabsorption syndromes, hereditary hemorrhagic telangiectasia, idiopathic pulmonary hemosiderosis, paroxysmal nocturnal hemoglobinuria, congenital atransferrinemia
Dietary Sources:	Nutritional supplements, enriched flour products, meat, fish, chicken, legumes, green leafy vegetables
	Heme iron (meats) and vitamin C (orange juice) eaten with vegetable foods increase iron uptake
	Tea, coffee, clay, phytates, high-dose calcium carbonate, achlorhydria, and hypochlorhydria decrease iron uptake

Zinc

Roles:	Metalloenzymes, membrane complexes, protein complexes
Functions:	Numerous (over 60 enzymes from each enzyme class): DNA, RNA, protein synthesis; regulatory roles in every cellular system; transcription regulation; membrane functions; metallothionein induction; antioxidant activity (superoxide dismutase); pH balance (carbonic anhydrase), cellular energy production (lactate dehydrogenase); cell motility and internal transport
Dietary Needs:	The 1995 RDI for zinc is 15 mg for adults
Deficiency Symptoms:	Growth retardation, depressed immune function, anorexia, dermatitis, eczema, skin ulcers, acne, seborrhea, rashes, hypogeusia (impaired taste), night blindness, impaired reproductive processes, bone abnormalities, diarrhea, alopecia, impaired wound healing, gastrointestinal symptoms
Deficiency Risk:	Malnourished, elderly, pregnancy, children, lower socioeconomic groups
Dietary Sources:	Nutritional supplements; oysters, red meats, grain germs, seeds, nuts, soybean products, legumes, potatoes, zinc-fortified cereals
	Phytates (whole grains), excess calcium, iron, copper, oxalates (rhubarb, spinach), fiber all decrease zinc uptake. Cow milk zinc is poorly available.
	Red meat (heme?), EDTA, citrate, methionine, cysteine, histidine, lysine, glycine, picolinate all increase zinc uptake

Copper

Roles:	Metalloenzymes

TABLE 2 Roles, Functions, Deficiency Symptoms, and Dietary Sources Of Trace Minerals (continued)

Functions:	Metallothenein induction, antioxidant activity (superoxide dismutase, ceruloplasmin), cellular energy production (cytochrome c oxidase), collagen synthesis (lysyl oxidase), (catecholamine and neurotransmitter synthesis (monoamine oxidases), melanin formation (tyrosinase), blood clotting (Factor IV), disulfide bond formation (thiol oxidase), hemoglobin synthesis
Dietary Needs:	The 1995 RDI for copper is 2.0 mg (0.6 to 0.7 mg/1000 kcal) for adults
Deficiency Symptoms:	Sideroblastic anemia, neutropenia, depressed immune function, abnormal electrocardiograms, skeletal abnormalities (osteoporosis, fractures, subperiosteal hemorrhages), cardiovascular disease, aneurysms, skin and hair depigmentation, hypothermia, hypotonia
Deficiency Risk:	Infants, Menke's disease, females, long-term TPN, malnourished, elderly, pregnancy, Ehlers-Danlos Syndrome V & IX
Dietary Sources:	Nutritional supplements, oysters, shellfish (lobsters, shrimp, crab, clams, mussels), soybean products, legumes, nuts, seeds, grain brans, liver, potatoes
	Excess calcium, phosphate, iron, zinc, cellulose fiber, vitamin C, fructose, uncooked meat all decrease copper uptake
	Breast milk, histidine, other single amino acids all increase copper uptake

Manganese

Roles:	Activation of glycosyltransferases, manganese superoxide dismutase, pyruvate carboxylase, arginase, phosphoenolpyruvate carboxykinase, glutamine synthetase
Functions:	Glycosaminoglycan and proteoglycan synthesis for bone, cartilage, connective tissue growth and repair; glycoprotein synthesis (immune function, cell recognition, mucus production); antioxidant activity (superoxide dismutase); gluconeogensis; carbohydrate metabolism; urea production
Dietary Needs:	The 1995 RDI for manganese is 2.0 mg for adults
Deficiency Symptoms:	Skeletal and cartilage abnormalities (osteoarthritis, osteoporosis, fractures), impaired wound healing
Deficiency Risk:	Females, malnourished (hospitalized patients, dieters, anorexics, many elderly), malabsorption syndromes, Down's Syndrome, lupus erythematosus, epileptics, chronic antacid use
Dietary Sources:	Nutritional supplements, tea, coffee, chocolate, whole grains (except corn), nuts, seeds, soybean products, legumes, liver, fruits
	Excess calcium, phosphate, iron, zinc, fiber (cellulose, pectin, phytate), oxalate, antacids (alkalinity), achlorhydria all decrease manganese uptake.
	Vitamin C, heme (meats) all increase manganese uptake.

Iodine

Roles:	Thyroid hormone component
Functions:	Activity of thyroid hormones (thyroxine and triiodothyronine)
Dietary Needs:	The 1995 RDI is 150 µg for adults
Deficiency Symptoms:	Iodine Deficiency Disorders (IDD), including: goiter, cretinism (mental deficiency, deaf mutism, spastic diplegia), hypothyroidsim, myxedema, apathy, fatigue, cardiovascular disease, hypothermia
Deficiency Risk:	Mostly Papua New Guinea, Zaire, South American Andes, India, Indonesia, certain regions of China
Dietary Sources:	Iodized salt, iodized salt in prepared foods, nutritional supplements, kelp, seafoods
	Cassava and excess maize, bamboo shoots, sweet potatoes, lima beans, millet contain goitrogenic thiocyanates

Selenium

Roles:	Component of glutathione peroxidase (major cellular antioxidant)
Functions:	Activates glutathione peroxidase, removes peroxides, recharges other antioxidants (vitamin E, vitamin C, thioredoxin), inactivates heavy metals, biological transformation of xenobiotics

TABLE 2   **Roles, Functions, Deficiency Symptoms, and Dietary Sources Of Trace Minerals (continued)**

Dietary Needs:	The 1995 RDI is 70 µg for adults
Deficiency Symptoms:	Keshan and Kashin-Beck diseases (cardiomyopathy and osteoarthritis partly attributable to selenium deficiency), increased cancer risk, increased cardiovascular disease risk, depressed immune functions; muscular weakness
Deficiency Risk:	Malnourished, long-term TPN, certain areas of China
Dietary Sources:	Nutritional supplements (selenomethionine, sodium selenite, high-selenium yeast), water and food selenium levels based on local soil and water levels

Chromium

Roles:	Glucose tolerance factor
Functions:	Potentiates insulin actions
Dietary Needs:	The 1995 RDI is 120 µg for adults
Deficiency Symptoms:	Impaired glucose tolerance, hyperglycemia and hypoglycemia, hyperinsulinism, hyperlipidemia, fatigue, carbohydrate (sweets) craving, irritability, facile weight gain, mature-onset diabetes, cardiovascular diseases
Deficiency Risk:	Malnourished, long-term TPN, intense exercise, trauma, pregnancy, high consumption of simple sugars, many persons in U.S. consume <50 µg/d
Dietary Sources:	Nutritional supplements (picolinate, polynicotinate, chloride, high chromium yeast), whole grains; meats

Other Trace Minerals:

Essential:	Molybdenum (1995 RDI is 75 µg for adults)
Possibly Essential:	Arsenic, boron, fluoride, nickel, silicon, vanadium
Unknown Essentiality:	Cesium, cobalt (apart from being a component of vitamin B_{12}), germanium, lithium, rubidium, strontium
Toxic Minerals:	Aluminum, antimony, arsenic, beryllium, bismuth, cadmium, lead, mercury, nickel, silver, tin, radioactive isotopes, certain valences of chromium, manganese, vanadium

conflicting evidence for other vitamins and trace minerals at this time to ascertain whether a deficiency reduces exercise performance.

V. EFFECT OF SUPPLEMENTATION WITH MULTIPLE VITAMINS AND/OR MINERALS ON NUTRIENT STATUS AND PHYSICAL PERFORMANCE

Others chapters are concerned with individual vitamins and minerals; therefore, a brief review of the effects of *multiple* vitamin/mineral supplementation on exercise parameters will be presented. At present, there is considerable controversy over the use and need of nutrient supplementation for exercising humans (see Table 4). On the one hand, regulatory agencies, most research scientists, many physician groups, and many health care professional groups all steadfastly maintain that essential micronutrient needs for exercising humans are, can be, and should be met by dietary intake of foods alone, except in cases of clear-cut nutrient deficiency conditions (such as iron-deficiency anemia).[41,42] On the other hand, the public (consumers), especially exercising humans, are consuming dietary supplements at a higher rate than ever before. In a recent review, Sobal and Marquart[43] reported an overall mean prevalence of athletes' use of vitamin/mineral supplements to be 46%. Subsets of athletes, such as weightlifters, have shown prevalences of 60 to 100% for consumption of vitamin/mineral supplements.[44] This disparity of views has increased as more data accumulate, which begs the question: Why?

Are millions of consumers falling prey to quacks and hyperbole? Or are millions of people feeling or experiencing something that cannot be easily measured in exercise physiology studies?

TABLE 3   Methods of Assessment for Vitamin and Trace Mineral Status

Functional Assays	Quantitative Tests
	Vitamin A (Retinol)
Relative dose response	Serum levels of retinols and carotenoids (colorimetric, fluorescent, HPLC)
Conjunctival impression cytology	Serum levels of retinol-binding protein
Night blindness determination	Tear analysis
	Vitamin B_1 (Thiamin)
Erythrocyte transketolase activity coefficient (ETKAC)	Serum levels of thiamin (colorimetric, HPLC)
Ex vivo lymphocyte growth response	Urinary excretion
	Microbial assays of body fluids
	Vitamin B_2 (Riboflavin)
Erythrocyte glutathione reductase enzyme activation coefficient (EGRAC)	Serum, urine, body fluid levels (fluorometric, HPLC)
Ex vivo lymphocyte growth response	Urinary excretion
	Microbial assays of body fluids
	Niacin, Niacinamide
Ex vivo lymphocyte growth response	Urinary excretion of N^1-methylnicotinamide and 2-pyridone
	Erythrocyte NAD levels
	Erythrocyte NAD/NADP ratio
	Microbial assays of body fluids
	Vitamin B_6 (Pyridoxine, Pyridoxal, Pyridoxamine)
Erythrocyte enzyme activation coefficients for ALT, AST enzymes	Serum or erythrocyte pyridoxal-5-phosphate (PLP) levels
Ex vivo lymphocyte growth response	Serum vitamin B_6 vitamer levels
Urinary xanthurenic and kynurenic acid levels after tryptophan load	Serum or urinary 4-pyridoxic acid levels
Plasma or urinary homocysteine levels after methionine load	Microbial assays of body fluids
Plasma or urine amino acid levels and ratios	
	Vitamin B_{12} (Cobalamins)
Serum or urinary levels of homocysteine ± oral methionine load	Serum or erythrocyte levels of cobalamins (RIA)
Serum or urinary levels of methyl malonic acid	Microbial assays of body fluids
Ex vivo lymphocyte growth response	
Schilling test or dual-isotope variation (for vitamin B_{12} absorption)	
	Folate
Urinary formiminoglutamate (FIGLU) levels ± oral histidine load	Serum and erythrocyte levels of folates (RIA)
Ex vivo lymphocyte growth response	Microbial assays of body fluids
Neutrophil hypersegmentation	

**TABLE 3   Methods of Assessment for Vitamin and Trace
Mineral Status (continued)**

Functional Assays	Quantitative Tests
	Pantothenate
Ex vivo lymphocyte growth response	Whole blood and urine levels (colorimetric, HPLC) Microbial assays of body fluids
	Biotin
Ex vivo lymphocyte growth response	Whole blood and urine levels (colorimetric, HPLC) Microbial assays of body fluids
	Vitamin C (Ascorbate)
Oral loading tests	Serum, leukocyte, platelet levels of ascorbate (HPLC)
	Vitamin D (Calciferol)
Clinical trial of supplementation	Serum levels of 25- and 1,25-dihydroxycholecalciferol (RIA, EIA)
	Vitamin E (Tocopherol)
Erythrocyte hemolysis by peroxide	Serum, platelet, adipose levels of tocopherols (colorimetric, HPLC) in relation to serum triglyceride levels
	Vitamin K (Phylloquinone)
Bleeding and clotting time Prothrombin time	Plasma des-γ-carboxyprothrombin levels (RIA) Urinary Gla protein level
	Iron
Bone marrow aspirate histology Iron tolerance test (plasma levels pre, post p.o. iron load) Zinc protoporphyrin levels in erythrocytes Complete blood count Clinical trial of supplementation	Serum ferritin levels (RIA, EIA) Serum iron levels (colorimetric, atomic absorption, ICP spectrometry) Total Iron Binding Capacity (TIBC) represents transferrin saturation
	Zinc
Clinical trial of supplementation *Ex vivo* lymphocyte growth responses Zinc tolerance test (plasma levels pre, post p.o. load) Alkaline phosphatase activity in neutrophils Zinc taste test (no taste from a 0.1% solution of zinc sulfate suggests a deficiency)	Serum, erythrocyte, hair, urine levels of zinc are unreliable Leukocyte zinc levels (atomic absorption, ICP spectrometry) Erythrocyte metallothionein levels Serum levels of retinol-binding protein
	Copper
Erythrocyte superoxide dismutase activity d-penicillamine challenge (urinary copper levels pre, post)	Whole blood, erythrocyte levels of copper (atomic absorption, ICP spectrometry) Serum copper and ceruloplasmin levels are not reliable indicators

TABLE 3   Methods of Assessment for Vitamin and Trace Mineral Status (continued)

Functional Assays	Quantitative Tests
Manganese	
Activation of isocitrate dehydrogenase	Serum, blood, lymphocyte, hair levels of manganese (atomic absorption, ICP spectrometry)
Electron paramagnetic resonance	
Clinical trial of supplementation	
Selenium	
Clinical trial of supplementation	Serum, hair, urine levels of selenium (graphite furnace atomic absorption, ICP spectrometry)
Blood, erythrocyte glutathione peroxidase activity	
Chromium	
Clinical trial of supplementation	Serum, blood, hair levels of chromium are unreliable indicators

Note: ALT = alanine aminotransferase (SGPT); AST = aspartate aminotransferase (SGOT); EIA = enzyme immuno assay; HPLC = high-pressure (performance) liquid chromatography; ICP = inductively coupled plasma spectrometry; NAD = nicotinamide adenine dinucleotide; NADP = nicotinamide adenine dinucleotide phosphate; RIA = radioimmunoassay.

After careful analysis of the existing human studies on multiple vitamin/mineral supplementation and physical performance, the reader will understand that *both* viewpoints are relying on scant data, insensitive techniques, statistically inadequate study designs, and conflicting results.

A.   STUDIES BEFORE 1960

The prevailing opinion of scientists and medical experts that micronutrient supplementation is unjustified relies heavily on data generated during the 1940s. This time period exhibited improved study designs (double-blind) and simultaneous determination of nutrient intake or status with performance. Clearly, supplementation of single or multiple B vitamins (and vitamin C) did not significantly affect physiological parameters or physical exercise performance in well-controlled studies.[26] However, only incomplete mixtures of B vitamins were studied (folate and vitamin B_{12} had yet to be characterized), and most of the trace minerals now known to be essential were thought to be coincidental contamination, or toxic, and therefore completely overlooked. Thus, all of these studies were incomplete in terms of nutrients examined and lacked dose-response data. It is possible that a deficiency of an unknown essential nutrient could have affected the results, negating effects of the supplemented nutrient. However, the prevailing attitude among researchers in exercise physiology was that vitamins in general had no effect on physical performance in the absence of a prolonged or severe deficiency. Newly discovered vitamins and trace minerals were infrequently examined for possible effects on exercise performance. Relatively few multiple combinations were subsequently examined, and which were always incomplete with regard to containing amounts of all known essential micronutrients at doses known or shown to improve status (see comparison of doses to current RDIs in Tables 5 and 6).

B.   B COMPLEX STUDIES

Previous scrutiny of human exercise performance trials after supplementation with one or more B complex vitamins found a dose-response effect.[45] For some vitamins (thiamin and

TABLE 4   Disparate Views on Vitamin and Trace Mineral Supplementation for Sports and Exercise: A Sampling of Published Quotations

"Considering these results under the most extreme physical work conditions that humans can tolerate, one can conclude that megadoses therapy in athletes can be classified as nutritional quackery."

Saris, W.H.M., Schrijver, J., Baart, M.-A.E., and Brouns, F., Adequacy of vitamin supply under maximal sustained workloads: the Tour de France, *Int. J. Vitam. Nutr. Res.*, 30S, 205, 1989.

"After 12 years of work, I firmly conclude that if others tell you that nutrients have little effect on athletic performance, do not believe them."

Colgan, M., Effects of multinutrient supplementation on athletic performance, in *Sport, Health, and Nutrition*, Katch, F.I., Ed., Human Kinetics, Champaign, IL, 1986, chap. 3.

"There is little if any evidence that nutritional supplements have any effect on performance or muscle mass in athletes consuming a balanced diet; some of these products have the potential to induce adverse effects, however."

Beltz, S.D. and Doering, P.L., Efficacy of nutritional supplements used by athletes, *Clin. Pharmacol.*, 12, 900, 1993.

"These natural medicines can make a significant impact on the performance levels of athletes as well as active persons."

Reaves, W., Herbs and supplements that go the distance, *Health Foods Bus.*, 37, 56, 1991.

"Only with high-quality, controlled research may we obtain data to answer some of the questions that still remain relative to vitamins and physical performance and possibly reduce the magnitude of the quackery that now exists in this area."

Williams, M.H., Vitamin supplementation and athletic performance, *Int. J. Vitam. Nutr. Res.*, 30S, 163, 1989.

"Does vitamin supplementation in large amounts to adequately nourished subjects increase performance? This is a difficult question to answer. Several studies do suggest an ergogenic effect of vitamin megadoses. However, in most well-controlled studies in which subjects' initial vitamin status was adequate, no effects of vitamin megadoses on performance were seen."

Keith, R.E., Vitamins and physical activity, in *Nutrition in Exercise and Sport*, 2nd ed., Wolinsky, I. and Hickson, J.F., Eds., CRC Press, Boca Raton, FL, 1994, 177.

"A final conclusion from the brief overview of research on nutritional ergogenic acids is that there is no question that dietary manipulation or supplements can improve human exercise performance in certain settings. A prevailing opinion that supplementation of athletes with nutrients is useless, harmful, or quackery is rapidly melting under the heat of scientific findings."

Bucci, L.R., Nutritional ergogenic aids, in *Nutrition in Exercise and Sport*, 2nd ed., Wolinsky, I. and Hickson, J.F., Eds., CRC Press, Boca Raton, FL, 1994, 330.

pantothenate), more does seem to be better; for some vitamins, more is definitely worse (niacin and vitamin B_6). Since individual B vitamins will be covered in subsequent chapters, Table 5 lists the doses and results for combinations of B vitamins from several studies.[30,37,46-55] Obviously, thresholds of effect for enhancement of physical performance by increased B complex vitamin intake are not clearly known, are not reproducible between populations, and multiple doses have been studied in only a few experiments. Notice that there are no studies that have examined a full complement of all eight B vitamins, and only two studies examined six B vitamins. Thus, every study listed is incomplete. Nevertheless, scrutiny of the available, but limited, data on mixtures of B complex vitamins reveals a pattern similar to individual vitamins — more may be better, especially for mental functions.

C. MULTIPLE VITAMIN/MINERAL MIXTURES

A series of studies from Europe, using a sugar, electrolyte, and multiple vitamin/mineral granulation (Beneroc®), were reported by Keul et al.,[56] Haralambie et al.,[57] and Dam[58] from 1974 to 1978 (Table 6). Acute administration was associated with improved work efficiency, lowered heart rate during exercise, increased speed in cross-country skiing, and improved reaction time with reduced neuromuscular irritability for fencers. However, the water, sugar, and electrolytes may have accounted for the observed results, rather than the vitamins per se. Low subject numbers and lack of placebo controls made results less trustworthy. The status of thiamin, riboflavin, and vitamin B_6 before supplementation was deficient,[58] meaning

TABLE 5 Correlation of Dose and Ergogenic Effects of Controlled Human Studies on B Vitamin Combinations

Investigators (year)	Ref.	Length of Admin.	Thiamin (mg)	Riboflavin (mg)	Niacin Equiv. (mg)	B_6 (mg)	B_{12} (mg)	Folate (mg)	Pantothenate (mg)	Biotin (mg)	Other Nutrients (mg)	Ergogenic Results[a]
Keys and Henschel (1941)	46	4 weeks	5		100						C (100)	—
Simonson et al. (1942)	47	15 weeks	6	8	80	0.3					80 units filtrate	—[b] / +
Foltz et al. (1942)	48	Acute i.v.[c]	3–15	0.3–1.6	10–50	1–5					C (100–200)	—
Keys and Henschel (1942)	49	4–6 weeks	5–17	0–10	100	0–10			0–20		C (100)	—
Frankau (1943)	50	4 days	5	5	50							+
Henschel et al. (1944)	51	3 days	5	10	100							+
Early and Carlson (1969)	52	6 days	100	8	100	5	25		30		C (70)	+
Buzina et al. (1982)[d]	30	3 months		2		2						+
Read and McGuffin (1983)	53	6 weeks	5	5	25	2	0.0005		12.5			—
Boncke and Nickel (1989)	54	8 weeks	90			60	0.12					+
Boncke and Nickel (1989)	54	8 weeks	300			600	0.60					+
van der Beek (1991)	37	8 weeks	2.5	4		4					e	—
Fogelholm et al. (1993)	55	5 weeks	15	15	20	10			25			—[f]

a A — indicates no significant effect on physiological or performance measurements; + indicates a significant improvement in physiological or performance measurements.

b No effects on physical performance, but significant improvement of mental fatigue and subjective feelings.

c Vitamins were administered by intravenous means.

d Large percentage of subjects exhibited clinical and biochemical signs of vitamin deficiencies.

e A supplement containing 2 × Dutch RDA for vitamins A, D, E, B_{12}, folate, biotin, niacinamide, pantothenate, plus 100 mg vitamin C were given to both the control and experimental groups.

f Only blood lactate levels were measured.

TABLE 6   Comparison of Multiple Vitamin/Mineral Formulas Studied for Effects on Exercise

	1995 RDI[a]	Keul 1974, Haralambie 1975, Dam 1978	Barnett 1984	Colgan 1986	Weight 1988	Guilland 1989	van der Beek 1991	Colgan 1991	Colgan 1991	Telford 1992[b]	Singh 1992[c]
Ref. no.		56,57,58	60	69	61	62	37	70	70	65,66	63,64
Total no.		12,14,40	20	16	30	75	77	23	23	82	22
Kleijnen scored[d]		60	52	50	67	55		56	56	75	68
Nutrients Per Serving											
Vitamin A (IU)	5,000		6,000	5,000–45,000	3,000		5,000	5,000	5,000	4,500	515
Vitamin D (IU)	400		600	200–2,480	400		400	400	400	400	
Vitamin E (IU)	30	100	15	200–1,600	516	15	150	15	15	151	51
Vitamin K (mcg)	80										
Ascorbate (mg)	60	1,000	135	2,000–16,000	850	200	500	60	500	550	169
Thiamin (mg)	1.5	20	15	40–600	60	7.5	12	1.5	1.5	75	54
Riboflavin (mg)	1.7	30	15	30–250	60	9	20	1.7	1.7	25	25
Niacin equiv. (mg)	20	40	75	100–1,000	70	35	210	20	20	100	35
Vitamin B_6 (mg)	2.0	50	21	10–300	60	11	20	2.0	152	100	135
Vitamin B_{12} (mg)	0.006		0.015	0.100–0.300	0.060		0.030	0.012	0.112	0.1	0.048
Folate (mg)	0.4		0.4	2.0–30	0.5		4.0	0.4		0.2	
Pantothenate (mg)	10	40	18	50–1,000	70	15	100		2.4	100	62
Biotin (mg)	0.3			2.0–100			2.0			0.1	0.4
Potassium (mg)		200	37.5	198–5,000	32					33	
Phosphorus (mg)	1,000	2,160(PO_4)		200–2,000	116					ND	
Calcium (mg)	1,000	500		1,000–3,500	230					115	57
Magnesium (mg)	400	340	52.5	1,000–2,000	116		100			7	57
Iron (mg)	18		37.5	30–60	13.4			18	48	1	
Zinc (mg)	15		15	50–150	5.2			15	60	3	14.6

Nutrient						
Copper (mg)	2.0	3	0–5	0.6		
Manganese (mg)	2.0	3	20–100	300?		0.01
Iodine (mg)	0.15	0.15	0.15–1.0	0.15		
Selenium (mg)	0.07		0.2–1.0	0.15	0.15	
Chromium (mg)	0.12		0.3–1.0	0.05	0.15	
Molybdenum (mg)	0.075		0.05–5			0.01
Bioflavonoids (mg)						50
Choline (mg)	97.5		200–2,000			75
Inositol (mg)	97.5		100–1,000			75
PABA (mg)	45		100–500			75
Betaine HCL (mg)	15					25
Others	Pancreatin, safflower oil, lecithin, wheat germ extract, rice bran extract, soya bean extract, liver		Potassium			Kelp, lecithin, glutamic acid

a RDI = Recommended Daily Intake, 1995.

b Amounts for minerals were calculated based on percentage of elemental mineral for each compound described.

c Only selected nutrients were analyzed for actual daily intakes. Only those nutrients analyzed were listed, although the supplement contained other nutrients. Analyzed amounts were frequently different from label claim.

d Kleijnen score = a rating of analyzing methodological quality of clinical trials, originally used to assess human trials with *Ginkgo biloba* preparations. Maximum score is 100, and 7 weighted criteria (patient characteristics, subject number, randomization, intervention description, double-blinding, effect measurements, and results accountability) were considered. See Kleijnen, J. and Knipschild, P., *Ginkgo biloba* for cerebral insufficiency. *Br. J. Clin. Pharmacol.,* 34, 352, 1992, for description of method.

that correction of vitamin deficiencies may have contributed to the observed results, rather than an ergogenic effect.

Another European study, by Ushakov et al.[59] in 1978, reported improved work capacity in 7 subjects after 20 days of supplementation with "nutrition correction supplements", an undescribed mixture of "... glutamic and aspartic acids, methionine, group B vitamins, ascorbic acid, vitamin A, rutin, nicotinamide, nucleic acids, organic K, Ca, Mg, and Ph salts." However, in addition to not describing the contents of the supplements, administration was not randomized, allowing for possible training effects. However, measurements of amino acid composition were reportedly improved after supplementation. Again, the low subject number and poor study design preclude trustworthy data.

In 1984, Barnett and Conlee[60] administered a commercial multiple vitamin/mineral formula for four weeks to nine subjects, while another nine subjects ingested placebos. A 1-h submaximal treadmill run was used to assess physiological and metabolic parameters ($\dot{V}O_2$max, R value, muscle glycogen, blood glucose, blood free fatty acids, and blood lactate), of which there was no significant differences between groups. There was no assessment of micronutrient status. The authors concluded "... the supplement had no beneficial effect on performance ..." even though performance was not directly measured. The authors correctly concluded that "... supplements of this nature are of no physiological value to the athlete who consumes a normal nutritionally balanced diet." However, dietary intakes were not analyzed. Also, amounts of each micronutrient were well below those which did change physiological or performance parameters in other studies (see Tables 5 and 6). Again, it must be stressed that this study extrapolated from a few (but important) physiological effects in a small number of subjects the fact that performance was not benefited, although actual exercise performance was never measured.

Weight and others[61] administered a more potent multiple vitamin/mineral supplement to 30 subjects in a randomized, double-blind crossover study for 3 months. Dietary analysis indicated low intakes for total calories, folate (66% of RDA), and vitamin B_6 (77% of RDA). Status of riboflavin (erythrocyte enzyme activation) and vitamin B_6 (serum levels) werethe only parameters that showed significant improvements after supplementation, and all nutrient status values for each study period were within normal limits, suggesting adequate nutrient status at the start of the experiment. Physiological measurements (sleep time, resting heart rate, maximum heart rate, body mass $\dot{V}O_2$max, and blood lactate levels during exercise) were unchanged. Peak treadmill speed during $\dot{V}O_2$max determinations was unchanged, as was a true measure of performance — 15-km race times (although some subjects dropped out before finishing, affecting the average time per group). This study strongly suggests that if micronutrient status is not improved (unchanged), race performance is not improved.

Another European study, by Guilland and others,[62] found that 30 days of multiple vitamin (but not mineral) supplementation to 55 athletes significantly improved status for vitamins A, thiamin, riboflavin, B_6, and C. This is not surprising, since a large proportion (28 to 80%) of athletes had intakes of vitamins B_6, C, and E below the RDA safety limit. Serum levels of gamma tocopherol and selenium were deficient throughout the study. Alpha tocopherol levels were unaffected by supplementation, and even significantly decreased after supplementation in sedentary males.

These results, taken together with the other European studies previously mentioned,[56-59] suggest that the micronutrient status of European athletes is inferior to athletes in the U.S., South Africa, or Australia. Thus, results of supplementation trials from European studies may simply reflect correction of deficiencies, and not enhancement of status or performance.

Beek[37] described an unpublished study of supplements containing 2 to 10 times the Dutch RDA for multiple vitamins with iron given to 77 sports students. Both placebo and supplemented groups exhibited similar training effects on aerobic power, indicating the supplement had no effect on physiological parameters during exercise.

Singh and others[63,64] described the effects of a multiple vitamin/mineral supplement on status[63] and performance[64] of 22 physically active males (11 per group), in a randomized, double-blind, placebo-controlled study. Dietary intakes showed no differences between the groups. The administered supplement was assayed for nutrient content, and found to be seriously subpotent (compared to label claim) for vitamin E, B vitamins, zinc, and magnesium, although the supplemental amounts were still considerable (between one and two orders of magnitude greater than the U.S. RDA). The supplement did not contain iron or copper.

Status (blood levels) for all B vitamins (except folate) was improved after supplementation, but the status of fat-soluble vitamins and minerals was not changed after supplementation. Importantly, the status was changed by the sixth week, indicating studies lasting for shorter time periods may not have reached full equilibration of micronutrient status. Physiological parameters during exercise, such as $\dot{V}O_2max$, heart rate, plasma lactate, ACTH, or glucose, were unchanged in each group after 12 weeks. Endurance performance (measured as the number of 30-s bouts to exhaustion at 100% $\dot{V}O_2max$ performed after 90 min of treadmill running at alternately 60 and 85% $\dot{V}O_2max$) was unchanged between groups. Measurements of muscular strength (power, peak torque, and peak work of resisted knee extensions) were unchanged in each group after 12 weeks.

The authors concluded that supplementation did not affect biochemical, physiological, or performance parameters. However, the supplement was not complete, and time to exhaustion for strictly aerobic activity was not directly measured. Although B vitamin status was significantly improved (although blood levels do not necessarily reflect intracellular function), doses were still below those shown to have significant effects (see Table 5).[45]

Telford and others,[65,66] in a study similar to that of Singh, et al. and published the same year (1992), studied the effect of a placebo or multiple vitamin/mineral supplement administered for 7 to 8 months to 86 athletes from various sports at the Australian Institute of Sport. The supplement had very small amounts of minerals, and large amounts (between one and two orders of magnitude) of most B vitamins. Compliance was measured and found to be low. Only 15/42 supplemented subjects and 19/44 placebo subjects consumed ≥70% of the administered pills, meaning the majority of subjects consumed less than half of the required doses. This unfortunate fact may have introduced large variability in measurements of status and performance. When only the high compliers were assessed the status of several B vitamins improved after supplementation, but mineral status was unaffected. Perhaps because of compliance issues, the status for other vitamins actually worsened in the supplemented group. Also, any subject in either group that exhibited a low ferritin level (checked every 8 weeks) was given iron supplements.

Performance was measured by a battery of tests specific for each sport, analyzed separately for each sport, and combined when possible. This practice severely curtailed subject number and statistical power. Instead of the approximately 25 subjects per group needed to detect a significant change (Bucci, L., StatMate Software, GraphPad Software, San Diego), at most 9 subjects per group were utilized, with the average subject number per group being 5.25. This is before the compliance issue, which would further reduce subject number and statistical power. Therefore, it is no surprise that no significant changes in physiological or performance values were found, except for increased body weight and skinfold measurements in male and female basketball players, and a higher vertical jump in female basketball players. Combined analysis of half the subjects did not find significant differences for vertical jump, cycle ergometer work, shoulder strength (Cybex), or $\dot{V}O_2max$. Combined analysis for all subjects showed a significant increase in total skinfold measurements for supplemented subjects. Overall, the results are difficult to interpret because of the large compliance problems, which reduced subject number and statistical power of the study.

Several double-blind, placebo-controlled studies did find significant improvements in physiological and performance values after supplementation with multiple vitamin/mineral products. Dragan and others[67] administered either a multiple vitamin supplement (control group, n = 10) or a supplement containing vitamins, minerals, amino acids, and selenium (experimental group, n = 10, Cantamega-2000®) to junior cyclists in Rumania. The Cantamega group exhibited faster recovery from fatigue and improved blood levels of hemoglobin, protein, calcium, and magnesium than the control group. However, these results may reflect repletion of deficiencies rather than a true ergogenic effect — a theme common to other European studies. On the other hand, this study allows a direct evaluation of the effects of mineral supplementation, since equivalent supplements were given to each group. Results suggest that multiple minerals may be more important than B vitamins for normalizing health and recovery from exercise.

Likewise, Pieralisi and others[68] administered a combination product containing ginseng, dimethylaminoethanol (DMAE), vitamins, minerals, and trace elements to 50 male sports teachers in a randomized, double-blind, crossover study lasting 6 weeks. Total work load and maximal oxygen consumption during exercise were significantly greater after the supplement. However, the presence of ginseng and DMAE means that results may not be attributable solely to vitamins and minerals.

Colgan[69,70] reported on results of individualized supplement protocols utilizing doses of vitamins and minerals considerably higher than other studies (see Table 6). In a randomized-order, double-blind crossover study, 22 subjects received supplements containing U.S. RDA amounts of vitamins and minerals for 12 weeks and showed declines in serum ferritin, iron, zinc, ascorbate, and vitamin B_6 status.[70] The same subjects crossed over to receive U.S. RDA amounts plus larger doses of iron (48 mg/d), zinc (60 mg/d), folate (2.4 mg/d), pyridoxine (150 mg/d), and ascorbate (500 mg/d) showed improvements in nutrient status, VO_2max, and time to exhaustion on a cycle ergometer.

Figures 1 to 3 illustrate the effects of individualized supplement protocols administered by Colgan[69] on the performance times for different athletes. It can be seen that although no statistical analysis was performed due to the low subject number, differences were large for most subjects, and amounted to very large improvements in race times. These results indicate that perhaps a dose-response effect is apparent for multiple vitamin/mineral supplementation, since the doses were considerably higher than those used in other studies, especially mineral intakes (see Table 6). These results have not been replicated by other investigators; however, these results have been consistent over a 10-year period with different subjects. Results of individualized or high-dose supplementation exceeding two orders of magnitude more than the U.S. RDA for selected micronutrients suggest that other studies simply were observing the lower end of dose-response curves for measured parameters. Studies by Colgan[69] demonstrated that athletes ingesting large amounts of vitamin/mineral supplements experienced tangible results in terms of personal best times, which would reinforce consumption of supplemental vitamins and minerals.

An excellent review by Fogelholm[71] has summarized data since 1980 on the effects of vitamin/mineral supplementation on micronutrient status and exercise performance in athletes. Conclusions were that most studies found similar status between athletes and untrained controls, but current indicators of micronutrient status may not reflect the status in muscles. Usually, supplementation with water-soluble vitamins and iron improved indicators of status, but fat-soluble vitamin and trace mineral supplementation usually did not change indicators of status in the blood. In general, supplementation did not improve physiological or physical performance, except that anemic subjects did realize improved performance after supplementation with iron.

However, several studies reviewed in this chapter were not considered by Fogelholm.[67-70] Also, significant study design weaknesses were found in *every* study examined, and suggestions for correction in future research include increased subject numbers, prospective designs, multiple indicators of status, training, and performance, and more standardization in data and specimen collections.

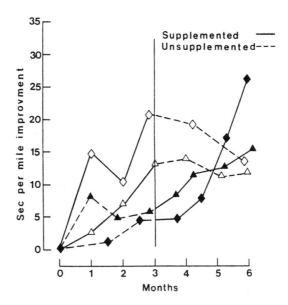

FIGURE 1 Seconds per mile improvement in time trials or races of 20+ miles (including marathons) for 4 experienced marathon runners with and without supplementation. (From Colgan, M., *Sports, Health, and Nutrition,* Katch, F.I., Ed., Human Kinetics, Champaign, IL, 1986. With permission.)

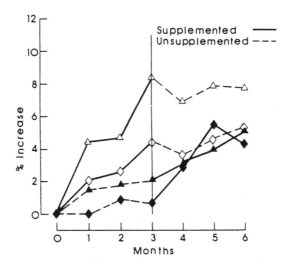

FIGURE 2 Percentage increases in poundage used in press and clean and jerk combined for four experienced weightlifters, with and without supplementation. (From Colgan, M., *Sports, Health, and Nutrition,* Katch, F.I., Ed., Human Kinetics, Champaign, IL, 1986. With permission.)

VI. OVERLOOKED OPPORTUNITIES FOR SPORTS NUTRITION RESEARCH ON VITAMINS AND MINERALS

Sports nutrition does not exist in a vacuum. Just because a substance does not alter $\dot{V}O_2$max does not mean it has no effect on sports performance. Effects of micronutrient deficiencies and supplementation on humans for several conditions have relevance for sports nutrition. These conditions include:

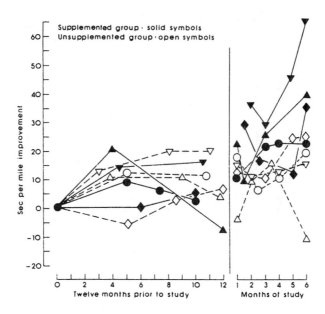

FIGURE 3   Seconds per mile improvement in time trials or races of 20+ miles (including marathons) for 8 athletes for 12 months prior to supplementation and for 6 months of supplementation of subjects. (From Colgan, M., *Sports, Health, and Nutrition,* Katch, F.I., Ed., Human Kinetics, Champaign, IL, 1986. With permission.)

- Mental fitness (subjective feelings of well-being, perception of fatigue, coordination, neurological parameters)
- Immune system function (resistance to infections and overtraining)
- Healing or prevention of musculoskeletal injuries

A brief perusal of the literature on these conditions outside of sports nutrition periodicals may illuminate why consumers insist on ingesting micronutrient supplements in spite of controversial scientific support.

A. MENTAL FITNESS (SUBJECTIVE FEELINGS OF FATIGUE, MOOD, CONCENTRATION, COORDINATION, NEUROLOGICAL PARAMETERS)

The physiological mechanisms for fatigue during exercise (cardiac output, oxygen delivery to tissues, fuel substrate availability, changes in neurotransmitters, dehydration, electrolyte depletion, ammonia and acidity increases, and other unidentified factors) have been well studied.[72] Although recognized as an important contributor to fatigue, psychological factors have been less-often studied.[72]

Often, the first signs of vitamin and mineral deficiencies appear as psychological alterations before other laboratory or clinical measures are able to demonstrate a deficiency.[47,73,74] These alterations include apathy, lethargy, reduced intelligence, depression, less ability to concentrate, reduced neuromuscular coordination, increased irritability, and fatigue.

One example of vitamin supplementation affecting mental but not physical performance is a report by Simonson et al. in 1942,[47] in which 12 subjects were given a supplement containing a few B vitamins in moderate doses (see Table 5), and 11 subjects were given a placebo. Measurements of physical performance (weight lifting, recovery period after exhaustion, maximum muscular force, heart rate) were unchanged by vitamin supplementation. However, fusion frequency of flicker, a validated test for central nervous system fatigue, was greatly improved by vitamin supplementation, but not by placebo. Furthermore, 8 of 12 supplemented subjects, but only 1 of 11 placebo subjects, felt more alert. Even more suggestive, "... all 12 [supplemented] subjects experienced a reduction of subjective fatigue and only 1 in the control group of 11 subjects."[47] These results demonstrate that moderate doses of some B vitamins, commonly found in multiple vitamin/mineral supplements, made people feel better, but not perform better.

Almost 50 years later, effects of a multiple vitamin/mineral supplement on intelligence was studied in Belgian children (13 years old).[75] After 5 months of supplementation, compared to placebo effects boys ingesting a "poor" diet showed a significant improvement in nonverbal intelligence, although boys eating a "good" diet, and girls, showed no significant effects. This study demonstrated that micronutrient supplementation, in doses consumed by the average athlete today, may affect mental functions which would not be measured by standard exercise physiology tests, but would still confer a potential competitive advantage for an individual.

Penland[76] fed diets with high and low boron intakes to healthy volunteers. Low boron intakes resulted in significantly poorer performance for manual dexterity tasks, eye-hand coordination, attention, perception, encoding, and both short- and long-term memory — all usual measures of IQ. However, in healthy athletes, boron supplementation did not affect physical parameters of strength, lean body mass, or testosterone levels.[77] Thus, a single trace mineral supplement has the potential to significantly improve mental fitness, but not physical fitness.

Bates and co-workers[78] described reduction of work performance in developing countries due to a *combination* of marginal micronutrient deficiencies. This finding is important because classical signs of nutrient deficiency for individual micronutrients were not seen. The findings correlate well with other reports describing improved physical performance after repletion of biochemical deficiencies.[30,79,80]

One of the most controversial (and unstudied) aspects of nutritional supplementation, both for athletes and nonathletes alike, is injection of vitamin B_{12} to relieve fatigue or provide a "boost" in energy levels. A sound biochemical mechanism for mood-elevating and antidepressant effects of vitamin B_{12} revolves around transmethylation processes in the brain increasing *S*-adenosyl-L-methionine (SAMe) levels.[81-84] In fact, SAMe is under investigation as a new antidepressant drug (Bucci, L., unpublished data). Furthermore, objective evidence from a randomized-order, placebo-controlled crossover study of vitamin B_{12} injections did find statistically significant ($p = .006$) increases in "general well-being" after vitamin B_{12} injections.[85]

Boncke and Nickel administered a supplement containing 300 mg thiamin, 600 mg vitamin B_6, and 600 mcg vitamin B_{12} (Neurobion Forte®, Merck Darmstadt and Cascan, Wiesbaden, Germany) for 8 weeks to 35 pentathlon marksmen in a double-blind, placebo-controlled study.[54] A statistically significant improvement in firing accuracy (hitting a small target with a pistol) was found for the supplemented group, but not for the placebo group, indicating improvement in physiological tremor mediated by neuromuscular motor control. This study used relatively large doses of a few B vitamins to subjects not suspected to be deficient to elicit a beneficial change in nervous system function affecting sports outcome. Few studies have used this range of doses[69,70] or have measured neurological parameters. Thus, there is evidence that micronutrient supplementation can beneficially affect neurological processes and have a positive impact on performance.

Taken together, these results suggest that consumers taking comprehensive, large doses of vitamins and minerals may be enhancing mental fitness parameters without affecting objective physical performance. Correction of even one micronutrient deficiency by a multiple vitamin/mineral product may lead to subjective improvement noticed by the user. Of course, studies measuring only physical parameters may not find evidence of an effect for micronutrient supplementation, leading to the incomplete conclusion that supplements have no benefits for exercising individuals. These results may help to explain the current disparity between consumers and researchers on the effectiveness of vitamin and/or mineral supplementation for exercise.

B. IMMUNE SYSTEM FUNCTION

A consensus in the literature indicates that acute, exhaustive exercise bouts or heavy chronic exercise is associated with increased risk of upper respiratory tract infections.[86,87] While the exact mechanisms are unclear, micronutrient deficiencies are one suspected culprit.[88-90] Micronutrient deficiencies are known to have adverse effects on immunocompetence,[88,91] and micronutrient supplementation to apparently healthy humans has resulted in improvements in immune function parameters and fewer infections.[88-90]

One study did find that 6 months of daily supplementation with 400 IU of vitamin E and 500 mg of vitamin C led to greater improvements in lymphocyte functions from fit subjects (exercisers) compared to sedentary subjects.[92] This suggests that the immune function of exercising subjects was less than ideal, and could be partially corrected by supplementation with only two micronutrients. In addition, incidence of infections was reported to be lessened after individualized, high-dose micronutrient supplementation.[69,70] The interaction of micronutrients with immune functions in athletes remains largely unexplored, but potentially large real-life impacts on ability to train or perform are suggested.

C. HEALING OR PREVENTION OF MUSCULOSKELETAL INJURIES

Again, little research has been applied to the role of micronutrient deficiencies or supplementation in the prevention of or recovery from musculoskeletal injuries in athletes.[93] If deficiencies of micronutrients exist, it is possible that healing or tissue repair can be delayed. An extensive review of the available literature has found that large doses of vitamin A, vitamin C, and/or zinc salts may accelerate healing of skin wounds.[93] However, no prospective trials of supplementation with a complete and potent multiple vitamin/mineral formula on injured athletes can be found. Animal and human data suggest that provision of additional micronutrients to healing tissues may accelerate connective tissue repair.[93] The interaction between nutrition, psychological state, and healing was explored in human surgical patients, and a clear improvement in mood and muscle metabolism was found in supplemented subjects.[94] Since injuries reduce training time and prevent participation in events, any reduction in healing time would greatly aid athletic endeavors.

Thus, several aspects of nutrition that do not relate directly to muscular performance may still greatly influence exercise performance via mental, immunological, and musculoskeletal mechanisms. Fertile areas for research into the effects of vitamins and trace minerals on sports performance abound.

VII. SUMMARY

Two diametrically opposed viewpoints with regards to vitamin and trace mineral supplementation for athletes have appeared. On the one hand, medical experts emphatically deny there is any need or advantage for supplementation and that such practices border on quackery.[41,42] On the other hand, athletes and exercising consumers are ingesting ever-increasing amounts of supplements, including essential vitamins and minerals.[43,44] The goal of this chapter was to review identity of vitamins and trace minerals, review studies of supplementation with combinations of vitamins and minerals, and point out some largely unexplored areas in sports nutrition that may account for the dichotomy of viewpoints.

Research into the efficacy of supplements continues to lag well behind availability and use. This position has increasingly put researchers into defensive postures to "debunk" popular fads or practices, generating a predominance of haphazard, negative data, and ultimately, a negative bias among researchers to disprove current practices rather than observe objectively.

The following list of experimental factors with less than ideal status in studies cited in this chapter illustrates opportunities for future research.[6] Experimental factors to carefully control include:

1. Adequate subject numbers to provide necessary statistical power given normal biological variability;
2. Doses that improve micronutrient status;
3. Multiple doses per study to explore dose-response relationships;
4. Subject compliance;
5. Verification of micronutrient content of dietary supplements;
6. Multiple measures of micronutrient status and intake, including functional assays;
7. Bioavailability of supplement studied;
8. Proper length of study;
9. Simultaneous measurement of performance, physiological, metabolic, psychological, immunological, neurological, and mental parameters;
10. Complete profile of all known essential vitamins and minerals;
11. Possible investigator bias in study design, execution, analysis, and presentation; and
12. Thorough, nonselective literature reviews for discussion in publications.

The available evidence indicates that relatively low doses of vitamins (at the 1995 U.S. Recommended Daily Intake [RDI] or one order of magnitude greater) will not alter physical performance except in individuals with deficient status.[33-37,60,61,63-66,71] The available evidence suggests that most athletes exhibit adequate vitamin and trace mineral status compared to the general population,[71] but assessment tools are not infallible.[20-25] These findings strongly suggest that beneficial changes in status or performance by vitamins and trace minerals can only be reproducibly accomplished by doses greater than one order of magnitude from the RDI. However, doses of some trace minerals greater than one or two orders of magnitude over the RDI are potentially toxic, compared to most vitamins, and should not be studied or condoned.

The available evidence suggests that relatively high doses of some B vitamins may beneficially affect a few parameters that indirectly affect performance (such as fine motor control[54]), or improve exercise under unusual conditions (heat[52]). Combinations of all essential trace minerals have been virtually unstudied, so it is premature to make any blanket statements regarding status or supplementation effects from multiple minerals. However, there is some evidence that when relatively high doses of comprehensive vitamin/mineral supplements are administered, improved exercise performance may be found.[67-70]

Available evidence strongly suggests that people simply feel better subjectively and mentally when taking supplements, *beyond a placebo effect*.[47,69,70,75,76,85] Near-universal use of psychoactive agents (caffeine, nicotine, alcohol, and illegal drugs of abuse) by humans convincingly demonstrates that people subjectively want to feel better. If multiple vitamin/mineral supplements make people feel better, then supplementation will continue whether there is a physiological benefit or not. Do people that feel better perform better? Widespread use of placebo controls argues for an affirmative answer.

A prudent, objective analysis of the available literature must conclude that the evidence is insufficient to conclusively state that supplementation with multiple vitamins and trace minerals will or will not alter exercise performance. In the absence of biochemical deficiencies, doses of multiple vitamins and minerals one order of magnitude or less than the current U.S. RDI will not benefit physical performance, but may benefit mental fitness. Apparent benefits from higher doses of multiple vitamins and minerals await further confirmation.

REFERENCES

1. Williams, M.H., Ed., *Ergogenic Aids in Sports*, Human Kinetics, Champaign, IL, 1983.
2. American College of Sports Medicine, Position stand on prevention of thermal injuries during distance running, *Med. Sci. Sports Exercise*, 16, ix, 1984.
3. Williams, M.H., *Nutritional Aspects of Human Physical and Athletic Performance*, Charles C Thomas, Champaign, IL, 1985.
4. Lamb, D.R. and Williams, M.H., Eds., *Perspectives in Exercise Science and Sports Medicine*, Vol. 4, Ergogenics - Enhancement of Performance in Exercise and Sport, Wm. C. Brown, Carmel, IN, 1991.
5. Bucci, L.R., *Nutrients as Ergogenic Aids for Sports and Exercise*, CRC Press, Boca Raton, FL, 1993.
6. Wolinsky, I. and Hickson, J.F., *Nutrition in Exercise and Sport*, 2nd ed., CRC Press, Boca Raton, FL, 1994.
7. Machlin, L.J., Ed., *Handbook of Vitamins*, 2nd ed., Marcel Dekker, New York, 1991.
8. Marks, J., *The Vitamins. Their Role in Medical Practice*, MTP Press, Lancaster, U.K., 1985.
9. Alpers, D.H., Clouse, R.E., and Stenson, W.F., Eds., *Manual of Nutritional Therapeutics*, 2nd ed., Little, Brown, Boston, 1988.
10. Bender, D.A., *Nutritional Biochemistry of the Vitamins*, Cambridge University Press, Cambridge, U.K., 1992.
11. Combs, G.F., *The Vitamins. Fundamental Aspects in Nutrition and Health*, Academic Press, San Diego, 1992.
12. Brown, M.L., Ed., *Present Knowledge in Nutrition*, 6th ed., International Life Sciences Foundation, Washington, D.C., 1990.
13. Shils, M.E., Olson, J.A., and Shike, M., Eds., *Modern Nutrition in Health and Disease*, 8th ed., Lea & Febiger, Philadelphia, 1994.
14. Prasad, A.S. and Oberleas, D., Eds., *Trace Elements in Human Health and Disease*, Vol. 2, Essential and Toxic Elements, Academic Press, New York, 1976.
15. Frieden, E., Ed., *Biochemistry of the Ultratrace Elements*, Plenum Press, New York, 1984.
16. Underwood, E. and Mertz, W., Eds., *Trace Elements in Human Health and Animal Nutrition*, Academic Press, New York, 1987.
17. Hurley, L.S., Keen, C.L., Lönnerdal, B., and Rucker, R.B., Eds., *Trace Elements in Man and Animals*, Vol. 6, Plenum Press, New York, 1988.
18. Tomita, H., Ed., *Trace Elements in Clinical Medicine*, Springer-Verlag, Tokyo, 1990.
19. Karcioğlu, Z.A. and Sarper, R.M., Eds., *Zinc and Copper in Medicine*, Charles C Thomas, Springfield, IL, 1980.
20. Sauberlich, H.E., Skala, J.H., and Dowdy, R.P., *Laboratory Tests for the Assessment of Nutritional Status*, 2nd ed., CRC Press, Boca Raton, FL, 1977.
21. Wright, R.A. and Heymsfield, S., *Nutritional Assessment*, Blackwell Scientific, Boston, 1984.
22. Baker, H., Frank, O., and Hutner, S.H., B-complex vitamin analyses and their clinical value, *J. Appl. Nutr.*, 41, 3, 1989.
23. Fogelholm, M., Vitamin and Mineral Status in Physically Active People. Dietary Intake and Blood Chemistry in Athletes and Young Adults, Social Insurance Institution, Turku, Finland, 1992.
24. Werbach, M.R., *Nutritional Influences on Illness*, 2nd ed., Third Line Press, Tarzana, CA, 1993.
25. Bucci, L.R., A Functional Analytical Technique for Monitoring Nutrient Status and Repletion. *Townsend Letter for Doctors*, July, 728–730, 1994.
26. Keys, A., Physical performance in relation to diet, *Fed. Proc.*, 2, 164, 1943.
27. Barborka, C.J., Foltz, E.E., and Ivy, A.C., Relationship between vitamin B-complex intake and work output in trained subjects, *J. Am. Med. Assoc.*, 122, 717, 1943.
28. Keys, A., Henschel, A., Taylor, H.L., Mickelsen, O., and Brozek, J., Experimental studies on man with a restricted intake of the B vitamins, *Am. J. Physiol.*, 144, 5, 1945.
29. Viteri, F.E. and Torun, B., Anemia and physiological work capacity, *Clin. Haematol.*, 3, 609, 1974.
30. Buzina, R., Grgic, Z., Jusic, M., Sapunar, J., Milanovic´, N., and Brubacher, G., Nutritional status and physical working capacity, *Hum. Nutr. Clin. Nutr.*, 36C, 429, 1982.
31. van der Beek, E.J., van Dokkum, W., Schrijver, J., Wesstra, J.A., and Hermus, R.J.J., Effect of marginal vitamin intake on physical performance of man, *Int. J. Sports Med.*, 5S, 28, 1984.
32. van der Beek, E.J., van Dokkum, W., Schrijver, J., Wedel, M., Gaillard, A.W.K., Wesstra, A., van der Weerd, H., and Hermus, R.J.J., Thiamin, riboflavin, and vitamins B-6 and C: impact of combined restricted intake on functional performance in man, *Am. J. Clin. Nutr.*, 48, 1451, 1988.
33. Brouns, F. and Saris, W., How vitamins affect performance, *J. Sports Med.*, 29, 400, 1989.
34. Williams, M.H., Vitamin supplementation and athletic performance, *Int. J. Vitam. Nutr. Res.*, S30, 163, 1989.
35. Haymes, E.M., Vitamin and mineral supplementation to athletes, *Int. J. Sport Nutr.*, 1, 146, 1991.
36. Clarkson, P.M., Minerals: exercise performance and supplementation in athletes, *J. Sports Sci.*, 9, 91, 1991.
37. van der Beek, E.J. Vitamin supplementation and physical exercise performance, *J. Sports Sci.*, 9, 77, 1991.
38. van der Beek, E.J., van Dokkum, W., Wedel, M., Schrijver, J., and van den Berg, A., Thiamin, riboflavin and vitamin B-6. Impact of restricted intake on physical performance in man, *J. Am. Coll. Nutr.*, 13, 629, 1994.

39. Haymes, E.M., Trace minerals and exercise, in *Nutrition in Exercise and Sport*, 2nd ed., Wolinsky, I. and Hickson, J.F., Eds., CRC Press, Boca Raton, FL, 1994, 223.

40. Weaver, C.M. and Rajaram, S., Exercise and iron status, *J. Nutr.*, 122, 782, 1992.

41. American Dietetic Association, Position of the American Dietetic Association and the Canadian Dietetic Association: nutrition for physical fitness and athletic performance for adults, *J. Am. Diet. Assoc.*, 93, 691, 1993.

42. Beltz, S.D. and Doering, P.L., Efficacy of nutritional supplements used by athletes, *Clin. Pharmacol.*, 12, 900, 1993.

43. Sobal, J. and Marquart, L.F., Vitamin/mineral use among athletes. A review of the literature, *Int. J. Sport Nutr.*, 4, 320, 1994.

44. Bazzare, T.L., Nutrition and strength, in *Nutrition in Exercise and Sport*, 2nd ed., Wolinsky, I. and Hickson, J.F., Eds., CRC Press, Boca Raton, FL, 1994, 417.

45. Bucci, L.R., Nutritional ergogenic aids, in *Nutrition in Exercise and Sport*, 2nd ed., Wolinsky, I. and Hickson, J.F., Eds., CRC Press, Boca Raton, FL, 1994, 330.

46. Keys, A. and Henschel, A.F., High vitamin supplementation (B1, nicotinic acid and C) and the response to intensive exercise in U.S. Army infantryman, *Am. J. Physiol.*, 133, 350, 1941.

47. Simonson, E., Enzer, N., Baer, A., and Braun, R., The influence of vitamin B (complex) surplus on the capacity for muscular and mental work, *J. Ind. Hyg. Toxicol.*, 24, 83, 1942.

48. Foltz, E.E., Ivy, A.C., and Barborka, C.J., Influence of components of the vitamin B complex on recovery from fatigue, *J. Lab. Clin. Med.*, 27, 1396, 1942.

49. Keys, A. and Henschel, A.F., Vitamin supplementation of U.S. Army rations in relation to fatigue and the ability to do muscular work, *J. Nutr.*, 23, 259, 1942.

50. Frankau, I.M., Acceleration of co-ordinated muscular effort by nicotinamide, *Br. Med. J.*, 13, 601, 1943.

51. Henschel, A., Taylor, H.L., Mickelsen, O., Brozek, J.M., and Keys, A., The effect of high vitamin C and B vitamin intakes on the ability of man to work in hot environments, *Fed. Proc.*, 3, 18, 1944.

52. Early, R.G. and Carlson, R.B., Water-soluble vitamin therapy in the delay of fatigue from physical activity in hot climactic conditions, *Int. Z. Angew. Physiol.*, 27, 43, 1969.

53. Read, M.H. and McGuffin, S.L., The effect of B-complex supplementation on endurance performance, *J. Sports Med.*, 23, 178, 1983.

54. Boncke, D. and Nickel, B., Improvement of fine motoric movement control by elevated dosages of vitamin B_1, B_6, and B_{12} in target shooting, *Int. J. Vitam. Nutr. Res.*, 30S, 198, 1989.

55. Fogelholm, M., Ruokonen, I., Lakso, J.T., Vuorimaa, T., and Himberg, J.-J., Lack of association between indices of vitamin B_1, B_2, and B_6 status and exercise-induced blood lactate in young adults, *Int. J. Sport Nutr.*, 3, 165, 1993.

56. Keul, J., Haralambie, G., Winker, K.H., Baumgartner, A., and Bauer, G., Die Wirkung eines Multivitamin-Elektrolytgranulats auf Kreislauf und Stoffwechsel bei langwährender Körperarbeit, *Schweiz. Z. Sportmed.*, 22, 169, 1974.

57. Haralambie, G., Keul, J., Baumgartner, A., Winker, K.H., and Bauer, G., Die Wirkung eines Multivitamin-Elektrolytpräparates auf Elektrodermalreflex une neuromuskuläre Erregbarkeit bei langwährender Körperarbeit, *Schweiz. Z. Sportmed.*, 23, 113, 1975.

58. van Dam, B., Vitamins and sport, *Br. J. Sports Med.*, 12, 74, 1978.

59. Ushakov, A.S., Myasnikov, V.I., Shestkov, B.P., Agureev, A.N., Belakovsky, M.S., and Rumyantseva, M.P., Effect of vitamin and amino acid supplements on human performance during heavy mental and physical work, *Aviat. Space Environ. Med.*, 49, 1184, 1978.

60. Barnett, D.W. and Conlee, R.K., The effects of a commercial dietary supplement on human performance, *Am. J. Clin. Nutr.*, 40, 586, 1984.

61. Weight, L.M., Noakes, T.D., Labadarios, D., Graves, J., Jacobs, P., and Berman, P.A., Vitamin and mineral status of trained athletes including the effects of supplementation, *Am. J. Clin. Nutr.*, 47, 186, 1988.

62. Guilland, J.C., Penaranda, T., Gallet, C., Boggio, V., Fuchs, F., and Klepping, J., Vitamin status of young athletes including the effects of supplementation, *Med. Sci. Sports Exercise*, 21, 441, 1989.

63. Singh, A., Moses, F.M., and Deuster, P.A., Vitamin and mineral status in physically active men: effects of a high-potency supplement, *Am. J. Clin. Nutr.*, 55, 1, 1992.

64. Singh, A., Moses, F.M., and Deuster, P.A., Chronic multivitamin-mineral supplementation does not enhance physical performance, *Med. Sci. Sports Exercise*, 24, 726, 1992.

65. Telford, R.D., Catchpole, E.A., Deakin, V., McLeay, A.C., and Plank, A.W., The effect of 7 to 8 months of vitamin/mineral supplementation on the vitamin and mineral status of athletes, *Int. J. Sport Nutr.*, 2, 123, 1992.

66. Telford, R.D., Catchpole, E.A., Deakin, V., Hahn, A.G., and Plank, A.W., The effect of 7 to 8 month vitamin/mineral supplementation on athletic performance, *Int. J. Sport Nutr.*, 2, 135, 1992.

67. Dragan, G.I., Ploesteanu, E., and Selejan, V., Studies concerning the ergogenic value of Cantamega-2000 supply in top junior cyclists, *Rev. Roum. Physiol.*, 28, 13, 1991.

68. Pieralisi, G., Ripari, P., and Vecchiet, L., Effects of a standardized ginseng extract combined with dimethy-laminoethanol bitartrate, vitamins, minerals, and trace elements on physical performance during exercise, *Clin. Ther.*, 13, 373, 1991.

69. Colgan, M., Effects of multinutrient supplementation on athletic performance, in *Sport, Health, and Nutrition*, Katch, F.I., Ed., Human Kinetics, Champaign, IL, 1986, chap. 3.

70. Colgan, M., Micronutrient status of endurance athletes affects hematology and performance, *J. Appl. Nutr.*, 43, 16, 1991.

71. Fogelholm, M., Indicators of vitamin and mineral status in athletes' blood: a review, *Int. J. Sport Nutr.*, 5, 267, 1995.

72. Atlan, G., Beliveau, L., and Bouissou, P., Eds., *Muscle Fatigue: Biochemical and Physiological Aspects*, Masson, Paris, 1991.

73. Chomé, J., Paul, T., Pudel, V., Bleyl, H., Hesker, H., Hüppe, R., and Kübler, W., Effects of suboptimal vitamin status on behavior, *Bibl. Nutr. Dieta*, 38, 94, 1986.

74. Werbach, M.R., *Nutritional Influences on Mental Illness. A Sourcebook of Clinical Research*, Third Line Press, Tarzana, CA, 1991.

75. Benton, D. and Buts, J.-P., Vitamin/mineral supplementation and intelligence, *Lancet*, 1, 1158, 1990.

76. Penland, J.G., Dietary boron, brain function, and cognitive performance, *Environ. Health Perspect.*, 102(Suppl. 7), 65, 1994.

77. Green, N.R. and Ferrando, A.A., Plasma boron and the effects of boron supplementation in males, *Environ. Health Perspect.*, 102(Suppl. 7), 73, 1994.

78. Bates, C.J., Powers, H.J., and Thurnham, D.I., Vitamins, iron, and physical work, *Lancet*, 2, 313, 1989.

79. Buzina, R. and Suboticanec, K., Significance of vitamins in child health, *Int. J. Vitam. Nutr. Res.*, Suppl. 26, 9, 1984.

80. Powers, H.J., Bates, C.J., Lamb, W.H., Singh, J., Gelman, W., and Webb, E., Effects of a multivitamin and iron supplement on running performance in Gambian children, *Hum. Nutr. Clin. Nutr.*, 39, 427, 1985.

81. Herbert, V. and Das, K.C., Folic acid and vitamin B_{12}, in *Modern Nutrition in Health and Disease*, 8th ed., Shils, M.E., Olson, J.A., and Shike, M., Eds., Lea & Febiger, Philadelphia, 1994, 402.

82. Metz, J., Pathogenesis of cobalamin neuropathy: deficiency of nervous system S-adenosylmethionine?, *Nutr. Rev.*, 51, 12, 1993.

83. Bressa, G.M., S-adenosyl-l-methionine (SAMe) as antidepressant: meta-analysis of clinical studies, *Acta Neurol. Scand.*, Suppl. 154, 7, 1994.

84. Bottiglieri, T., Hyland, K., and Reynolds, E.H., The clinical potential of ademetionine (S-adenosylmethionine) in neurological disorders, *Drugs*, 48, 137, 1994.

85. Ellis, F.R. and Nasser, S., A pilot study of vitamin B12 in the treatment of tiredness, *Br. J. Nutr.*, 30, 277, 1973.

86. Nieman, D.C., Exercise, infection, and immunity, *Int. J. Sports Med.*, 15, S131, 1994.

87. Hoffman-Goetz, L. and Watson, R.R., Immune functions in exercise, sport, and inactivity, in *Nutrition in Exercise and Sport*, 2nd ed., Wolinsky, I. and Hickson, J.F., Eds., CRC Press, Boca Raton, FL, 1994, 475.

88. Chandra, R.K., 1990 McCollum award lecture. Nutrition and immunity: lessons from the past and new insights into the future, *Am. J. Clin. Nutr.*, 53, 1087, 1991.

89. Nieman, D.C. and Nelson-Cannarella, S.L., Exercise and infection, in *Exercise and Disease*, Eisinger, M. and Watson, R.R., Eds., CRC Press, Boca Raton, FL, 1992.

90. Nieman, D.C., Physical activity, fitness and infection, in *Exercise, Fitness and Health: A Consensus of Current Knowledge*, Bouchard, C., Ed., Human Kinetics, Champaign, IL, 1993.

91. Myrvik, Q.N., Immunology and nutrition, in *Modern Nutrition in Health and Disease*, 8th ed., Shils, M.E., Olson, J.A., and Shike, M., Eds., Lea & Febiger, Philadelphia, 1994, 623.

92. Ismail, A.H., Petro, T.M., and Watson, R.R., Dietary supplementation with vitamin E and C in fit and nonfit adults: biochemical and immunological changes, *Fed. Proc.*, 42, 335, 1983.

93. Bucci, L.R., *Nutrition Applied to Injury Rehabilitation and Sports Medicine*, CRC Press, Boca Raton, FL, 1994.

94. Hill, G.L., Effects of nutritional therapy, in *Disorders of Nutrition and Metabolism in Clinical Surgery*, Churchill Livingstone, Edinburgh, U.K., 1992, 85.

Chapter 2

ASCORBIC ACID

Robert E. Keith

CONTENTS

I. INTRODUCTION

Vitamin C (ascorbic acid) has been one of the most widely studied vitamins in relation to sports performance and exercise. Several previous review articles have addressed this topic area.[1-3] The present chapter will attempt to expand knowledge concerning vitamin C and exercise. Basic functions and deficiency symptoms of ascorbic acid as related to exercise will be covered along with specific articles related to exercise and vitamin C requirements, vitamin C supplementation and sports performance, and intakes/needs of physically active persons for the vitamin.

0-8493-8192-4/97/$0.00+$.50

A. HISTORY

While the existence of vitamin C has been known for only a relatively short time, the fact that a vitamin C deficiency could adversely affect physical performance has been documented for centuries.[1,4] There are reports from the British Navy in the late 1700s concerning sailors with scurvy (vitamin C deficiency).[4] These reports describe sailors who had good appetites and were cheerful, yet collapsed and died on deck upon the initiation of physical activity. During the Crimean War (1854-1856) and the American Civil War, scurvy was reported among the soldiers. Soldiers with scurvy were reported to have shortness of breath upon exertion and greatly reduced energy and powers of endurance.[4] These are just a couple of examples of how ascorbic acid deficiency has adversely affected the physical ability of sailors and soldiers in the last several centuries. Thus, while the study of vitamin C and physical performance is a relatively new area, the fact that scurvy has caused decreases in physical performance has existed for centuries.

B. GENERAL PROPERTIES AND STRUCTURE

Vitamin C is a water-soluble vitamin required by humans, primates, and guinea pigs. Most other animal species can make ascorbic acid from glucose. Humans lack an enzyme necessary to convert glucose to ascorbic acid. Vitamin C exists in humans in two biologically active forms, ascorbic acid and dehydroascorbic acid. It is the ability to interconvert between these two forms that gives vitamin C its antioxidant capabilities. The structures of glucose, ascorbic acid and dehydroascorbic acid are shown in Figure 1.[5-8]

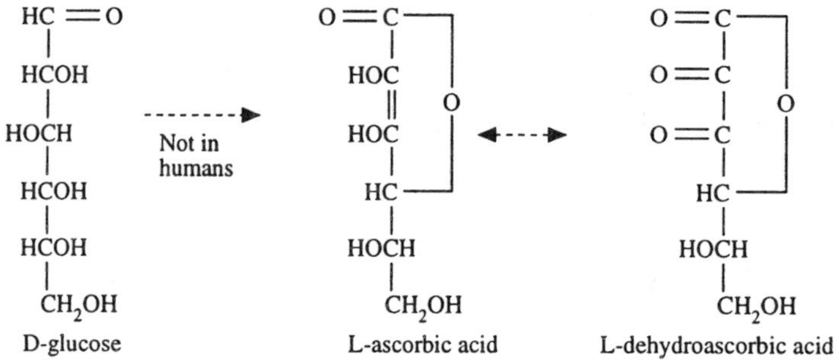

FIGURE 1   The structure and interconversions of glucose, ascorbic acid, and dehydroascorbic acid.

Vitamin C is absorbed in the upper small intestine by active transport mechanisms at physiological dietary intakes (50 to 200 mg/day). Large intakes (gram doses) of the vitamin may be absorbed by passive diffusion. Most (80 to 90%) of a physiological dose will be absorbed. However, this absorbance value may drop to 10 to 20% for megadoses. Vitamin C is found in high concentrations in the adrenal glands, pituitary gland, white blood cells, the lens of the eye, and brain tissue.[5-8]

C. FUNCTIONS

Ascorbic acid has several important functions as related to physical activity. The vitamin has long been known to be necessary for normal collagen synthesis. Collagen is one of the most abundant proteins in the body and is a vital component of cartilage, ligaments, tendons, and other connective tissues. Vitamin C is needed for the formation of the vitamin-like compound, carnitine. Carnitine is necessary for the transport of long-chain fatty acids into the mitochondria — the fatty acids can then be used as an energy source. The neurotransmitters, norepinephrine and epinephrine, also require vitamin C for their synthesis. Ascorbic acid seems to be needed for the proper transport of nonheme iron, the reduction of folic acid intermediates, and for the proper synthesis and/or release of the stress hormone, cortisol. Finally, vitamin C acts as a powerful water-soluble antioxidant. The vitamin seems to exert antioxidant functions in plasma and probably interfaces at the lipid membrane level with vitamin E to regenerate vitamin E from the vitamin E radical. Table 1 describes some of these functions in more detail.[5-8]

TABLE 1 Selected Functions of Vitamin C that Could Affect Physical Performance

Chemical Reaction Requiring Vitamin C	Body Function
Lysine → hydroxylysine Proline → hydroxyproline	Needed for normal collagen (cartilage, connective tissue, ligaments, tendons)
Lysine → carnitine (liver, kidney)	Necessary for normal fatty oxidation in muscle cell mitochondria
Phenylalanine → dopamine, norepinephrine, epinephrine	Needed for normal neurotransmitter formation
Ascorbic acid ↔ dehydroascorbic acid	Normal antioxidant function

Through these various functions vitamin C can interface with physical activity at several levels. For example, poor development of connective tissues could result in increased numbers of ligament and tendon injuries and poor healing of these injuries. Inadequate production of carnitine would decrease a person's ability to utilize fatty acids as an energy source. This would force increased use of glycogen stores, thus exhausting these stores earlier during exercise and causing fatigue and decreased performance.

With decreased production of norepinephrine and epinephrine an athlete might not be able to properly stimulate the neural and metabolic systems necessary for optimal performance. Poor iron and folate metabolism would result in anemia, impairing the transport of oxygen to tissues. This would be a definite hindrance to optimal performance in aerobic endeavors.

Through its various functions, vitamin C has ample opportunity to interface with physical performance at several metabolic sites.

D. DEFICIENCY AND PHYSICAL PERFORMANCE

It should follow from the previous section that a vitamin C deficiency (scurvy) would cause a decrease in physical performance. This point is not controversial. Table 2 lists the major symptoms of vitamin C deficiency and how each symptom could decrease a certain aspect of physical activity.

TABLE 2 Vitamin C Deficiency Symptoms and Physical Performance

Deficiency Symptom	Effect on Performance
Poor connective tissue development, poor injury healing, swelling, bleeding in joints	Strains, sprains may increase, heal poorly. Poor range of motion.
Subcutaneous hemorrhages, increased bruising	Hemorrhages due to contact would be worse, more extensive
Anemia	Decreased aerobic performance.
Fatigue	Decreased aerobic and anaerobic performance due to decreased fatty acid use and neurotransmitter function
Muscular weakness, pain	Decreased force production, decreased performance due to pain when moving
Anorexia	Decreased performance due to low energy intake

A marginal status for ascorbic acid probably also exerts some detrimental effects on performance. Ratsimamanga[9] reported that guinea pigs on a vitamin C-deficient diet, and undergoing forced exercise, became more fatigued than control animals, and muscle glycogen content of the deficient guinea pigs was lower than the healthy control animals. Wachholder[10] reported growth failure in young guinea pigs that were deficient in vitamin C and had to perform prolonged exercise. Lemmel[11] studied 110 children receiving a diet low is ascorbic acid. The addition of 100 mg daily of ascorbic acid over a 4-month period improved the work capacity and liveliness of 48% of the children as compared with 12% in a control group. Babadzanjan et al.[12] studied 40 train engine drivers and crew. These individuals had an initially low vitamin C status. The administration of 200 mg of vitamin C per day normalized blood concentrations and reduced fatigue in these subjects. More recently, Buzina and Suboticanec[13] reported that $\dot{V}O_2$max values were improved in young adolescents with low plasma concentrations of vitamin C when these adolescents were supplemented with vitamin C. The improvement in the $\dot{V}O_2$max stopped when plasma C concentrations were normalized. Van der Beek et al.[14,15] produced marginal vitamin C status in subjects by feeding them 32.5 to 50% of the Dutch recommended dietary allowance for vitamin C for 3 to 8 weeks. In one study,[15] an increased heart rate was seen at the "onset of blood lactate" level during the time of reduced vitamin C intake. In addition, reduced vitamin C status may have been partly responsible for a significant reduction in aerobic power seen in the other study.[14]

E. RECOMMENDED INTAKES AND FOOD SOURCES

The current adult Recommended Dietary Allowance (RDA) for vitamin C is 60 mg/day.[16] This level of intake is known to maintain adequate tissue levels of the vitamin and prevent signs of scurvy in most individuals. However, these guidelines were developed for lightly active to moderately active people, not specifically for athletes or persons engaged in strenuous or prolonged physical activity.

Various forms of physiological stress are known to increase the need for vitamin C. These stresses include infections,[5] cigarette smoking,[17,18] extreme environmental temperature,[19,20] and altitude,[20] among others. Recently, the RDA for cigarette smokers was increased to 100 mg/day.[16] Strenuous and/or prolonged exercise is a form of physiological stress[21] and could possibly increase the requirements and, thus, the recommended intakes of the vitamin in physically active individuals. However, to date, no official recommendations for vitamin C intake for physically active individuals have been made.

Vitamin C is found naturally and almost exclusively in fruits and vegetables. Some vitamin C can be found in milk and liver, but these values are minimal.[7] In addition to natural sources of the vitamin, many foods, such as breakfast cereals, are now vitamin C fortified. Thus, it is more likely today than ever before that significant vitamin C intake could be obtained from foods other than fruits and vegetables. Nonetheless, vitamin C is different in terms of intake as compared with many other vitamins, particularly the B complex vitamins. B complex vitamin intake tends to correlate well with the total energy intake of an athlete. Thus, if an athlete is consuming sufficient energy it is reasonably likely that the B vitamin intake also is sufficient. However, because ascorbic acid is found principally in some fruits and vegetables, the possibility exists that the athlete could have an otherwise adequate diet but one that is low in vitamin C. This would occur if the athlete did not consume sufficient servings of fruits and vegetables. The vitamin C content of selected fruits and vegetables can be found in Table 3.

II. REQUIREMENTS FOR ASCORBIC ACID AS AFFECTED BY EXERCISE

Two questions can be addressed when evaluating the literature relevant to vitamin C and exercise. One question is: What effects do physical activity have on the requirements for

TABLE 3   Vitamin C Content of Selected Fruits and Vegetables

Fruits	Vitamin C (mg/100 g)	Vegetables	Vitamin C (mg/100 g)
Strawberries	65	Peppers	163
Oranges	50	Greens	130
Tangerines	30	Brussels sprouts	120
Pineapple	30	Broccoli	115
Melons	25	Spinach	70
Apples	20	Cauliflower	70
Cherries	10	Cabbage	45
Peaches	10	Asparagus	22
Bananas	7	Potatoes	20
		Beans/Peas	20
		Onions	20
		Tomatoes	20

Adapted from Moser, U. and Bendich, A., *Handbook of Vitamins*, 2nd ed., Machlin, L.J., Ed., Marcel Dekker, New York, 1991.

vitamin C? A possible answer to this question can be deduced by looking at changes in tissue concentrations, enzymes, hormones, and other biochemical markers. This question is addressed in the present section. Another question would be: What effects do taking extra vitamin C beyond requirement amounts have on exercise performance? This question will be addressed in Section III.

A. ANIMAL STUDIES

Several animal studies have been conducted that attempted to determine the effects of exercise on vitamin C requirements. Animal studies have the advantage of being able to evaluate various tissue concentrations of vitamin C or other biochemical markers following the death of exercised and sedentary animals.

Stojan et al.[22] swam rats to exhaustion on a single occasion. The vitamin C concentrations in various tissues were then compared with those of a sedentary baseline control group. The exercised rats had adrenal vitamin C concentrations that were 50 to 65% of the baseline values. The same swimming stress, but at a simulated altitude, reduced adrenal ascorbic acid content even more than at nonaltitude.

Hughes et al.[23] used guinea pigs as their animal model. Guinea pigs were forced to swim 1 h/day for 18 days. A nonswimming control group was used for comparison of tissue concentrations. All animals received 1.0 mg of vitamin C per 100 g of body weight per day. Exercised guinea pigs had lower vitamin C concentrations in the adrenal glands, brain, and spleen.

Akamatsu et al.[24] studied rats subjected to a swimming stress at a high environmental temperature. These authors reported that adrenal vitamin C concentrations were reduced in the exercised rats.

In a study by Keith and Lee,[25] 40 guinea pigs were divided into 4 groups: exercise, no exercise, vitamin C at requirement level, or five times requirement. Animals were maintained on the diets for 3 weeks and the exercised animals were killed 24 h following a single bout of treadmill running to exhaustion. Results indicated that ascorbic acid concentrations were significantly lower in the livers of the exercised guinea pigs and nonsignificantly lower ($p < .1$) in the plasma and adrenal glands. The authors also reported that exercised animals on the higher vitamin C intake had lower TBARS values (a marker of oxidative damage) for liver, kidney, adrenal, and skeletal muscle tissue as compared with animals receiving a requirement level of vitamin C. However, none of the differences reached significance. The authors concluded that a single bout of exhaustive exercise could reduce vitamin C tissue concentrations.

In another animal study, Keith and Pomerance[26] exercised guinea pigs on a treadmill (20 m/min, 5 day/week, 1 h/day). This training program was continued for eight weeks. A sedentary control group was included and all animals received vitamin C at 0.75 mg/100 g body weight per day. Exercised guinea pigs had significantly reduced liver and adrenal gland vitamin C concentrations.

In a somewhat different study,[27] exercised guinea pigs had improved muscle and liver glycogen concentrations as the vitamin C content of their diet was increased.

Thus, five animal studies are all in agreement that exercise reduces the vitamin C content of various tissues. This would seem to indicate that exercise increased the need for vitamin C in these animals.

B. HUMAN STUDIES

Research studies investigating the effect of exercise on ascorbic acid needs in humans are greater in number and more diverse in their approach as compared with animal studies. Human studies have been performed that have addressed the relationship between exercise and vitamin C for blood concentrations of the vitamin, excretion in the urine, immune function, hormonal status, muscle soreness/blood enzymes, heat stress adaptation, and markers of free radical damage. These papers are reviewed in the following paragraphs.

Several papers have evaluated blood/plasma vitamin C changes with exercise or in athletes at rest. Namyslowski and Desperak-Secomska[28] found decreased blood vitamin C levels in a group of physical culture students. Even though diets of the students may not have been adequate in vitamin C, the authors concluded that strenuous exercise had caused an additional decrease in these blood concentrations. Namyslowski[29] followed the first paper with a second study. This study found that blood vitamin C levels decreased in athletes ingesting 100 mg of vitamin C per day. Dietary intakes of 300 mg/day (5 times the RDA) were required to maintain or increase blood concentrations of ascorbic acid in the athletes.

Several recent studies[30-36] have reported normal mean vitamin C concentrations in the plasma of athletes and physically active individuals, although at least one study[36] reported 12% of their subjects with low plasma vitamin C concentrations while another[32] had mean ascorbic acid concentrations for their subjects at the low end of the normal range. Blood vitamin C concentrations above 0.6 mg/ 100 ml are usually considered adequate.[37] Mean plasma vitamin C concentrations in active, mostly male, subjects have been reported to range from a low of 0.6 mg/100 ml to a high of 1.50 mg/100 ml. One study with female ballet dancers reported a plasma vitamin C concentration of 0.81 mg/100 ml.[33] Thus, for the most part, plasma concentrations in physically active individuals appear to be normal. However, some care must be taken in interpreting these values as compared with a sedentary population. Several papers have reported that physical activity can increase plasma vitamin C concentrations for up to 24 h.[30-32,38] Thus, plasma values for vitamin C in some of the reported studies could possibly be falsely elevated if they were obtained within 24 h of strenuous exercise. This could be a mitigating factor in evaluating plasma vitamin C in athletes. Plasma vitamin C values in various athletic groups are given in Table 4.

One study evaluated changes in leukocyte ascorbic acid in 31 professional soccer players before and after a vigorous 2-h training session.[39] The leukocyte vitamin C content decreased in these athletes following the training session. The authors likened this fall with the fall in leukocyte vitamin C seen following other stressful events such as myocardial infarction and the common cold.

Three studies have reported decreased urinary excretion of vitamin C with increased physical activity.[29,30,40] Bacinskij[40] studied 30 young sedentary male medical students and 33 physical culture students who participated in various forms of exercise on a daily basis. The physical culture students excreted only about 50% of the vitamin C of the medical students. The author concluded that persons engaged in physical activity need extra vitamin C.

TABLE 4   **Resting or Baseline Plasma Ascorbic Acid Concentrations (mg/100 ml) in Various Athletic Groups**

Athletic Group	Subject Number	Ascorbic Acid Value	Ref.
Various athletes	50 M, 36 F	0.98	36
Runners	4 M	1.39, 1.50	30
Runners	7 M	0.6	32
Runners	9 M	0.93	31
Runners	30 M	1.01	34
Various athletes	55 M	1.29	35
Ballet dancers	10 M, 12 F	1.04 M, 0.81 F	33

Note: Normal plasma ascorbic acid concentration range = 0.6–2.0 mg/dl.[37]

Namyslowski[29] also reported decreased urine vitamin C in a group of skiers. The author suggested that the skiers needed 200 to 250 mg of vitamin C each day. Fishbaine and Butterfield[30] studied four healthy, male trained runners and seven matched sedentary controls housed for eight weeks in a metabolic ward. All food intake was controlled. Subjects consumed 315 mg of vitamin C each day. Runners excreted less vitamin C in their urine as compared with sedentary subjects. However, this difference was not significant.

Several papers have examined the relationships among exercise, vitamin C needs, and adaptation to heat stress in humans.[41-45] An early study[41] found no effect from 500 mg of vitamin C on rectal temperature, sweat rate, recovery heart rate, or strength in subjects working in a hot environment. However, studies since then have found some improvement in the ability of humans to exercise in a hot environment when they were given additional vitamin C.[42-45]

Strydom et al.[44] studied the effects of vitamin C ingestion (250 or 500 mg/day for 21 days vs. placebo) in a group of 60 mine workers undergoing heat acclimatization. Subjects were not exposed to heat for at least six months prior to the study. Exercise consisted of a 4-h step test in a comfortable environment (20 to 22°C) vs. repeated testing in a hot environment. (32.2°C wet bulb and 33.9°C dry bulb). Results indicated no differences among groups for heart rate or total sweat rate. However, rectal temperatures were significantly lower in the groups receiving vitamin C. The authors concluded that the rate and degree of heat acclimatization was enhanced by vitamin C supplementation.

Kotze et al.[45] also investigated heat acclimatization in 13 male volunteers. Subjects exercised 4-h each day for 10 days in a manner and under conditions previously described by Strydom et al.[44] Volunteers were placed into diet groups receiving 250 or 500 mg vitamin C daily or a placebo. Groups receiving vitamin C had a reduction in total sweat output and rectal temperature. The authors concluded that vitamin C may be effective in reducing heat strain in unacclimatized persons.

In another study, Peters et al.[46] evaluated the effects of a vitamin C supplement (600 mg/day for 21 days or a placebo) on the incidence of upper respiratory tract infections (URTI) in a group of ultramarathoners following an ultramarathon race. All subjects had a normal dietary vitamin C intake of approximately 500 mg/day. Thus, supplemented subjects were ingesting 1100 mg of vitamin C each day. Runners were monitored for 14 days following the race. A total of 68% of the runners in the placebo group had symptoms of URTI following the race. Only 33% of the vitamin C-supplemented subjects had symptoms of URTI. This difference was significant. The authors concluded that vitamin C supplementation may enhance resistance to postrace URTI that frequently occur in competitive long-distance runners.

Two papers[47,48] have reported on the effect of vitamin C on postexercise muscle soreness/damage with mixed results. An earlier study by Staton[47] showed no differences in delayed muscle soreness as measured by a sit-up test between subjects receiving 100 mg of vitamin C and those receiving a placebo. However, in a recent study by Jakeman and Maxwell[48] postexercise maximal voluntary isometric contraction of an eccentrically exercised leg was determined over a period of seven days. In general, retention of force production was better in a group of subjects receiving 400 mg of vitamin C each day for 21 days prior to exercise as compared with a group receiving vitamin E. The authors concluded that vitamin C may offer protection from eccentric exercise-induced muscle damage.

Vitamin C is a potent water-soluble antioxidant.[5-8] However, to date, research on the effects of oxidative stress associated with exercise and vitamin C metabolism/requirements have not been extensively investigated in humans. One preliminary study[49] reported on the effects that oxidant stress had in humans during consecutive days of exercise (cycle ergometry, 90 min/day at 65% $\dot{V}O_2$max for 3 days). The authors stated that the reactive oxidant species formed during the exercise were metabolized by blood glutathione and plasma vitamin C. Currently, few other papers, if any, have been published that report on the effects of exercise, oxidative damage, and ascorbic acid.

In summarizing the animal and human data on the effects of exercise on vitamin C requirements, the data would seem to support the concept that strenuous exercise does increase the need for the vitamin. Several animal studies are all in agreement, showing reduced tissue concentrations of ascorbic acid with exercise. Plasma ascorbic acid concentrations in exercising humans appear to be normal. However, several human studies report decreased urinary excretion of vitamin C with exercise, improved adaptation to exercise in the heat, and reduced incidence of upper respiratory tract infection (one study). While ascorbic acid might provide some increased antioxidant protection to exercising persons, there are few data to support or refute this point.

From the studies that have been cited in this section, intakes of vitamin C in the range of 100 to 500 mg/day would appear to be acceptable under most conditions for person engaged in strenuous physical activity. Extremely strenuous exercise (as in ultramarathons) might move up this range of intake. Doses of 100 to 500 mg/day are safe and can be obtained in the diets of athletes without supplementation. Data to support this point can be found in Section IV of this chapter. The actual need for ascorbic acid for an individual athlete would probably vary due to such factors as the duration or volume of training, how strenuous the activity might be, as well as the environmental conditions under which the activity is performed.

III. EFFECTS OF SUPPLEMENTAL ASCORBIC ACID ON VARIOUS ASPECTS OF PHYSICAL PERFORMANCE

Numerous studies have been performed over the last 50 years concerning the relationship between ascorbic acid intake and improvement of physical performance. Many of these reports have found positive effects and an equal number have found no effect. It should be noted that many positive studies were performed early in the investigation of vitamin C. These studies suffer from poor control and dubious statistics. In addition, the initial vitamin C status of the subjects was usually not ascertained and could have been low. However, several "no effect" articles could be criticized for giving ascorbic acid doses that were probably too low to have possible ergogenic effects.

A. POSITIVE FINDINGS

Studies finding positive effects of vitamin C on performance have been reported for both animal and human subject groups. These papers are reviewed in the following sections.

1. Animal Studies

Through the years, a few animal studies have been performed with ascorbic acid. In an early study, Basu and Biswas[50] reported that the contractions of frog gastrocnemius muscle were larger in amplitude, and the development of fatigue delayed, when ascorbic acid was present in the Ringer's solution bathing the frog muscle. Later, Bushnell and Lehmann[51] showed that large doses of ascorbic acid (125 and 500 mg/kg body weight) could prevent swimming impairment in mice exposed to ethanol. Richardson and Allen[52] supplemented rats for 30 days with vitamin C. The added vitamin C increased muscle contraction time by almost 20% but had no effect on strength as compared with control rats. Lang et al.[53] also reported increased endurance capacity in guinea pigs supplemented with ascorbic acid.

2. Human Studies

Several studies prior to 1950 did show a positive effect of vitamin C in the diet on physical performance. Sieburg[54] reported that the physical condition of athletes undergoing training was improved with the addition of dietary ascorbic acid. Wiebel[55] showed that students receiving a vitamin C supplement had an improved capacity for sports as compared with students receiving a placebo. Basu and Ray[56] gave 4 subjects 600 mg of ascorbic acid and reported that the onset of fatigue in the finger muscles of the subjects was delayed as compared with a group of control subjects. Harper et al.[57] conducted a study with 69 cadets for a period of 21 weeks. Two groups were used: a group receiving ascorbic acid at 50 mg/day and a placebo group. Treatment was continued for 10 weeks at which time the treatment groups were reversed. Cadets receiving the vitamin C had a greater endurance in breath holding but they also had a faster resting pulse rate. Hoitink[58] exercised subjects on a cycle ergometer before, during, and after giving them 300 mg of ascorbic acid a day for 1 to 2 weeks. Hoitink reported that the administration of vitamin C increased the amount of work done and reduced the resting pulse and respiratory rates of the subjects.

Several studies performed since 1960 also have reported positive performance changes in subjects given additional ascorbic acid. Hoogerwerf and Hoitink[59] worked 33 male, untrained students on a cycle ergometer at 120 W for 10 min. The study was performed in a double-blind manner with 15 students receiving 1000 mg of ascorbic acid a day for 5 days while the rest of the students received a placebo. Blood ascorbate concentrations in the subjects were within the normal range at the beginning of the study. The authors found that excess metabolism due to work decreased and mechanical efficiency increased significantly in the group receiving ascorbic acid as compared with the placebo group. Margolis[60] studied 40 adult male workers; half of the subjects received a vitamin C supplement of 100 mg while the other subjects served as controls. The authors concluded that the vitamin C supplement was helpful in reducing fatigue and in increasing or preventing a decrease in muscular endurance.

Spioch et al.[61] gave 30 healthy men 500 mg of ascorbic acid intravenously prior to a 5-min step test. Oxygen consumption was reduced by 12%, oxygen debt by 40%, total energy output by 18%, and pulse rate by 11% compared to the same test without ascorbic acid. Mechanical efficiency also improved in the subjects receiving the ascorbic acid. Meyer et al.[62] investigated the effect of a predominantly fruit diet containing 500 to 1000 mg of vitamin C on the athletic performance of 6 male and 3 female university and high school students. All students performed 1 h of exercise and a 20-km run each day. Measurements were taken before, during, and after the diet, which was continued for 14 days. Running times of the students were reduced following the diet but no changes were noted for resting heart rate.

Howald et al.[63] studied 13 athletes undergoing a moderately intense, continuous training program. The athletes were initially given a placebo for 14 days. This was followed by a vitamin C supplement of 1000 mg/day for the next 14 days. Exercise tests were performed at the end of each dietary period. The exercise test was a progressive cycle ergometer test starting at a workload of 30 W and increasing in 40-W increments every 4 min until the subject reached exhaustion. Subjects exhibited a significantly greater physical working capacity at a heart rate of 170 beats per minute. In addition, heart rates were consistently lower at each workload throughout the progressive test when the subjects were receiving vitamin C. Finally, the addition of vitamin C to the diets of a group of trained Indian university women also resulted in an improvement in their $\dot{V}O_2$max and work efficiency in the Harvard step test.[64]

B. STUDIES SHOWING NO EFFECT

While many studies do report an ergogenic effect of ascorbic acid, almost as many studies have found that supplementing the vitamin produced no effect on performance. All of these studies involved human subjects.

Several studies prior to 1960 found no effect of vitamin C. Jetzler and Haffler[65] found no difference in endurance capabilities in a 50-km ski race between athletes who had been supplemented with 300 mg of vitamin C and those who had not. Fox et al.[66] and Jokl and Suzman[67] gave 40 mg of vitamin C each day to a group of mine workers and no supplements to a control group. There was a total of 572 subjects. No differences were noted in putting the shot, a 100 yd (110 m) sprint, a 1-mi (1620 m) run, or in various strength measures between the two groups. Keys and Henschel[68] added 100 to 200 mg of vitamin C or a placebo to the diets of 26 young soldiers (13 per group). All soldiers received both treatments in a crossover design and exercised vigorously on a motor-driven treadmill. The ascorbic acid supplement had no effect on pulse rate, oxygen consumption, respiratory quotient, or blood lactic acid concentrations. Jenkins and Yudkin[69] found no differences in resting pulse rate, breath holding time, or endurance abilities in 87 children supplemented with 25 mg of vitamin C daily vs. a group of 91 children acting as a control. In another study,[70] no differences were found in running times or 7-month training records of 2 identical twins when 1 received a supplement of 300 mg of vitamin C per day and the other twin received a placebo.

Several studies, conducted since 1960, also reported no effect of ascorbic acid on performance. Rasch[71] found no differences in performance of cross-country runners receiving either 500 mg of vitamin C per day or a placebo. The experiment lasted one cross-country season and diets during this time were not controlled.

Margaria et al.[72] administered 240 mg of vitamin C to subjects 90 min before exercise. These authors found no effects of the vitamin on treadmill run time to exhaustion or $\dot{V}O_2$max as compared with control conditions. Snigur[73] studied school children for a period of two years. Half of the children were given an ascorbic acid supplement of 100 mg/day and the rest of the children acted as controls. Normal dietary vitamin C intake of the children was calculated at 40 mg/day. No differences between groups were seen for fatigability as estimated by strength of the wrist muscles or vital capacity of the lungs. Another investigator[74] gave subjects a vitamin C supplement or a placebo in a double-blind protocol and exercised them on a motor-driven treadmill. No differences were noted for oxygen consumption, respiratory quotient, or pulse or respiratory rate.

Gey et al.[75] used 286 soldiers as subjects. The experiment lasted for 12 weeks and subjects were administered 1000 mg of vitamin C or a placebo in a double-blind manner. No differences were seen for endurance performance or overall improvement as measured by the mean distance covered on a 12-min walk/run test. Bailey et al. conducted two studies.[76,77] Young male subjects were exercised on a level motor-driven treadmill at various speeds. The experiments were conducted in a double-blind manner with subjects receiving either 2000 mg of ascorbic acid or a placebo for 5 days. No differences were noted for minute ventilation, oxygen uptake, oxygen pulse, or respiratory variables. In another study,[78] the effects of giving 250 to 1000 mg of ascorbic acid, either as a supplemental tablet or by drinking orange juice, were evaluated in normal athletic subjects. A placebo and untreated control group were included. No differences were noted among groups for sprint times, long-distance running, or work efficiency as measured by the Harvard step test. Horak and Zenisek[79] gave two groups of well-trained athletes either 200 mg of ascorbic acid daily as a supplement or a diet high in foods containing vitamin C. These authors reported no significant relationship between resting vitamin C concentrations and work efficiency.

The few studies on vitamin C and exercise performed since 1980 have shown no effects. Keren and Epstein[30] reported on the effects of a vitamin C supplement on both anaerobic and aerobic performance. Ascorbic acid at 1000 mg/day or a placebo were given in a double-blind manner for 21 days to a group of male subjects undergoing training. No differences were noted for $\dot{V}O_2$max or anaerobic performance. Keith and Merrill[81] reported no differences in maximum grip strength or in muscular endurance in 15 male subjects receiving either a single dose of 600 mg of vitamin C or a placebo given 4 h prior to exercise. Mean muscular endurance values were actually worse in those on the vitamin C supplement although this value was not significantly different. The experiment was performed using a double-blind, crossover protocol. Normal vitamin C intake of the subjects was calculated to be 140 mg/day.

Keith and Driskell[82] found no differences in forced expiratory volume, vital capacity, treadmill workload, resting heart rate, or postexercise lactic acid in a group of male subjects receiving 300 mg of ascorbic acid vs. a group receiving a placebo for 21 days. The study was conducted in a double-blind, crossover manner with a three-week washout period between treatments. Subjects had normal plasma ascorbic acid concentrations at the beginning of the study. In a final study for this section, Driskell and Herbert[83] gave 1000 mg of ascorbic acid or a placebo daily to male subjects undergoing treadmill testing. The experiment lasted six weeks. No significant differences were noted for a variety of performance measures.

Summarizing the data on ascorbic acid as a possible ergogenic aid is difficult. Several studies report an ergogenic effect while just as many studies cite no effect. Weaknesses can be found in studies taking both points of view. However, several of the latest studies, in which the initial vitamin C status was apparently adequate, seemed to show no ergogenic effects of additional vitamin C. While exceptions may be found, it is the opinion of this writer that supplemental ascorbic acid, when given to well-nourished subjects, has no pronounced and/or consistent ergogenic effects.

IV. DIETARY INTAKES OF ASCORBIC ACID IN PHYSICALLY ACTIVE PERSONS

Numerous studies have reported on the vitamin C intake of different types of male and female athletes.[33,35,84-104] These studies are summarized in Table 5. Generally, mean vitamin intakes in these groups were above the RDA, with males having larger intakes than females. The range of mean vitamin C intakes for males was 95 to 529 mg/day, while female athletes had intakes of 55 to 234 mg/day. As previously mentioned, the RDA for vitamin C is 60 mg/day.[16] Thus, almost all studies reported mean vitamin C intakes in athletes to be above the RDA and at levels that would probably be considered adequate, under most conditions, for athletes.

However, while mean intakes for the athletic groups were generally adequate, several studies did report that a portion of their athletic population consumed ascorbic acid in suboptimal amounts. Steen and McKinney[103] reported that 23% of their male wrestlers consumed less than two thirds of the RDA for vitamin C. Other papers have indicated similar figures: Hickson et al.,[86] 12 to 20% of football players below 2/3 RDA; Guilland et al.,[35] 25% with low intakes; Cohen et al.,[33] 10% of dancers below the RDA; and DeBolt et al.[97] reported that 10% of Navy SEALS were below the RDA. Female athletes show similar figures: Nowak et al.[87] reported mean intakes of a group of basketball players to be below the RDA; Hickson et al.[100] found 13 to 22% of basketball players and gymnasts to be below 2/3 RDA; Keith et al.[101] showed that 25% of the cyclists in their study consumed less than 2/3 RDA; Loosli et al.[104] found 10% of

TABLE 5   Mean Daily Dietary Intakes of Vitamin C in Various Athletic Groups

Athletic Group	Subject Number	Vitamin C Intake (mg/day)	Ref.
Males			
Endurance runners	15	219	84
Marathon runners	291	147	85
High school football	134	180	86
Competitive runners	30	109	34
Basketball players	16	184	87
Elite triathletes	20	275	88
Competitive bodybuilders	13	272	89
Various athletes	55	95	35
Cross-country runners	12	262	90
Swimmers	22	186	91
Ice hockey players	48	161	92
Elite Nordic skiers	5	282	93
Elite ballet dancers	10	170	33
Ultramarathoners	82	520	46
Elite Nordic skiers	13	232–371 (R)	94
College athletes	—	97–433 (R)	95
College soccer	18	252,529	96
Navy SEALS	267	353	97
Females			
Marathon runners	56	115	85
University dancers	21	148	98
College basketball	10	55	87
High school gymnasts	13	84	99
College basketball	13	106	100
College gymnasts	9	207	100
Competitive bodybuilders	11	196	89
Swimmers	21	188	91
Adolescent gymnasts	42	112	92
Trained cyclists	8	80	101
Elite Nordic skiers	7	234	93
Elite ballet dancers	12	162	33
Adolescent ballerinas	92	148	102
Elite Nordic skiers	14	173–210 (R)	94
Various college athletes	—	84–223 (R)	95

Note: R = range, instead of mean.

gymnasts to be below 2/3 RDA; and Cohen et al.[33] and Benson et al.[102] found 8 to 25% of surveyed dancers to be consuming vitamin C at less than the RDA. Thus, while group means for intake of vitamin C appear to be acceptable, anywhere from about 10 to 25% of an athletic group may be consuming suboptimal levels of the vitamin as compared with the RDA. Improved dietary intakes would be needed in these athletes to assure adequate physical performance.

V. SUMMARY AND RECOMMENDATIONS

Historical and scientific evidence demonstrate that vitamin C deficiency or even marginal vitamin C status can adversely affect physical performance.[1,4,9-14] Ascorbic acid can adversely affect physical functioning at several different metabolic sites, such as impaired collagen formation leading to increased ligament and tendon problems, decreased synthesis of carnitine which would impair the use of fatty acids as an energy source, decreased synthesis of epinephrine and norepinephrine resulting in improper metabolic responses to exercise, as well as improper folate metabolism possibly resulting in anemia and fatigue with consequential decreases in aerobic performance. Thus, all physically active persons should strive to maintain optimal vitamin C status through the intake of generous servings of fruits and vegetables high in ascorbic acid content, or if this is not possible, through proper supplementation with the vitamin.

Several animal[22-26] and human studies[28,29,42-46] do seem to indicate that strenuous physical activity increases the need for vitamin C. Animal studies consistently show reduced tissue levels of ascorbic acid with exercise. Human studies have shown reduced urinary excretion and white blood cell content of vitamin C with exercise, increased adaptation to exercise in the heat with additional ascorbic acid, as well as possible favorable changes in immune status in athletes undergoing strenuous exercise. Vitamin C intake in these studies generally ranged from 100 to 500 mg/day and this would seem to be a reasonable range of intake for physically active individuals. Numerous other data from dietary intake studies with athletes[33,35,84-104] also show mean vitamin C intakes of most athletic groups to be in the 100 to 500 mg/day range. However, several of these studies[33,35,87,97,100,101,104] report that 10 to 25% of the athletes consumed vitamin C at less than RDA levels. Thus, while mean ascorbic acid intakes appear to be adequate, a large percentage of athletes may be consuming suboptimal amounts of the vitamin.

Numerous studies have been conducted in an attempt to find possible ergogenic effects of ascorbic acid. The results of these studies are mixed. Many studies[56-64] report possible ergogenic effects of vitamin C, while just as many studies[65-83] find no effect of ascorbic acid supplementation on subsequent performance. Most of the more recent and generally better-controlled studies do not seem to indicate an ergogenic effect of vitamin C. At the present time the data do not seem to support a clear and/or consistent ergogenic effect of vitamin C.

While a wealth of knowledge does exist concerning ascorbic acid and exercise, many areas remain understudied. The relationship between exercise and vitamin C requirements/needs is one such area. The effect that exercise has on white blood cell ascorbic acid concentrations, how ascorbic acid alters heat adaptation to exercise, the effects of strength/power exercise on ascorbic acid status, and the effects of exercise, ascorbic acid metabolism, and immune function and hormonal changes are all areas that need future research. Little, if any, work has been performed evaluating how exercise might alter ratios of ascorbic acid and dehydroascorbic acid in tissues. For example, this ratio may be altered in some disease states.

Finally, while the relationships among exercise, oxidative damage, and vitamin E have been studied to some extent, very few studies have been performed in this area with vitamin C. All of these subjects need to be explored in the future to further our understanding of vitamin C and physical activity.

REFERENCES

1. Gerster, G., Review: The role of vitamin C in athletic performance, *J. Am. Coll. Nutr.*, 8, 636, 1989.
2. Clarkson, P.M., Vitamins and trace minerals, ergogenics: enhancement of performance in exercise and sport, in *Perspectives in Exercise Science and Sports Medicine,* Lamb, D.R. and Williams, M.H., Eds., Vol. 4, Wm. C. Brown, Dubuque, Iowa, 1991, 123.
3. Keith, R.E., Vitamins and physical activity, in *Nutrition in Exercise and Sport,* 2nd. ed., Wolinsky, I. and Hickson, J.F., Eds., CRC Press, Boca Raton, FL, 1993, 159.
4. Carpenter, K.J., *The History of Scurvy & Vitamin C,* Cambridge University Press, London, 1986.
5. Basu, T.K. and Schorah, C.J., *Vitamin C in Health and Disease,* AVI Publishing, Westport, CT, 1982.

6. Davies, M.B., Austin, J., and Partridge, D.A., *Vitamin C: Its Chemistry and Biochemistry,* The Royal Society of Chemistry, Cambridge, England, 1991.

7. Moser, U. and Bendich, A., Vitamin C, in *Handbook of Vitamins,* 2nd ed., Machlin, L.J., Ed., Marcel Dekker, New York, 1991, 195.

8. Groff, J.L., Gropper, S.S., and Hunt, S.M., *Advanced Nutrition and Human Metabolism,* 2nd ed., West Publishing, Minneapolis, 1995, 222.

9. Ratsimamanga, A.R., Relationship between ascorbic acid and muscular activity, *C.R. Soc. Biol.,* 126, 1134, 1937.

10. Wacholder, K., Rise in the turnover and destruction of ascorbic acid (vitamin C) during muscle work, *Arbeitsphysiologie,* 14, 342, 1951.

11. Lemmel, G., Vitamin C deficiency and general capacity for work, *Muench. Med. Wochenschr.,* 85, 1381, 1938.

12. Babadzanjan, M.G., Kalnyn, V.R., Koslynn, S.A., and Kostina, E.I., Effect of vitamin supplements on some physiological functions of workers in electric locomotive teams, *Vopr. Pitan.,* 19, 18, 1960.

13. Buzina, R. and Suboticanec, K., Vitamin C and physical working capacity, *Int. J. Vitam. Nutr. Res.,* S27, 157, 1985.

14. Van der Beek, E.J., van Dokkum, W., Schrijver, J., Wesstra, J.A., van der Weerd, H., and Hermus, R.J.J., Effect of marginal vitamin intake on physical performance of man, *Int. J. Sports Med.,* 5, 28, 1984.

15. Van der Beek, E.J., van Dokkum, W., Schrijver, J., Wesstra, A., Kistemaker, C., and Hermus, R.J.J., Controlled vitamin C restriction and physical performance in volunteers, *J. Am. Coll. Nutr.,* 9, 332, 1990.

16. National Research Council, *Recommended Dietary Allowances,* 10th ed., National Academy of Sciences, Washington, D.C., 1989.

17. Keith, R.E. and Mossholder, S.B., Ascorbic acid status of smoking and nonsmoking adolescent females, *Int. J. Vitam. Nutr. Res.,* 56, 363, 1986.

18. Schectman, G., Byrd, J.C., and Gruchow, H.W., The influence of smoking on vitamin C status in adults, *Am. J. Public Health,* 79, 158, 1989.

19. Thaxton, J.P. and Pardue, S.L., Ascorbic acid and physiological stress, in *Ascorbic Acid in Domestic Animals,* Wegger, I., Tagwerker, F.J., and Moustgaard, J., Eds., The Royal Danish Agriculture Society, Copenhagen, 1984, 25.

20. Askew, W.A., Environmental and physical stress and nutrient requirements, *Am. J. Clin. Nutr.,* Suppl. 61, 631, 1995.

21. Stone, M.H., Keith, R.E., Kearney, J.T., Fleck, S.J., Wilson, G.D., and Triplett, N.T., Overtraining: A review of the signs and symptoms and possible causes, *J. Appl. Sport Sci. Res.,* 5, 35, 1991.

22. Stojan, B., Pfefferkorn, B., and Schmieder, J., Studies on the ascorbic acid content of the adrenals of the rat after muscular work under normal and lowered oxygen partial pressure, *Acta Biol. Med. Ger.,* 18, 369, 1967.

23. Hughes, R.E., Jones, P.R., Williams, R.S., and Weight, P.F., Ascorbic acid and cholesterol in the tissues of the guinea pig, *Life Sci.,* 10, 661, 1971.

24. Akamatsu, A., Whan, Y.W., Yamada, K., and Hosoya, N., The effect of high environmental temperature and exercise on the metabolism of ascorbic acid in rats, *Vitamins (Jpn.),* 60, 199, 1986.

25. Keith, R.E. and Lee, S., Effects of dietary ascorbic acid and exercise on tissue ascorbic acid, lactate dehydrogenase and thiobarbituric acid reactive substances in guinea pigs, *FASEB J.,* 7, A611, 1993.

26. Keith, R.E. and Pomerance, G.M., Exercise and tissue ascorbic acid content in guinea pigs, *Nutr. Res.,* 15, 423, 1995.

27. Altenburger, E., Relationship of ascorbic acid to the glycogen metabolism of the liver, *Klin. Wochenschr.,* 15, 1129, 1936.

28. Namyslowski, L. and Desperak-Secomska, B., The vitamin C content of the blood in a selected group of students during 1952 and 1953, *Rocz. Panstw. Zakl. Hig.,* 6, 289, 1955.

29. Namyslowski, L., Investigations of the vitamin C requirements of athletes during physical exertion, *Rocz. Panstw. Zakl. Hig.,* 7, 97, 1956.

30. Fishbaine, B. and Butterfield, G., Ascorbic acid status of running and sedentary men, *Int. J. Vitam. Nutr. Res.,* 54, 273, 1984.

31. Gleeson, M., Robertson, J.D., and Maughn, R.J., Influence of exercise on ascorbic acid status in man, *Clin. Sci.,* 73, 501, 1987.

32. Duthie, G.G., Robertson, J.D., Maughn, R.J., and Morrice, P.C., Blood antioxidant status and erythrocyte lipid peroxidation following distance running, *Arch. Biochem. Biophys.,* 282, 78, 1990.

33. Cohen, J.L., Potosnak, L., Frank, O., and Baker, H., A nutritional and hematologic assessment of elite ballet dancers, *Phys. Sportsmed.,* 5, 43, 1985.

34. Weight, L.M., Noakes, T.D., Labadarios, D., Graves, J., Jacobs, P., and Berman, P.A., Vitamin and mineral status of trained athletes including the effects of supplementation, *Am. J. Clin. Nutr.,* 47, 186, 1988.

35. Guilland, J.-C., Penaranda, T., Gallet, C., Boggio, V., Fuchs, F., and Klepping, J., Vitamin status of young athletes including the effects of supplementation, *Med. Sci. Sport Exercise,* 21, 441, 1989.

36. Telford, R.D., Catchpole, E.A., Deakin, V., McLeay, A.C., and Plank, A.W., The effect of 7 to 8 months of vitamin/mineral supplementation on the vitamin and mineral status of athletes, *Int. J. Sport Nutr.,* 2, 123, 1992.

37. Zeman, F.J., *Clinical Nutrition and Dietetics,* 2nd ed., Macmillan, New York, 1991, 760.
38. Garry, P.J. and Appenzeller, O., Vitamins A and C and endurance races, *Ann. Sports Med.,* 1, 82, 1983.
39. Boddy, K., Hume, R., King, P.C., Weyers, E., and Rowan, T., Total body, plasma and erythrocyte potassium and leucocyte ascorbic acid in "ultra-fit" subjects, *Clin. Sci. Mol. Med.,* 46, 449, 1974.
40. Bacinskij, P.P., Effect of physical activity on the vitamin C and B1 supply of the body, *Vopr. Pitan.,* 18, 53, 1959.
41. Henschel, A., Taylor, H.L., Brozek, J., Mickelsen, O., and Keys, A., Vitamin C and the ability to work in hot environments, *Am. J. Trop. Med.,* 24, 259, 1944.
42. Visagie, M.E., du Plessis, J.P., and Laubscher, N.F., Effect of vitamin C supplementation on black mine-workers, *S. Afr. Med. J.,* 49, 889, 1975.
43. Karnaugh, N., Effect of physical work and heat microclimate on the excretion of 17-hydroxycorticosteroids and ascorbic acid, *Vrach. Delo,* 3, 134, 1976.
44. Strydom, N.B., Kotze, H.F., van der Walt, W.H., and Rogers, G.G., Effect of ascorbic acid on rate of heat acclimatization, *J. Appl. Physiol.,* 41, 202, 1976.
45. Kotze, H.F., van der Walt, W.H., Rogers, B.B., and Strydom, N.B., Effects of plasma ascorbic acid levels on heat acclimatization in man, *J. Appl. Physiol.,* 42, 771, 1977.
46. Peters, E.M., Goetzsche, J.M., Grobbelaar, B., and Noakes, T.D., Vitamin C supplementation reduces the incidence of postrace symptoms of upper-respiratory-tract infection in ultramarathon runners, *Am. J. Clin. Nutr.,* 57, 170, 1993.
47. Staton, W.M., The influence of ascorbic acid in minimizing post-exercise muscle soreness in young men, *Res. Q. Am. Assoc. Health Phys. Educ. Recreat.,* 23, 356, 1952.
48. Jakeman, P. and Maxwell, S., Effect of antioxidant vitamin supplementation on muscle function after eccentric exercise, *Eur. J. Appl. Physiol.,* 67, 426, 1993.
49. Viguie, C.A., Frei, B., Shigenaga, M.K., Ames, B.N., Packer, L., and Brooks, G.A., Oxidant stress in humans during consecutive days of exercise, *Med. Sci. Sport Exercise,* 22, S86, 1990.
50. Basu, N.M. and Biswas, P., The influence of ascorbic acid on contractions and the incidence of fatigue of different types of muscles, *Indian J. Med. Res.,* 28, 405, 1940.
51. Bushnell, R.G. and Lehmann, A.G., Antagonistic effect of sodium ascorbate on ethanol-induced changes in swimming of mice, *Behav. Brain Res.,* 1, 351, 1980.
52. Richardson, J.H. and Allen, R.B., Dietary supplementation with vitamin C delays onset of fatigue in isolated striated muscle of rats, *Can. J. Appl. Sport Sci.,* 8, 140, 1983.
53. Lang, J., Gohil, K., and Packer, L., Effect of dietary vitamin C on exercise performance and tissue vitamin C, vitamin E and ubiquinone levels, *Fed. Proc.,* 45, 1747, 1986.
54. Sieburg, H., Redoxon as a tonic for sportsmen, *Dtsch. Med. Wochenschr.,* 63 (Arzt. und Sport), 13, 11, 1937.
55. Wiebel, H., Studies of dosage with vitamin C in athletic female students, *Dtsch. Med. Wochenschr.,* 65, 60, 1939.
56. Basu, N.M. and Ray, G.K., The effect of vitamin C on the incidence of fatigue in human muscles, *Indian J. Med. Res.,* 28, 419, 1940.
57. Harper, A.A., MacKay, I.F.S., Raper, H.S., and Camm, G.L., Vitamins and physical fitness, *Br. Med. J.,* i, 243, 1943.
58. Hoitink, A.W., Vitamin C and work. Studies on the influence of work and of vitamin C intake on the human organism, *Verh. Ned. Inst. Praevent. Geneesk.,* 4, 176, 1946.
59. Hoogerwerf, A. and Hoitink, A.W., The influence of vitamin C administration on the mechanical efficiency of the human organism, *Int. Z. Angew. Physiol. Arbeitsphysiol.,* 20, 164, 1963.
60. Margolis, A.M., Vitamin C status of miners and some other population groups in the Don basin, *Vopr. Pitan.,* 23, 78, 1964.
61. Spioch, F., Kobza, R., and Mazur, B., Influence of vitamin C upon certain functional changes and the coefficient of mechanical efficiency in humans during physical effort, *Acta Physiol. Pol.,* 17, 204, 1966.
62. Meyer, B.J., deBruin, E.J., Brown, J.M., Bieler, E.U., Meyer, A.C., and Grey, P.C., The effect of a predom-inately fruit diet on athletic performance, *Plant Foods Man,* 1, 223, 1975.
63. Howald, H., Segesser, B., and Korner, W.F., Ascorbic acid and athletic performance, *Ann. N.Y. Acad. Sci.,* 258, 458, 1975.
64. Samanta, S.C. and Biswas, K., Effect of supplementation of vitamin C on the cardiorespiratory endurance capacity of college women, *Snipes J.,* 8, 55, 1985.
65. Jetzler, A. and Haffler, C., Vitamin C-bedarf bei einmaliger sportlicher dauerleistung, *Wein. Med. Wochenschr.,* 89, 332, 1939.
66. Fox, F.W., Dangerfield, L.F., Gottlich, S.F., and Jokl, E., Vitamin C requirements of native mine labourers. An experimental study, *Br. Med. J.,* ii, 143, 1940.
67. Jokl, E. and Suzman, H., A study of the effects of vitamin C upon physical efficiency, *Transvaal Mine Med. Off. Assoc. Proc.,* 19, 292, 1940.
68. Keys, A. and Henschel, A.F., Vitamin supplementation of U.S. Army rations in relation to fatigue and the ability to do muscular work, *J. Nutr.,* 23, 259, 1942.

69. Jenkins, G.N. and Yudkin, J., Vitamins and physiological function, *Br. Med. J.,* ii, 265, 1943.
70. Vinarickij, R., An attempt to improve the efficiency of medium distance runners by large doses of vitamin B1, B2 and C, *Scr. Sci. Med.,* 27, 1, 1954.
71. Rasch, P., Effects of vitamin C supplementation on cross country runners, *Sportzarztliche Praxis,* 5, 10, 1962.
72. Margaria, R., Agheno, P., and Rovelli, E., The effect of some drugs on the maximal capacity of athletic performance in man, *Int. Z. Angew. Physiol.,* 20, 281, 1964.
73. Snigur, O.I., Signs of fatigue in school children in different states of ascorbic acid supply, *Gig. Sanit.,* 7, 117, 1966.
74. Kirchhoff, H.W., Effect of vitamin C on energy expenditure and circulatory and ventilatory function in stress studies, *Nutr. Diet.,* 11, 184, 1969.
75. Gey, G.O., Cooper, K.H., and Bottenberg, R.A., Effect of ascorbic acid on endurance performance and athletic injury, *J. Am. Med. Assoc.,* 211, 105, 1970.
76. Bailey, D.A., Carron, A.V., Teece, R.G., and Wehner, H.J., Vitamin C supplementation related to physiological response to exercise in smoking and nonsmoking subjects, *Am. J. Clin. Nutr.,* 23, 905, 1970.
77. Bailey, D.A., Carron, A.V., Teece, R.G., and Wehner, H.J., Effect of vitamin C supplementation upon the physiological response to exercise in trained and untrained subjects, *Int. J. Vitam. Res.,* 40, 435, 1970.
78. Bender, A.E. and Nash, A.H., Vitamin C and physical performance, *Plant Foods Man,* 1, 217, 1975.
79. Horak, J. and Zenisek, A., Vitamin C blood level before and after laboratory load and its relation to cardiorespiratory performance parameters in top sportsmen, *Cas. Lek. Cesk.,* 116, 679, 1977.
80. Keren, B. and Epstein, Y., Effect of high dosage vitamin C intake on aerobic and anaerobic capacity, *J. Sports Med. Phys. Fitness,* 20, 145, 1980.
81. Keith, R.E. and Merrill, E., The effects of vitamin C on maximum grip strength and muscular endurance, *J. Sports Med. Phys. Fitness,* 23, 253, 1983.
82. Keith, R.E. and Driskell, J.A., Lung function and treadmill performance of smoking and nonsmoking males receiving ascorbic acid supplements, *Am. J. Clin. Nutr.,* 36, 840, 1982.
83. Driskell, J.A. and Herbert, W.G., Pulmonary function and treadmill performance of males receiving ascorbic acid supplements, *Nutr. Rep. Int.,* 32, 443, 1985.
84. Peters, A.J., Dressendorfer, R.H., Rimar, J., and Keen, C.L., Diets of endurance runners competing in a 20-day road race, *Phys. Sportsmed.,* 14, 63, 1986.
85. Nieman, D.C., Butler, J.V., Pollett, L.M., Dietrich, S.J., and Lutz, R.D., Nutrient intake of marathon runners, *J. Am. Diet. Assoc.,* 89, 1273, 1989.
86. Hickson, J.F., Duke, M.A., Risser, W.L., Johnson, C.W., Palmer, R., and Stockton, J.E., Nutritional intake from food sources of high school football athletes, *J. Am. Diet. Assoc.,* 87, 1656, 1987.
87. Nowak, R.K., Knudsen, K.S., and Schulz, L.O., Body composition and nutrient intakes of college men and women basketball players, *J. Am. Diet. Assoc.,* 88, 575, 1988.
88. Burke, L.M. and Read, R.S.D., Diet patterns of elite Australian male triathletes, *Phys. Sportsmed.,* 15, 140, 1987.
89. Bazzarre, T.L., Kleiner, S.M., and Ainsworth, B.E., Vitamin C intake and lipid profiles of competitive male and female bodybuilders, *Int. J. Sport Nutr.,* 2, 260, 1992.
90. Niekamp, R.A. and Baer, J.T., In-season dietary adequacy of trained male cross-country runners, *Int. J. Sport Nutr.,* 5, 45, 1995.
91. Berning, J.R., Troup, J.P., van Handel, P.J., Daniels, J., and Daniels, N., The nutritional habits of young adolescent swimmers, *Int. J. Sport Nutr.,* 1, 240, 1991.
92. Rankinen, T., Fogelholm, M., Kujala, U., Rauramaa, R., and Uusitupa, M., Dietary intake and nutritional status of athletic and nonathletic children in early puberty, *Int. J. Sport Nutr.,* 5, 136, 1995.
93. Fogelholm, M., Rehenen, S., Gref, C.-G., Laakso, J.T., Lehto, J., Ruokonen, I., and Himberg, J.-J., Dietary intake and thiamin, iron, and zinc status in elite Nordic skiers during different training periods, *Int. J. Sport Nutr.,* 2, 351, 1992.
94. Ellsworth, N.M., Hewitt, B.F., and Haskell, W.L., Nutrient intake of elite male and female Nordic skiers, *Phys. Sportsmed.,* 13, 78, 1985.
95. Short, S.H. and Short, W.R., Four-year study of university athletes' dietary intake, *J. Am. Diet. Assoc.,* 82, 632, 1983.
96. Hickson, J.F., Schrader, J.W., Pivarnik, J.M., and Stockton, J.E., Nutritional intake from food sources of soccer athletes during two stages of training, *Nutr. Rep. Int.,* 34, 85, 1986.
97. DeBolt, J.E., Singh, A., Day, B.A., and Deuster, P.A., Nutritional survey of the US Navy SEAL trainees, *Am. J. Clin. Nutr.,* 48, 1316, 1988.
98. Evers, C.L., Dietary intake and symptoms of anorexia nervosa in female university dancers, *J. Am. Diet. Assoc.,* 87, 66, 1987.
99. Moffat, R.J., Dietary status of elite female high school gymnasts: inadequacy of vitamin and mineral intake, *J. Am. Diet. Assoc.,* 84, 1361, 1984.
100. Hickson, J.F., Schrader, J., and Trischler, L.C., Dietary intakes of female basketball and gymnastics athletes, *J. Am. Diet. Assoc.,* 86, 251, 1986.

101. Keith, R.E., O'Keeffe, K.A., and Alt, L.A., Dietary status of trained female cyclists, *J. Am. Diet. Assoc.*, 89, 1620, 1989.
102. Benson, J., Gillien, D.M., Bourdet, K., and Loosli, A.R., Inadequate nutrition and chronic calorie restriction in adolescent ballerinas, *Phys. Sportsmed.*, 13, 79, 1985.
103. Steen, S.N. and McKinney, S., Nutrition assessment of college wrestlers, *Phys. Sportsmed.*, 14, 100, 1986.
104. Loosli, A.R., Benson,J., Gillien, D.M., and Bourdet, K., Nutrition habits and knowledge in competitive adolescent female gymnasts, *Phys. Sportsmed.*, 14, 118, 1986.

Chapter 3

THIAMIN

_____ James J. Peifer

CONTENTS

I. INTRODUCTION

Anorexia, progressive weakness of leg muscles, loss of tendon reflexes, peripheral and cerebral neuropathies, mental disorientation, and possible cardiomyopathy are symptomatic of beriberi, a deficiency disease resulting from severe depletion of thiamin.[1-3] A major concern is that the dietary habits and physical activities of athletes might induce mild depletions of thiamin that could compromise their neuromuscular activities. Significant numbers of athletes and other young people from the wealthier nations are reported to have marginal to more serious depletions of thiamin.[4-7] Increased physical exertion has been linked to increased demands for thiamin by beriberi victims and athletes,[8-11] and vigorous exercise is reported to induce a transient increase in protein catabolism and the related thiamin-dependent catabolism of branched-chain amino acids (BCAA).[12-14] High caloric intakes of carbohydrates and increased intakes of BCAA have also been linked to increased metabolic demands for

0-8493-8192-4/97/$0.00+$.50

thiamin.[15-17] Severe caloric restrictions and the limiting of food selection to thiamin-poor foods[18] are additional dietary factors that increase the risks of mild to more severe depletions of thiamin. Despite the multiple links cited for thiamin and physical activities, contradictory results are also reported for participants involved in physical activities.[10,11,19,20] One goal of this review is to identify possible reasons for some of these reported discrepancies, and another is to determine whether there is sufficient available information to recommend changes in dietary intakes of thiamin for those participating in physical activities.

II. METABOLIC FUNCTIONS OF THIAMIN

Key roles of thiamin in energy metabolism and biosynthetic processes are briefly outlined in the seven metabolic pathways of Figure 1. Thiamin diphosphate (TDP), also referred to as thiamin pyrophosphate (TPP) , is required for energy transformations (pathways 1 to 5) and transketolases of the pentose phosphate pathway (6 and 7).[1,2] In the citric acid cycle (CAC) (pathways 1 and 2), TDP is required for oxidative decarboxylation of pyruvic and α-keto-glutaric acids. TDP is also required for catabolism of BCAA (pathways 3 to 5). Catabolism of BCAA is initiated through transamination to their respective ketoacids (BCKA), and these BCKA are then catabolized by TDP-dependent oxidative decarboxylation. The BCKA derived from leucine, valine, and isoleucine, respectively, are α-ketoisocaproic, α-ketoisovaleric, and α-keto-ß-methylvaleric acids. In each case, BCKA is further degraded to metabolites that can enter the CAC. Only the dephosphorylated form of the BCKA-dehydrogenase complex (BCKAD) is active for these oxidative decarboxylations.[21]

The obligatory roles of TDP for generating NADPH and pentoses are shown in pathways 6 and 7. Biosynthesis of fatty acids is one example of a NADPH-dependent reductive-biosynthetic process. Pentoses generated by this pathway are utilized for biosynthesis of tissue nucleotides.[1-3]

III. THIAMIN IN BRAIN AND NEURAL TISSUES

The obligatory role of glucose catabolism in brain and other neural tissues emphasizes the importance of maintaining TDP-dependent metabolic pathways for optimal functioning of the nervous system. Thiamin appears to have an additional functional role in neural tissues. This vitamin is bound, possibly as TDP or thiamin triphosphate (TTP), to axonal membranes, and conduction of nerve impulses is accompanied by the release of free thiamin from these biomembranes.[22-24] Rats depleted of thiamin have a reduced conduction of nerve impulses in their peripheral nerves.[25] Displacement of thiamin from peripheral nerves leads to aberrations in nerve impulse spike potentials characteristic of altered sodium channels in axonal membranes.[26-28] These and other observations[29] suggest that a phosphorylated ester of thiamin plays a central role in regulating sodium transport during conduction of nerve impulses. The possibility that a mild depletion of thiamin from neural tissues might directly affect neuro-muscular functions should be investigated with experimental animals. Further details on the role of thiamin in the nervous system are included in an excellent review by Haas.[29]

IV. ASSESSMENT OF THIAMIN STATUS

Measurements of the relative urinary excretion of thiamin have been used to establish dietary requirements for this vitamin as well as the thiamin status of population groups.[30-34] Depletion of thiamin reserves is accompanied by a decreased urinary excretion of thiamin.[34,35] Blood levels of the vitamin have also been used to evaluate thiamin status,[33,36] but this is

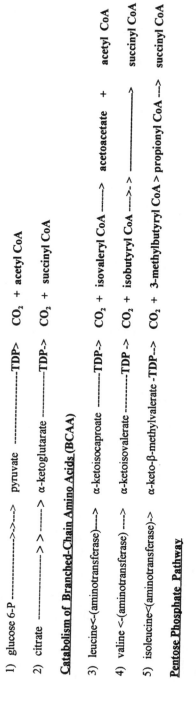

FIGURE 1 Thiamin diphosphate (TDP)-dependent metabolic pathways. TDP requirements for oxidative decarboxylations in CAC are shown in pathways 1 and 2. TDP requirements for catabolism of branched-chain amino acids (BCAA) are illustrated in pathways 3 to 5. BCAA are transaminated to their respective branched-chain ketoacids (BCKA), and these BCKA undergo TDP-dependent decarboxylation to CoA metabolites which enter CAC. TDP-dependent transketolase activities of the pentose phosphate pathway are summarized in pathways 6 and 7.

more commonly evaluated on the basis of TDP and/or TDP-dependent transketolase activity in erythrocytes (ETKA).[35,37-39] Young healthy men, depleted of thiamin for eight weeks, experience progressive decreases in their ETKA and daily urinary excretion level of thiamin.[35] ETKA measurements reflect differences in TDP-dependent transketolase activity at the time of collecting the blood samples. Urinary excretion of thiamin and its multiple derivatives is a reflection of the reserves of this vitamin during 24 h to several days prior to the collection of urine.[34] High pressure liquid chromatography (HPLC) techniques[39,40] may prove to be a more sensitive and reliable method for evaluating the thiamin status in population groups. One HPLC study suggests that loss of TDP precedes detectable changes in ETKA.[41]

V. DIETARY ALLOWANCES AND TOXICITIES

Dietary guidelines for thiamin are based on its central role in energy metabolism. Recommended allowance for the general public is an intake of 0.5 mg thiamin per 1000 kcal. The specific recommended daily dietary allowances (RDA) are 1.1 and 1.5 mg/day for 15- to 51-year-old females and males, respectively.[42] This guideline suggests that common daily energy expenditures of up to 5000 kcal would not increase demands for thiamin beyond the range of 2.5 mg. Continued studies are needed to determine whether this same guideline applies to athletes involved in frequent bouts of vigorous physical activity

Thiamin absorption occurs by both passive diffusion and a sodium-dependent active-transport system.[3,43,44] Because of the human's limited capacity to absorb this vitamin, mega amounts of thiamin (500 mg/day) can be tolerated for short periods of time.[2] However, intravenous and intramuscular injections of megadoses of thiamin can induce serious toxic effects including convulsions and cardiac arrhythmia.[45,46] Daily intakes of megadoses of thiamin and other nutrients have little scientific support, and athletes should be warned about the potential hazards of injecting megadoses of this vitamin.

VI. DIETARY SOURCES OF THIAMIN

Thiamin is widely distributed among the different food groups , but many foods provide very limited amounts of this vitamin.[18] Best sources of thiamin are pork, whole grain cereals, enriched breads, and other thiamin-supplemented foods. Beans, peas, and orange juice are good sources of thiamin, but most other vegetables and fruits contain very limited amounts of thiamin.[18]

VII. THIAMIN, PHYSICAL ACTIVITY AND SPORT

A. EXPERIMENTAL ANIMAL STUDIES

The use of animal models has provided much of our basic knowledge about the physiological and metabolic roles of thiamin.[29] Results from some preliminary studies in our laboratory illustrate how rats depleted of thiamin exhibit many of the signs of thiamin depletion reported for beriberi victims.[1-3] Rats deprived of thiamin for 1 month eat sub-normal amounts of food, have elevated blood levels of pyruvate, lose approximately 95% of thiamin from their liver, and only limited amounts of residual thiamin are excreted in their urine.[47,48] Thiamin-deficient rats also have depressed TDP-dependent transketolase activity in their brains, and have a significantly reduced conduction velocity in their peripheral nerves.[25,49]

The earlier observation that increased physical activity accelerates depletion of thiamin in beriberi subjects[8,9] has been demonstrated in experimental animals. Repeated bouts of vigorous physical activity are reported to deplete thiamin reserves of rats.[50] Although a single bout of exhaustive swimming did not significantly alter tissue levels of thiamin of rats, repeated (10 days) daily bouts of vigorous swimming led to significant losses of this vitamin from their blood, liver, and kidneys.[50] Depletion of glycogen reserves, rather than dramatic losses of thiamin reserves, is probably the immediate cause of muscle fatigue from a single bout of exhaustive exercise. Other studies suggest that the transient increased metabolic demands for TDP during vigorous exercise may be compensated for by supplements of thiamin. Mice, trained to swim vigorously for daily intervals of 30 min, swam 40% longer when their high-carbohydrate diet was augmented with an injection of 100 times the minimal daily requirement (MDR) of thiamin.[51] However, the megadose of thiamin had no influence on delaying fatigue in mice fed a high-fat diet. Further studies should investigate the possibility that dietary intakes of 5 to $10 \times$ MDR of thiamin may afford the same degree of protection against the early onset of muscle fatigue in mice or rats fed high-carbohydrate diets.

Rats subjected to vigorous physical activity experience an increased net catabolism of BCAA (leucine) and muscle protein,[52,53] and this introduces an additional transient demand for TDP-dependent catabolism of BCAA (pathways 3 to 5, Figure 1).

B. HUMAN STUDIES

Various reports suggest a definitive link between high-carbohydrate intakes, physical exertion, and nutritional-metabolic demands for thiamin in humans. Increased physical exertion accelerates further depletion of thiamin reserves in beriberi subjects consuming high-carbohydrate diets,[8,9] and carbohydrate loading accelerates the onset of Wernicke's syndrome in subjects depleted of their reserves of thiamin.[16] The study of Sauberlich et al.[15] further demonstrated that human requirements for thiamin are greatest with high caloric intakes of carbohydrates. Nijakowski reported that energy expenditures resulting from repeated bouts of vigorous skiing led to significant decreases in blood levels of thiamin.[10] A report by Early and Carlson[11] suggests that multivitamin supplements which include thiamin (100 mg), pantothenic acid (30 mg), and other B vitamins are effective in delaying the onset of fatigue in young men participating in 50-yd dash events in hot climates. These investigators speculated that the multivitamin supplement was compensating for sweat losses of thiamin and pantothenic acid, but further controlled studies are needed to test the validity of this speculation.

Vigorous exercise is accompanied by an increased demand for thiamin because of increased TDP-dependent CAC activities and an increased catabolism of BCAA in muscle protein. The link between vigorous exercise and a transient increase in protein catabolism is illustrated by the study of Rennie et al.[13] In their study, men participating in prolonged vigorous exercise (50% $\dot{V}O_2$max /3.8 h) on a treadmill experienced a transient depression of protein synthesis (14%) coupled with a 54% increased catabolism of proteins. Because of the abundance of BCAA in proteins,[21] an increased catabolism of proteins is accompanied by an increased demand for TDP needed for the catabolism of BCAA in these proteins. Wolfe et al.[55,56] reported that less-strenuous exercise (30% $\dot{V}O_2$max /105 min) on a bicycle ergometer induced some transient inhibition of protein synthesis without a major change in protein catabolism. Young[54] reports that high intakes of proteins also increases catabolism of protein, but further studies are needed to demonstrate how high protein intakes may affect nutritional demands for thiamin in participants of vigorous exercise events.

Moderate physical activities do not appear to significantly deplete thiamin reserves of healthy adults. The controlled studies of Keys et al.[19] suggest that a limited intake of thiamin (0.23 mg thiamin per 1000 kcal) is adequate for young men participating in repeated (10 to 12 weeks) 60- to 90-min sessions on a treadmill. A fourfold increase of thiamin intake (1.0 mg/1000 kcal) did not significantly alter leg muscle strength or the blood levels of glucose, pyruvate, and lactate of their participants. A more recent study by Fogelholm[20] suggests that repeated bouts of short-term (30 to 60 min) aerobic exercises does not significantly alter thiamin reserves of healthy young Finnish women. In this study, an exercise session was either a 30-min interval of sufficient intensity to induce a 70 to 80% increase in heart rate, or a 60-min interval of sufficient intensity to induce 60 to 65% increases in heart rate. Equivalent levels of TDP-dependent ETKA were found in the control subjects (n = 18) and experimental group (n = 21) participating in 1 to 24 (30 min to 12 hs) aerobic exercising sessions per week. The report by Caster and Mickelsen[57] suggests that 1500 kcal/day energy expenditure on a treadmill induced a marginal depletion of thiamin. The initial study induced decreases in urinary excretion of thiamin (indicative of depleted thiamin reserves), but a repeat of the study failed to yield the same correlation between treadmill exercise and urinary excretion of thiamin.

The increased metabolic demands of pregnancy are accompanied by increased dietary requirements for thiamin and most other nutrients.[42] The effect of superimposing mild aerobic expenditures of energy on the energy demands for pregnancy was investigated by Lewis et al.[58] Healthy pregnant women participated in this study during their 22nd to 30th week of gestation. The aerobic exercise sessions were 30-min intervals (3 times weekly) of walking on a treadmill with sufficient intensity to induce a 70% maximum of their age-predicted heart rate. At the end of 8 weeks of these aerobic energy expenditures, the walking group (n = 18) and the nonwalking control group (n = 10) had equivalent erythrocyte transketolase activities.

Many reports on thiamin and physical activities do not include detailed information about daily intakes of thiamin by the participants, but reports by Wolfe et al.,[55,56] Keys et al.,[19] Fogelholm,[20] and Lewis et al.[58] suggest that thiamin intakes in the range of one to two times its RDA (i.e., 1.5 to 3.0 mg/day) is adequate for the increased energy demands of moderate aerobic physical activities. Some of the conflicting reports in the literature may be related to the dietary habits of the participants. Aerobic exercise studies carried out in individuals consuming diets containing high levels of fat and only moderate levels of carbohydrate (35% fat calories and 48 to 50% carbohydrates)[19,20] have less demands on their thiamin reserves than those generating energy expenditures from higher carbohydrate intakes.[15] McNeil and Mooney[51] failed to find thiamin supplements effective in improving the endurance of exercising mice fed high-fat diets.

VII. SUMMARY

Although thiamin intakes are not clearly stated in many of the reported physical activity studies, available data suggest that thiamin intakes in the range of one to two times its RDA (1.5 to 3.0 mg/day) adequately meets the requirement for this vitamin in moderate aerobic physical activities by healthy men and women. Experimental animal studies and limited reports on human subjects suggest that repeated bouts of vigorous exercise significantly increase nutritional-metabolic demands for thiamin, but further studies are needed to determine optimal intakes of thiamin for such physical activities. The greatest demand for thiamin occurs during the course of vigorous physical activity when carbohydrates are the major source of energy expenditure and there is an additional demand for TDP-dependent catabolism of BCCA.

It is recommended that further human studies include standardization of thiamin intakes (i.e., 1.5 to 2.5 mg/day) and the consumption of a nonvitamin-supplemented high-carbohydrate mixture (i.e., 400 to 1000 kcal) 3 to 4 h before initiating a physical activity event. These double-blind controlled studies should be designed to establish optimal levels of thiamin (i.e., 5, 10, or 50 × RDA) needed to significantly delay the onset of fatigue caused by repeated bouts of vigorous physical activities. The use of sensitive measurements of ETKA and/or

HPLC-determined TDP in erythrocytes provides an opportunity to demonstrate thiamin demands during the peak of vigorous physical activity.

Further studies are also recommended to determine how high vs. moderate intakes of proteins may affect thiamin demands of experimental animals and human subjects subjected to frequent bouts of vigorous physical activity.

ACKNOWLEDGMENT

I wish to acknowledge my great indebtedness to Dr. Richard Lewis for his considerable assistance in collecting literature required for this review.

REFERENCES

1. **Tanphaichitr, V.,** Thiamin, in *Modern Nutrition in Health and Disease,* 8th ed., Shils, M. E. and Olson, J. A., Eds., Lea & Febiger, Philadelphia, 1994, 359.
2. **Groff, J. J., Grooper, S. S., and Hunt, S. A.,** Thiamin, in *Advanced Nutrition and Human Metabolism,* 2nd ed., West Publishers, New York, 1995, 237.
3. **Brown, M. L.,** Thiamin, in *Present Knowledge in Nutrition,* 6th ed., Brown, M. L., Ed., International Life Science Institute, Nutrition Foundation, Washington, D.C., 1990, chap. 16.
4. **Wood, B. and Pennington, D. G.,** The thiamin status of Australians, *Food Technol. Aust.,* 26, 278, 1974.
5. **Hatanaka, Y. and Ueda, K.,** High incidence of subclinical hypovitaminosis of B_1 among university students found by a field study in Ehime, Japan, *Med. J. Osaka Univ.,* 31, 83, 1981.
6. **Hickson, J. F., Jr., Schrader, J. W., Pivarnik, J. M., and Stockton, J. E.,** Nutritional intake from food sources of soccer athletes during two stages of training, *Nutr. Rep. Int.,* 34, 85, 1986.
7. **Guilland, J.-C., Penaranda, T., Gallet, C., Boggio, V., Fuchs, F., and Klepping, J.,** Vitamin status of young athletes including the effects of supplementation, *Med. Sci. Sports Exercise,* 21, 441, 1989.
8. **Burgess, R. C.,** Beriberi. I. Epidemiology, *Fed. Proc.,* 17(Suppl. 2), 3, 1958.
9. **Platt, B. S.,** Beriberi, II. Clinical features of endemic beriberi, *Fed. Proc.,* 17(Suppl. 2), 8, 1958.
10. **Nijakowski, F.,** Assay of some vitamins of the B complex group in human blood in relation to muscular effort, *Acta Physiol. Pol.,* 17, 397, 1966.
11. **Early, R. and Carlson, B.,** Water soluble vitamin therapy on the delay of fatigue from physical activity in hot climatic conditions, *Int. Z. Angew. Physiol.,* 27, 43, 1969.
12. **Henderson, S. A., Black, A. L., and Brooks, G. A.,** Leucine turnover and oxidation in trained rats during exercise, *Am. J. Physiol.,* 249, E137, 1985.
13. **Rennie, M. J., Edwards, R. N. T., Krywawych, S., Davies, C. T. M., Halliday, D., Waterlow, J. C., and Millward, D. J.,** Effect of exercise on protein turnover in man, *Clin. Sci.,* 61, 627, 1981.
14. **Layman, D. K., Paul, G., and Olken, M. H.,** Amino acid metabolism during exercise, in *Nutrition in Exercise and Sport,* 2nd ed., Wolinsky, I. and Hickson, J. F., Eds., CRC Press, Boca Raton, FL, 1994.
15. **Sauberlich, H. E., Herman, Y. F., and Stevens, Y. F.,** Thiamin requirement of the adult human, *Am. J. Clin. Nutr.,* 23, 671, 1970.
16. **Watson, A. J. S., Walker, J. F., Tomkin, G. H., Finn, M. M. R., and Keogh, J. A. B.,** Acute Wernicke's encephalopathy precipated by glucose loading, *Ir. J. Med. Sci.,* 150, 301, 1981.
17. **Harper, A. E. and Benjamin, E.,** Relationship between intake and rate of oxidation of leucine and α-ketoisocaproate in vivo in the rat, *J. Nutr.,* 114, 431, 1984.
18. **Block, A. S. and Shills, M. E.,** in *Nutrition Facts Manual: A Quick Reference,* Williams & Wilkins, Baltimore, 1996.
19. **Keys, A., Henschel, A. F., Mickelsen, O., and Brozek, J. M.,** The performance of normal young men on controlled thiamin intakes, *J. Nutr.,* 26, 399, 1943.
20. **Fogelholm, M.,** Micronutrient status in females during a 24-week fitness-type exercise program, *Ann. Nutr. Metab.,* 36, 209, 1992.
21. **Harper, A. E., Miller, R. H., and Block, K. P.,** Branched-chain amino acid metabolism, *Annu. Rev. Nutr.,* 4, 1984, 409.
22. **Cooper, J. R. and Pincus, J. H.,** The role of thiamin in nervous tissue., *Neurochem. Res.,* 4, 223, 1979.
23. **Tanaka, C. and Cooper, J. R.,** The fluorescent microscopic localization of thiamin in nervous tissue, *J. Histochem. Cytochem.,* 16, 362, 1968.
24. **Matsuda, T. and Cooper, J. R.,** Thiamin as an integral component of brain symptosomal membranes, *Proc. Natl. Acad. Sci. U.S.A.,* 78, 5886, 1981.

25. **McLane, J. A., Kahn, T., and Held, I. R.,** Increased axonal transport in peripheral nerves of thiamine-deficient rats, *Exp. Neurol.,* 95, 482, 1987.

26. **Itokawa, Y. and Cooper, J. R.,** Thiamine release from nerve membranes by tetrodotoxin, *Science,* 166, 759, 1969.

27. **Goldberg, D. J. and Cooper, J. R.,** Effects of thiamine antagonists on nerve conduction. I. Actions of antimetabolites and fern extract on propagated action potentials, *J. Neurobiol.,* 6, 435, 1975.

28. **Schoffeniels, E.,** Thiamin phosphorylated derivatives and bioelectrogenesis, *Arch. Int. Physiol. Biochim.,* 91, 233, 1983.

29. **Haas, R. H.,** Thiamin and the brain, *Annu. Rev. Nutr.,* 8, 483, 1988.

30. **Mickelsen, O., Caster, W. D., and Keys, A. A.,** A statistical evaluation of the thiamine and pyramin excretions of normal young men on controlled intakes of thiamine, *J. Biol. Chem.,* 168, 415, 1947.

31. **Stearns, G., Adamson, L., McKinley, J. B., Lenner, T., and Jeans, P. C.,** Excretion of thiamine and riboflavin by children, *Am. J. Dis. Child.,* 95, 185, 1958.

32. **Ziporin, Z. Z., Nunes, W. T., Powell, R. C., Waring, P. P., and Sauberlich, H. E.,** Thiamine requirements in the adult human as measured by urinary excretion of thiamin metabolites, *J. Nutr.,* 85, 297, 1965.

33. **Pearson, W. N.,** Blood and urinary vitamin levels as potential indices of body stores, *Am. J. Clin. Nutr.,* 20, 514, 1967.

34. **Sauberlich, H. E., Dowdy, R. R., and Skala, J. H.,** Thiamin (Vitamin B₁) in *Laboratory Tests for the Assessment of Nutritional Status,* CRC Press, Boca Raton, FL, 1974, 22.

35. **van der Beek, E. J., van Dokkum, W, Schrijver, J., Wedel, M., Gaillard, A. W. K., Wesstra, A., van de Weerd, H., and Hermus, R. J. J.,** Thiamin, riboflavin and vitamins B-6 and C: impact of combined restricted intake on functional performance in man, *Am. J. Clin. Nutr.,* 48, 1451, 1988.

36. **Kawai, C. and Wakabayashi, A.,** Reappearance of beriberi heart disease in Japan. A study of 23 cases, *Am. J. Med.,* 69, 383, 1980.

37. **Brin, M.,** Erythrocyte as a biopsy tissue for functional evaluation of thiamin adequacy, *J. Am. Med. Assoc.,* 187, 762, 1964.

38. **Warnock, L. G.,** Transketolase activity of blood hemolysate, a useful index for diagnosing thiamin deficiency, *Clin. Chem.,* 21, 432, 1975.

39. **Warnock, L. G.,** The measuremnet of erythrocyte thiamin pyrophosphate by high performance liquid chromatography, *Anal. Biochem.,* 126, 394, 1982.

40. **Kimura, M. and Itokawa, Y.,** Determination of thiamin and its phosphorylated esters in human and rat blood by high-performance liquid chromatography with post-column derivatization, *J. Chromatogr.,* 181, 332, 1985.

41. **Warnock, L. G., Prudhomme, C. R., and Wagner, C.,** The determination of thiamin pyrophosphate in blood and other tissues, and its correlation with erythrocyte transketolase activity, *J. Nutr.,* 108, 421, 1979.

42. **National Research Council,** *Recommended Dietary Allowances,* 10th ed., National Academy Press, Washington, D.C., 1989.

43. **Rindi, G. and Ventura, V.,** Thiamin intestinal transport, *Physiol. Rev.,* 52, 821, 1972.

44. **Hoyumpa, A. M., Strickland, R., Sheehan, J. J., Yarborough, G., and Nochols, S.,** Dual systems of intestinal transport in humans, *J. Lab. Clin. Med.,* 99, 701, 1982.

45. **AMA,** *Drug Evaluation,* American Medical Association, Chicago, 1980, 833.

46. **Combs, G. F.,** *The Vitamins,* Academic Press, San Diego, CA, 1992, 251.

47. **Peifer, J. J. and Cleland, G.,** Elevated blood pyruvate levels and decreased retention of thiamin in rats mildly depleted of vitamin B₁₂, *Nutr. Res.,* 7, 1179, 1987.

48. **Peifer, J. J. and Clelland, G.,** Metabolic demands for coenzyme B₁₂ - dependent mutase increased by thiamin deficiency, *Nutr. Res.,* 7, 1197, 1987.

49. **McCandles, D. W., Curley, A. D., and Cassidy, C. E.,** Thiamin deficiency and the pentose phosphate cycle in rats: intracerebral mechanisms, *J. Nutr.,* 106, 1144, 1976.

50. **Bialek, M. and Nijakowski, F.,** Influence of physical effort on the level of thiamin in tissues and blood, *Acta Physiol. Pol.,* 15, 192, 1964.

51. **McNeill, A. W. and Mooney, T. J.,** Relationship among carbohydrate loading, elevated thiamine intake and cardiovascular endurance of conditioned mice, *J. Sports Med.,* 23, 257, 1983.

52. **Henderson, S. A., Black, A. L., and Brooks, G. A.,** Leucine turnover and oxidation in trained rats during exercise, *Am. J. Physiol.,* 249, E137, 1985.

53. **Layman. D. K., Paul, G. L., and Olken, M. H.,** Amino acid metabolism during exercise, in *Nutrition in Exercise and Sport,* 2nd ed., Wolinsky I. and Hickson, J. F., Jr., Eds., CRC Press, Boca Raton, FL, 1994, chap. 6.

54. **Young, V. R.,** Metabolic and nutritional aspects of physical exercise, *Fed. Proc.,* 44, 341, 1985.

55. **Wolfe, R. R., Goodenough, R. D., Wolfe, M. H., Royle, G. T. and Nadle, E. R.,** Isotopic analysis of leucine and urea in exercise in humans, *J. Appl. Physiol.,* 52, 27, 1982.

56. **Wolfe, R. R., Wolfe, M. H., Nadel, E. R., and Shaw, J. H. F.,** Isotopic determination of amino acid-urea interactions in exercise in humans, *J. Appl. Physiol.,* 56, 221, 1984.

57. **Caster, W. O. and Mickelsen, O.,** Effect of diet and stress on the thiamin and pyramin excretion of normal young men maintained on controlled intakes of thiamin, *Nutr. Res.,* 11, 549, 1991.

58. **Lewis, R. D., Yates, Y. Y., and Driskell, J. A.,** Riboflavin and thiamin status and birth outcome as a function of maternal aerobic exercise, *Am. J. Clin. Nutr.,* 48, 110, 1988.

Chapter 4

RIBOFLAVIN AND NIACIN

_____ Richard D. Lewis

CONTENTS

I. INTRODUCTION

Carbohydrate, fat, and to a limited extent, protein, are necessary substrates for physical work. The degree to which each macronutrient is utilized depends on several factors including the training and nutritional status of an individual and the duration and intensity of an exercise bout. Riboflavin and niacin, in their respective coenzyme forms, are intimately involved in metabolic reactions necessary for the utilization of these fuels. One could hypothesize that because of their multiple roles as cofactors in glycolysis, the tricarboxylic acid cycle (TCA), electron transport and ATP synthesis (oxidative phosphorylation), and lipid oxidation, nutritional requirements for these vitamins would be elevated with rigorous physical training. This chapter will attempt to address this hypothesis by reviewing each vitamin's metabolic roles, methodologies used for status assessment, recommended and usual intakes, dietary sources, and the literature regarding the impact of exercise on riboflavin and niacin status. In addition, the metabolic and performance responses to supplementation will be discussed.

0-8493-8192-4/97/$0.00+$.50
© 1997 by CRC Press, Inc.

II. RIBOFLAVIN

A. STRUCTURE AND METABOLIC ROLES

The water-soluble vitamin B_2, or riboflavin, is composed of an isoalloxazine ring and is chemically referred to as 7,8-dimethyl-10-(1'-D-ribityl).[1] Free riboflavin is not the active form of the vitamin, but serves as the precursor in the synthesis of the two coenzymatically active forms, flavine mononucleotide (FMN) and the more prevalent flavine-adenine dinucleotide (FAD). FMN is synthesized from cellular riboflavin in an ATP-dependent flavokinase reaction and can then be converted to FAD, catalyzed by FAD synthetase. Biosynthesis of the flavin coenzymes is dependent on riboflavin status and is enhanced by thyroxine and triiodothyronine.[1]

The two coenzymes assist in a host of redox reactions classified as dehydrogenases, oxidases, and monooxygenases by serving as either one-electron (FMNH, FADH) or two-electron ($FMNH_2$, $FADH_2$) acceptors or donors.[1] Acetyl CoA, derived either from glucose via glycolysis or from fatty acids through β-oxidation, enters the TCA cycle within the mitochondrial matrix for oxidation. Figures 1, 2, and 3 highlight the key metabolic roles of the flavin coenzymes in glycolysis, the TCA cycle, and electron transport.[2] Within the TCA cycle the key enzymatic reaction assisted by FAD is succinate dehydrogenase, in which succinate is converted to fumarate and FAD is reduced to $FADH_2$. The electrons from $FADH_2$ are then transferred to ubiquinone via a succinate dehydrogenase complex. Also occurring associated with the electron transport chain, reduced nicotinamide adenine dinucleotide ($NADH_2$) is oxidized to NAD by the FMN-dependent NADH dehydrogenase.

In addition to the key roles of flavin coenzymes in the TCA cycle and the electron transport chain, FAD is reduced in a flavin-dependent acyl-CoA dehydrogenase reaction, the first step of β-oxidation in which acyl-CoA is converted to enoyl-CoA. The electrons generated are also transferred to ubiquinone within the electron transport system. Another key flavin-dependent reaction, one which is the basis for clinical riboflavin assessment, is the erythrocyte glutathione reductase (EGR) reaction:[3]

$$GSSG + NADPH + H^+ \xrightarrow[\text{EGR}]{\text{FAD}} 2\ GSH + NADP^+$$

FAD is reduced by NADPH and $FADH_2$ gives up electrons to form reduced glutathione (GSH). Both the conversion of pyridoxine to its active coenzyme of pyridoxal 5'-phosphate and the conversion of tryptophan to niacin are also flavin dependent.[1]

With increased energy expenditure there is an accelerated use of carbohydrate and fat for energy. Based on the above roles of the flavin coenzymes in respiratory metabolism, one might expect increased needs associated with the enhanced oxidative potential of skeletal muscle with aerobic training. Prior to addressing the issue of physical activity and riboflavin status, current dietary recommendations and typical intakes of the general population will be examined.

B. RECOMMENDED DIETARY ALLOWANCES AND DIETARY SOURCES

Recommendations for riboflavin intakes are based on long-term feeding trials in which clinical signs of riboflavin deficiency and urinary excretion of riboflavin were used as factors in determining the Recommended Dietary Allowance (RDA).[4] Riboflavin needs have been thought to be related to energy consumption[5] and to lean body mass.[6] The RDA committee suggests that an intake of 1.6 μmol/4184 kJ (0.6 mg/1000 kcal) will meet the needs of most healthy adults, or a minimum level of 3.2 μmol (1.2 mg) for those who are consuming less than 8368 kJ (2000 kcal).[4] The current RDA is 4.5 μmol (1.7 mg) for men, 23 to 50 years of age, and 3.5 μmol (1.3 mg) for women 23 to 50 years of age. The requirement is lower

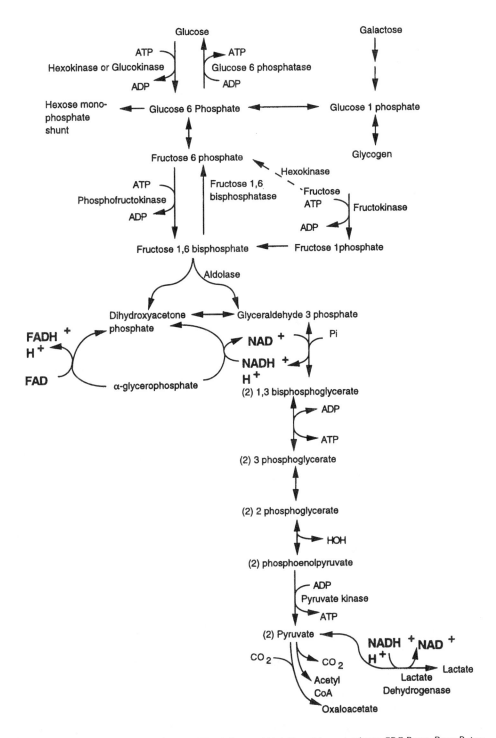

FIGURE 1 Glycolysis. (From Berdanier, C.D., *Advanced Nutrition: Macronutrients,* CRC Press, Boca Raton, FL, 1995.)

for the 50+ age group, based on the lower energy requirement for the older individual. Russell[7] suggests, however, that the requirements for the elderly should be increased because the breakpoint for urinary excretion of riboflavin in dose-response feeding trials occurs at levels of dietary riboflavin similar to the requirement for younger individuals. Data from the USDA Nationwide Food Consumption Survey[4] indicates that in 1985 in the U.S. men and women

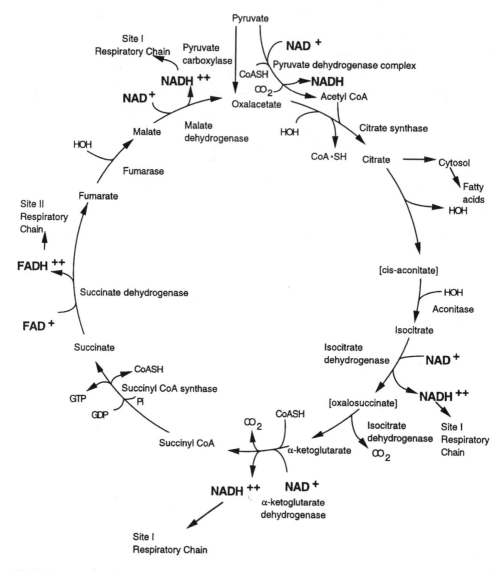

FIGURE 2   Tricarboxylic acid cycle. (From Berdanier, C.D., *Advanced Nutrition: Macronutrients*, CRC Press, Boca Raton, FL, 1995.)

consumed 5.5 μmol (2.08 mg) and 3.6 μmol (1.34 mg) of riboflavin per day, respectively. These data suggest that men and women are consuming adequate amounts of riboflavin. In a review of dietary intakes of different athletic groups, it appears as though most athletes are also consuming adequate amounts of riboflavin.[8]

Riboflavin is widely distributed in foods, with dairy products, eggs, meats, greens, and enriched grains providing the best sources.[9] The riboflavin content of some common foods are listed in Table 1.[9] Milk, which contains free riboflavin, is the best source for this water-soluble vitamin providing 0.9 μmol (0.34 mg) per cup of skim milk. However, consumption of milk products in the U.S. over a 12-year period from 1977–78 to 1989–90 decreased approximately 5%.[10]

While Short[8] indicated that most athletes consume adequate riboflavin, it is possible that subpopulations of athletes — those with concerns about body weight — may be at risk for lower intakes. In college gymnasts, it has been reported that milk and dairy product intake, in addition to overall caloric intake, is much lower than current recommendations.[11] Further

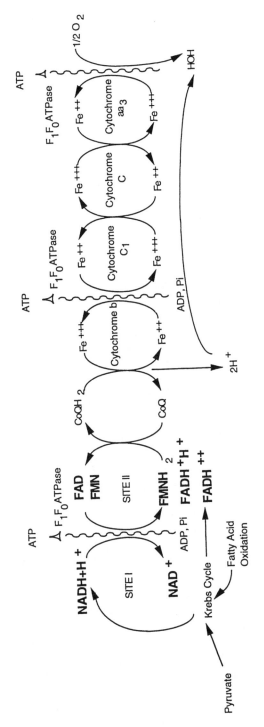

FIGURE 3 Electron transport. (From Berdanier, C.D., *Advanced Nutrition: Macronutrients*, CRC Press, Boca Raton, FL, 1995.)

TABLE 1 Riboflavin and Niacin Content in Common Foods

Food Item	Riboflavin μmol	Riboflavin mg	Niacin μmol	Niacin mg
1 Egg	0.67	0.25	0.30	0.04
1/2 c Bran flakes	0.77	0.29	28.1	3.43
1 slice Bread	0.21	0.08	7.70	0.94
1 oz Hamburger	0.16	0.06	12.0	1.46
1 oz Chicken	0.19	0.07	14.7	1.79
1 oz Tuna	0.08	0.03	28.7	3.50
3.5 fl oz Orange juice	0.08	0.03	2.80	0.34
1/2 c Sweet corn	0.21	0.08	9.80	1.20
1 Banana	0.29	0.11	5.10	0.62
1 c Milk	0.90	0.34	1.80	0.22

controlled dietary studies of low-body-weight athletes are needed to confirm this observation and to assess riboflavin status.

C. ASSESSMENT OF RIBOFLAVIN STATUS

As mentioned, oxidized glutathione (GSSG) is reduced to GSSH in an FAD-dependent glutathione reductase reaction.[3,12] This oxidation-reduction reaction is the basis for the most commonly used and most sensitive method for the assessment of riboflavin nutriture. A majority of studies examining the influence of physical activity on riboflavin status and requirements utilized the measurement of EGR activity as the primary indicator of status. This method is based on the *in vitro* assessment of EGR activity with and without added FAD, and is expressed as an activity coefficient (EGRAC):[3,12]

$$EGRAC = \frac{\text{Enzyme activity (with added FAD)}}{\text{Basal enzyme activity (without added FAD)}}$$

The numerator represents total stimulated EGR activity, or the degree of apoprotein saturation with FAD, while the denominator reflects changes in basal unstimulated EGR activity. Basal EGR activity appears more responsive to dietary intake.[3] For example, over a period of time with a diet low in riboflavin, EGRAC increases — primarily as the result of a decrease in basal activity.

While there are still some questions regarding acceptable values and interpretation of EGRAC, one investigator suggested that values below 1.20 be considered acceptable, 1.20 to 1.39 marginal, and >1.40 deficient.[3] Because of concerns with analytical variability, Belko et al.[13] recommended the use of a more conservative cutoff such that values <1.25 be regarded as normal. Campbell et al.[14] questions the guidelines for interpretation of EGRAC. They found that in a Chinese population a majority of those surveyed would be classified as deficient based on the 1.20 or 1.25 cutoff, without clear evidence of deficiency symptoms.[14] Horwitt,[15] in a letter to the editor of the *American Journal of Clinical Nutrition,* suggested that EGRAC be used only to distinguish those who are clearly deficient or have an EGRAC of >1.5. He further suggests using caution when interpreting EGRACs in nondeficient subjects because the glutathione reductase enzyme is not completely saturated with FAD even in normal subjects. Horwitt recommends that urinary excretion of riboflavin be used in conjunction with EGRAC for the most meaningful results.

Urinary excretion of riboflavin (24-h urinary collections) has been used for years to assess riboflavin nutriture and is a good indicator of recent intakes of riboflavin, but it is not a sensitive indicator of tissue stores.[16] In addition, urinary riboflavin values (milligrams per gram of creatinine) vary widely and are influenced by many factors including sleep, nitrogen balance, bed rest, environmental temperatures, and physical activity.[16,17] Gibson[16] recommends urinary excretion of riboflavin from 24-h urine samples be used to confirm the results of EGRAC. Serum riboflavin and erythrocyte or whole-blood riboflavin evaluations are not recommended as they appear to be insensitive indicators of riboflavin status.[16]

D. PHYSICAL ACTIVITY AND CHANGES IN RIBOFLAVIN STATUS

The relationship between physical activity and/or increased energy expenditure and riboflavin status was initially addressed several years ago as scientists were attempting to accurately estimate riboflavin requirements.[17] The question of whether physical activity influences the requirement for riboflavin has been addressed recently utilizing short- and long-term (5 to 40 weeks) exercise interventions in women[13,18-23] and men.[20,24,25] Methodological differences exist in some of these more current studies, with one key factor being whether riboflavin status was assessed by EGRAC alone[20-22] or in combination with urinary riboflavin excretion.[13,18,19,23,24] Another important methodological factor was whether dietary riboflavin intake was controlled[13,18,19,23,24] or assessed through the use of dietary records.[20-22]

In an effort to determine the effects of environmental factors, including work, on riboflavin excretion, Tucker et al.[17] examined the effects of acute (45 min) and chronic (3 and 9 days) treadmill walking in men under controlled dietary riboflavin conditions. In all three experiments there was a significant reduction in 24-h urinary riboflavin excretion with the hard work. While decreased excretion with the acute bout of exercise was most likely associated with decreased renal plasma flow, the authors hypothesized that the decreased excretion with chronic treadmill walking may have been associated with incorporation of riboflavin into newly synthesized muscle tissue.[17] These results seemed to agree with earlier reports of Delachaux and Ott[26] and Friedemann et al.,[27] who reported reduced urinary excretion of riboflavin with increased physical training.

Belko et al. conducted a series of often-cited studies examining the influence of exercise on riboflavin requirements in normal[13] and overweight women[18,19] under controlled intakes of riboflavin. In the first study of normal weight women[13] they determined that riboflavin intakes of 0.23 µg/kJ (0.96 µg/kcal) and 0.28 µg/kJ (1.16 µg/kcal) were necessary for women under sedentary and exercise conditions (6 weeks of running), respectively, to achieve EGRAC values under the 1.25 cutoff. The RDA of 0.15 µg/kJ (0.6 µg/kcal) was not satisfactory. In fact, during the nonexercise phase of the study, in which subjects were consuming the RDA level for riboflavin, 11 out of 12 subjects had EGRAC values >1.25, with a mean value of 1.41 ± 0.09. The exercise-induced increase in EGRAC was not associated with the small gains in lean body mass. Horwitt[15] recommended that urinary excretion of riboflavin should have been reported in conjunction with the EGRAC data for a more thorough assessment of the influence of excercise on riboflavin status. Roe and Belko[28] indicated that their use of EGRAC was based on the method being a more sensitive indicator of tissue stores of riboflavin, was less influenced by environmental factors, and, in their study, having a much lower coefficient of variability than the urinary excretion data.

In a follow-up to the first study, Belko et al.[18] examined the effects of exercise (aerobic dance) and weight loss on riboflavin status in sedentary, overweight women, in a crossover design, who were consuming 0.19 µg/kJ (0.8 µg/kcal) of riboflavin. The authors were interested in determining if substantial decreases in lean body mass with weight loss would be associated with riboflavin status. Both EGRAC and urinary riboflavin excretion were used as markers of riboflavin status and hydrodensitometry was used to estimate lean body mass. Regardless of exercise, 0.19 µg/kJ (0.8 µg/kcal) was not adequate, as mean baseline sedentary EGRAC values were 1.28 ± 0.11. Aerobic exercise increased EGRAC values significantly, from 1.40 ± 0.12 (nonexercise period) to 1.49 ± 0.16 and decreased urinary excretion of riboflavin from 30% of intake (nonexercise period) to 19% of intake. Changes in riboflavin status were not related to decreases in lean tissue mass. It is possible that more accurate estimates of lean tissue mass by including estimates of total body water in conjunction with hydrodensitometry, would have better clarified the lean body mass-riboflavin relationship.

Belko et al.,[19] in a third study, attempted to confirm in overweight, sedentary women the riboflavin requirements established in the first study, i.e., 0.23 µg/kJ (0.96 µg/kcal) (moderate) during nonexercise periods and 0.28 µg/kJ (1.16 µg/kcal) (high) during exercise. Similar to the earlier reports, exercise (bicycle ergometry) increased EGRAC significantly in both the high-riboflavin group (1.16 ± 0.03 to 1.20 ± 0.02) and the low-riboflavin group (1.31 ± 0.03 to 1.36 ± 0.02). EGRAC values were in the normal range for the high-riboflavin group during both the exercise and nonexercise periods, while EGRAC values were higher than 1.25 in the moderate-riboflavin group during either the exercise or nonexercise periods. Urinary excretion of riboflavin significantly declined with exercise, but only in the high-riboflavin group. The authors suggest that 0.23 µg/kJ (0.96 µg/kcal) was not adequate with or without exercise, while 0.28 µg/kJ (1.16 µg/kcal) brought EGRAC values to within biochemical normality. Referring back to the ratio for calculation of EGRAC, they suggested that the mechanism for exercise-induced increases in EGRAC may be different depending on the level of riboflavin in the diet. The high-riboflavin group had an increase in total stimulated enzyme activity while the moderate-riboflavin group had a decrease in basal enzyme activity. While there is some question regarding interpretation of EGRAC values and whether values >1.25 are riboflavin deficient, there still appeared to be a significant exercise effect over time.

The results from Belko's lab provided the rationale for an animal study conducted by Hunter and Turkki[29] to examine the effects of exercise on riboflavin status. Unlike the findings of Belko et al.,[13,18,19] Hunter and Turkki[29] found no effect of exercise on riboflavin status. Using marginal levels of dietary riboflavin — 5.3 µmol/kg bw (2.0 mg/kg bw) and 6.6 µmol/kg bw (2.5 mg/kg bw) and progressive treadmill running for 6 and 8 weeks — the authors found that exercise in rats did not increase EGRAC values. They did find that increasing the riboflavin content in the diet from 5.3 to 6.6 µmol/kg bw significantly reduced EGRAC regardless of exercise. Riboflavin content in the gastrocnemius and soleus muscles was increased with exercise at both 6 and 8 weeks when expressed as kilograms per muscle or kilograms per 100 g bw. Training adaptations appeared to occur as palmitoyl CoA dehydrogenase activity in the soleus muscle of the exercise groups increased when expressed as nanomoles per minute per gram of tissue or as whole muscle tissue. The authors were unsure why there were increases in muscle riboflavin content and oxidative enzyme activity with marginal intakes of the vitamin. They did suggest the possibilities of decreased turnover, decreased nonfunctional metabolism, and/or decreased excretion of riboflavin. Riboflavin excretion was measured, and while it appeared as though the exercised rats excreted less riboflavin, values were not statistically significant. It is possible that had riboflavin content and EGRAC been assessed earlier in the training program (short-term), with intakes at 5.3 µmol/kg (2.0 mg/kg) bw, differences may have been apparent. With extended training there may be adaptive conservation of riboflavin for the increased oxidative potential of the animal.

Older population groups are becoming increasingly aware of the importance of physical fitness, and that the health benefits of participating in a regular exercise program are not limited to younger adults and children. Winters et al.[23] extended some of the earlier work of Belko and co-workers[13,18,19] to assess the effects of exercise on riboflavin requirements in older women (50 to 67 years of age). The authors utilized a crossover design of nonexercise and exercise (cycle ergometry) with high (0.22 µg/kJ; 0.9 µg/kcal) and low (0.15 µg/kJ; 0.6 µg/kcal) levels of dietary riboflavin. The exercise intervention lasted 4 weeks. The low-riboflavin group had significantly higher EGRAC values than the high-riboflavin group (1.224 ± 0.079 vs. 1.070 ± 0.031) during the nonexercise period, suggesting that 0.15 µg/kJ (0.6 µg/kcal) may not be adequate in the diet for older women, regardless of exercise status. Exercise, similar to the previous reports from Belko's lab,[13,19] significantly increased EGRAC values in both the low- and high-riboflavin groups. Urinary excretion of riboflavin also decreased significantly in both groups with exercise. While exercise increased EGRAC in the high-riboflavin group from 1.070 ± 0.031 to 1.109 ± 0.045, dietary provision of 0.22 µg/kJ (0.9 µg/kcal) of riboflavin appeared adequate as the EGRAC values remained lower than their criterion coefficient value of 1.25.

The study by Winters et al.[23] was particularly relevant to the recent review by Russell[7] suggesting that riboflavin requirements should be increased for older populations. The value of 0.15 µg/kJ (0.6 µg/kcal) dietary riboflavin appeared marginal in these older women based on the mean EGRAC value of 1.224 ± 0.079. However, a riboflavin intake of 0.22 µg/kJ (0.9 µg/kcal), which is higher than the current RDA of 0.15 µg/kJ (0.6 µg/kcal), was adequate. The authors suggest that while older women may not require as much riboflavin as younger women, 0.22 µg/kJ (0.9 µg/kcal) vs. 0.28 µg/kJ (1.16 µg/kcal), requirements are still higher than the current RDA and adjustments for regular vigorous physical activity may be warranted.

Fogelholm[21] assessed riboflavin status in 18 to 33-year-old females before and after a 24-week aerobic fitness program. Riboflavin status determined by EGRAC was considered normal at the onset of the study. While the exercise subjects had a significant 10% increase in aerobic capacity as determined by a maximal ergometry test, EGRAC did not change. Mean intakes of riboflavin from 4-day food records were 5.1 µmol (1.9 µg) and 4.8 µmol (1.8 mg) per day for exercisers and controls, respectively. It is possible that the lack of exercise-induced changes in EGRAC may be the result of riboflavin intakes higher than the current recommendations.

Lewis et al.[22] trained previously sedentary women for 8 weeks during pregnancy and found that while aerobic fitness improved significantly in the exercise group, there was no change in EGRAC. Similar to the report by Folgelhom,[21] initial riboflavin status was normal and mean dietary intakes of riboflavin were high for both exercisers and controls, with intakes of approximately 7.3 µmol (2.7 mg) and 6.7 µmol (2.5 mg) per day, respectively, throughout the duration of the study.

While the relationship between exercise and riboflavin status has been examined more thoroughly in women, a few studies have investigated the influence of physical activity on riboflavin status in men.[20,24,25] In a crossover study[24] conducted at the National Institute of Nutrition in Hyderabad, India researchers confirmed the results of previous studies on women that exercise increases the need for riboflavin as determined by EGRAC and urinary riboflavin excretion. Six men in a metabolic ward were given a diet of 0.10 to 0.11 µg/kJ (0.42 to 0.46 µg/kcal) riboflavin (low, based on the RDA) and subjected to an 18-day exercise intervention consisting of 30 min of treadmill walking and 30 min of bicycle ergometry daily. Mean EGRAC values increased from 1.36 ± 0.21 during the maintenance period to 1.57 ± 0.31 following the exercise period. Urinary excretion of riboflavin as a percent of intake decreased from $26.2 \pm 9.2\%$ during maintenance to $18.1 \pm 5.4\%$ following exercise. Unlike the report of Belko et al.[19] in which overweight women consuming moderate intakes of riboflavin had a decrease in basal activity with exercise, the men had nonsignificant increases in both basal and stimulated activity. The authors speculate that because there was a slightly higher increase in stimulated EGR or total activity compared to basal activity, there was an increase in the EGR apoenzyme and consequently an increased need for FAD. Because the diet used in this study was low in riboflavin (as evidenced by baseline mean EGRAC values considerably higher than 1.25), decreases in basal activity would also have been expected over the course of the study.

Evelo et al.[20] trained sedentary men and women, 28 to 41 years of age, to run a half-marathon using a 40-week running program. EGRAC was assessed at baseline, 20, and 40 weeks. By 20 weeks of training EGRAC unexpectedly decreased. The EGRAC values of 1.03 to 1.08 were within the normal range, suggesting that long-term running did not compromise riboflavin status. Unfortunately, however, diet and/or supplementation was not reported and it is possible that as training increased, riboflavin intakes also increased, resulting in greater riboflavin availability and retention.

Ohno et al.[25] trained 7 sedentary men for 10 weeks using a running program. Like Evelo et al.,[20] dietary intake of riboflavin was not controlled or assessed. The 10-week running program increased $\dot{V}O_2$max and significantly increased EGRAC, the result of a significant increase in stimulated or total activity of EGR. There was no change in basal activity. The increases in total EGR activity with exercise are somewhat consistent with changes observed by Soares et al.[24] and Belko et al.,[19] such that apoprotein was responsive to FAD stimulation. As Soares et al.[24] indicated, increased synthesis of apoprotein associated with the exercise stimulus is possible.

E. RIBOFLAVIN STATUS IN ATHLETES AND PERFORMANCE

Intervention studies with controlled intakes of riboflavin seem to suggest that exercise alters biochemical indices of riboflavin status, such that EGRAC is elevated and urinary excretion of riboflavin is decreased.[13,18,19,23,24] Therefore, the hypothesis that athletes participating in vigorous activity may have compromised riboflavin status seems plausible. However, riboflavin status has been examined in various athletic groups[30-34] to determine whether trained athletes are at risk for riboflavin deficiency and the results do not support the findings from intervention studies. While Haralambie[30] reported that 45% of the athletes (8/18, all males) had EGRAC values indicative of inadequate riboflavin nutriture (>1.25), Guilland et al.[32] found that 55 male athletes and 20 controls had normal EGRAC values and that riboflavin intakes met the RDA of 0.15 μg/kJ (0.6 μg/kcal). Riboflavin intake and urinary excretion of riboflavin were not reported in the Haralambie study.

In a study of triathletes and tennis and track athletes, Keith and Alt[31] also found that riboflavin status determined by EGRAC was normal for all athletes. Compared to controls, there were trends in the data suggesting that EGRAC values were higher (1.06 ± 0.06 vs. 1.01 ± 0.07) and urinary excretion of riboflavin (milligrams per gram creatinine) lower (63 ± 26 vs. 86 ± 16). Riboflavin intakes were higher than the RDA for both athletes and controls, as intakes were 0.24 μg/kJ (1.0 μg/kcal) and 0.22 μg/kJ (0.9 μg/kcal), respectively. In the studies conducted by Belko et al.,[13,19] women consuming a diet of 0.23 μg/kJ (0.96 μg/kcal) riboflavin, which is similar to the intakes reported by Keith and Alt[31] and higher than those of Guilland et al.,[32] had an inadequate intake based on the 1.25 cutoff EGRAC value. The fact that Belko's subjects were initially deplete (EGRAC >1.25) and untrained (compared to athletes who have been training for years) may contribute to the discrepancies in EGRAC status between these studies.[35]

In a supplementation study Tremblay[33] found, as in the athletes studied by Keith and Alt[31] and Guilland et al.,[32] that all male and female elite swimmers (no controls) had EGRAC values below 1.25 at baseline. Supplementation with 160 μmol (60 mg) per day for 16 to 20 days did not change EGRAC values or improve performance as determined by 50-m freestyle swim tests. The authors concluded that when athletes consume adequate amounts of riboflavin and maintain normal riboflavin status, supplementation does not improve performance or alter EGRAC. These results agree with the finding of van Dokkum and van der Beek,[36] who found no effect of riboflavin supplementation on bicycle ergometry performance in subjects with normal riboflavin status.

While the primary aim of the studies by Belko et al.[13,18,19] was to assess the effects of exercise on riboflavin status, they were also interested in the relationship between increasing riboflavin intakes and aerobic performance. They found that aerobic capacity was not related to riboflavin status. There were no significant correlations between the change in aerobic capacity following 5 weeks of exercise training and the change in EGRAC or urinary riboflavin excretion.[18] In addition, they concluded that subjects fed a higher level of riboflavin — 0.28 μg/kJ (1.16 μg/kcal) — high enough to promote normal riboflavin status — did not improve performance or aerobic capacity.[19] Thus, riboflavin supplementation will probably not improve performance unless status is severely compromised by chronic undernutrition prior to supplementation.[37] Dietary restriction of several B vitamins to 33% of the Dutch RDAs over an 8-week period significantly reduced aerobic capacity.[37] While riboflavin status was clearly compromised by the 8th week (EGRAC = 1.46 ± 0.05), inadequate status of the other B vitamins, in combination with the riboflavin deficiency may have contributed to the decreased work capacity.

F. SUMMARY AND RECOMMENDATIONS FOR EXERCISE AND SPORT

Based on the findings of Belko et al.,[13,18,19] Winters et al.,[23] and Soares et al.,[24] who controlled riboflavin intake, it appears as though exercise in previously sedentary or nonathletic individuals alters indices of riboflavin status as evidenced by increases in EGRAC and decreases in urinary riboflavin excretion. Succinate dehydrogenase (SDH) activity in localized skeletal muscle increases with endurance training.[38] One would expect that increases in activity of SDH and other flavin-dependent enzymes associated with the enhanced oxidative potential of skeletal muscle with training[29] would increase the need for riboflavin in active muscle. However, riboflavin status, based on EGRAC, appears to be adequate in athletes and active individuals on free-living diets.[31-33] This may be the result of long-term training adaptations, and the fact that athletes may be consuming more riboflavin. It would be interesting to observe the biochemical responses of women and men on controlled intakes of riboflavin with more prolonged training (>5 months).

Belko and co-workers[13,18,19] recommend that the RDA for riboflavin be adjusted to account for regular physical activity. Whether these exercise-induced changes in biochemical parameters represent a need for greater dietary riboflavin and a need to adjust the RDA still needs further clarification. Regardless, most of the general population, as well as many athletes, consume considerably more riboflavin than the RDA. In addition, there is no evidence that supplementation enhances performance. In summary, physical activity alters biochemical indices of riboflavin status and this observation appears to be associated with initial training and riboflavin status and, possibly, the length of training. There is no need or advantage to supplement the diet of athletes or active individuals with riboflavin unless individuals are truly riboflavin deficient. Continued investigation into the long-term effects of exercise on riboflavin status is warranted. Further assessment of riboflavin intakes in athletes attempting to achieve or maintain a low body weight is needed.

III. NIACIN

A. STRUCTURE AND METABOLIC ROLES

Niacin or vitamin B_3, also referred to as nicotinic acid and nicotinamide, is a water-soluble vitamin with a basic structure of pyridine-3-carboxylic acid (nicotinic acid). The structure of nicotinamide is similar to nicotinic acid, with an amine group added. Like riboflavin, these free vitamins are not the active forms of the vitamin. Nicotinamide serves as a precursor of nicotinamide adenine dinucleotide (NAD) and NAD phosphate (NADP), the two active coenzyme forms.[39]

The coenzyme forms of nicotinamide have a major role in intermediary metabolism as they serve as carriers of reducing equivalents in glycolysis, the pentose shunt, the TCA cycle, and electron transport (Figures 1, 2, and 3),[2] and also in β-oxidation and fat and protein biosynthesis. In fact, there are at least 200 enzymes requiring NAD or NADP.[39] In glycolysis (Figure 1), once reducing equivalents are generated in the 3-phospho-glyceraldehyde dehydrogenase reaction, the hydrogens can be utilized for the synthesis of lactate under anaerobic conditions or transferred to the electron transport chain if oxygen is available. In the TCA cycle (Figure 2), several enzymes including pyruvate dehydrogenase, isocitrate dehydrogenase, α-ketoglutarate dehydrogenase, and malate dehydrogenase require NAD as an electron acceptor. The primary function of NAD in these cycles is to accept two electrons and a proton from intermediary substrates, becoming NADH. The hydrogens are then transferred to the electron transport system via the NADH complex, where NADH is reoxidized to NAD and ATP is generated (Figure 3). The regeneration of NAD is essential to continued ATP synthesis.

B. ASSESSMENT OF NIACIN STATUS, RECOMMENDED DIETARY ALLOWANCES, AND DIETARY SOURCES

Recommendations for niacin are based on older human depletion and repletion studies and from studies of individuals with pellagra, a niacin deficiency disease.[4] Urinary excretion of N1-methylnicotinamide (NMN) and N1-methyl-2-pyridone-5-carboxylamide (2-pyridone), the major end products of niacin metabolism, have been used to assess the adequacy of niacin and tryptophan in the diet.[16] The use of a ratio of urinary 2-pyridone to N1-methylnicotinamide is recommended for assessment of niacin status, even though excretion of these two metabolites are reduced with generalized malnutrition.[16] A ratio of less than 1.0 is considered to indicate niacin deficiency and 1.0 to 4.0 is considered acceptable. Others suggest the use of individual metabolite values and comparing them to urinary excretion criteria (<5.8 μmol [0.8 mg] per day is considered deficient for NMN). Measurement of NMN (milligrams per gram creatinine) over a period of 4 to 5 hours following a 410-μmol (50 mg) load of niacinamide is also commonly used as a measure of niacin nutriture.[16]

Niacin is unique among water-soluble vitamins in that part of the RDA for this vitamin can be met through its synthesis from the precursor amino acid tryptophan.[39] Therefore, recommendations take into account the preformed niacin provided in the diet as well as the contribution of dietary tryptophan. The term Niacin Equivalent (NE) is used as a factor to describe the niacin contribution in the diet from tryptophan, and 1 NE denotes the dietary provision of either 290 μmol (60 mg) of tryptophan or 8.2 μmol (1 mg) of niacin.[39] The conversion of tryptophan to niacin typifies the interrelationships of the B vitamins as both riboflavin and vitamin B_6 are required as cofactors for this conversion.

Because of the extensive roles of NAD and NADP in energy metabolism, RDAs are based on energy intakes and expressed per 4184 kJ (1000 kcal).[4] Requirements are 54 μmol (6.6 mg NE) per 4184 kJ for adults, with a minimum of 107 μmol (13 mg) NE for those consuming under 8368 kJ. RDAs for adult males and females, 23 to 50 years of age, are 156 μmol (19 mg) NE and 123 μmol (15 mg) NE, respectively.[4] Data from the 1977-1978 Nationwide Food Consumption Survey estimates that men and women in the U.S. are consuming 336 μmol (41 mg) NE and 221 μmol (27 mg) NE, respectively; far more than the 1989 RDAs.[4]

Niacin in most unprocessed food products is found in the coenzyme forms of NADP(H) and NAD(H). Meat, fish, and poultry contain high levels of both niacin and tryptophan. For example, 1-oz servings of hamburger, tuna, and chicken contain 12 μmol (1.46 mg), 29 μmol (3.50 mg), and 15 μmol (1.79 mg) niacin, respectively (Table 1).[9] In addition, these foods provide good-quality protein, of which approximately 1% could be estimated to contain tryptophan. For example, if 1 oz of chicken provides approximately 8 g of protein, then 387 μmol or 80 mg of tryptophan would be provided. Using the conversion factor of 290 μmol (60 mg) of tryptophan for 1 NE, the 1 oz of chicken provides another 1.3 NE from tryptophan for a total of 3.1 NE. Foods such as milk products and eggs are poor sources of niacin but provide sufficient tryptophan. Cereals, grains, and legumes are important sources of preformed niacin; however, bioavailability may be low as niacin can be bound to carbohydrates (niacytins) or peptides (niacinogens).[39]

Pharmacological doses of nicotinic acid are being used extensively for treatment of elevated serum cholesterol.[40] Nicotinic acid, ingested in large doses of approximately 3 g/day, can lower total serum cholesterol and low-density cholesterol, and elevate high-density cholesterol. Unfortunately, there are some undesirable side effects associated with such high intakes including increased histamine release causing vascular dilation or flushing, abnormal liver function related to elevation of some hepatic enzymes, elevated serum uric acid levels, and transient hyperglycemia.[39] Other metabolic effects include increased use of muscle glycogen and decreased release of fatty acids from adipose tissue during exercise.[44-48,51] In addition, there are cardiovascular responses to nicotinic acid administration, which may provide some rationale for why nicotinic acid could possibly enhance performance. Nicotinic acid administration has been shown to increase cardiac output[41] and increase myocardial oxygen consumption.[42]

C. NICOTINIC ACID ADMINISTRATION, SUBSTRATE AVAILABILITY, AND PERFORMANCE

Much of what we know about the role of niacin in exercise performance has been learned through studies investigating the relative contributions of fat and carbohydrate substrates during short-term and prolonged exercise. Nicotinic acid administration has been utilized in the experimental designs of these studies because of the pronounced effects the vitamin has on free fatty acid (FFA) availability at rest and during exercise. Because skeletal muscle tissue contains only a small amount of lipid, the majority of fatty acids available for energy during exercise are supplied by adipose tissue.[43] Hydrolysis of fatty acids from adipose tissue is under sympathetic nervous system control, via adenylate cyclase and cAMP stimulation of hormone-sensitive lipase.[43] The primary metabolic effect of nicotinic acid supplementation is inhibition of fatty acid release from adipocytes[44-48,51] and, presumably, this is related to inhibition of the adenylate cyclase cascade.[40]

Carlson et al.[44] investigated the effects of nicotinic acid administration in 2 young men on plasma FFA, the fractional rate of FFA removal from blood, oxidation of FFA, plasma glucose, and plasma glycerol at rest and during 2 h of cycling exercise. Nicotinic acid reduced the level of FFA in plasma at rest and during exercise and decreased plasma glycerol and glucose (n = 1) during exercise. Exercise had no influence on the rate of removal of FFA from blood or the oxidation of FFA. The combination of a decreased plasma glucose and elevated respiratory quotient (RQ) indicated a greater reliance on glucose as a substrate. Mechanical efficiency and heart rate in subjects given nicotinic acid were no different from controls.

Jenkins[45] followed up the work of Carlson's group to explore the metabolic responses of nicotinic acid administration during running. Three men performed two treadmill running trials, one without nicotinic acid and the other with 200 mg of nicotinic acid. They were asked to run for 1.5 h (n = 2) and 2.5 h (n = 1). Similar to the results of Carlson et al.,[44] plasma FFA was reduced and the RQ elevated during exercise. Unexpectedly, blood glucose was elevated. Jenkins speculated that the depressed plasma FFA resulted in decreased ketone body formation, with a concomitant reduction in insulin secretion and elevation of blood glucose.

In addition to studying the metabolic responses to nicotinic acid administration (1.6 g), Bergstrom et al.[46] wanted to focus on the influence of nicotinic acid on work capacity and muscle glycogen stores. Two exercise trials — a short-term, near-maximal cycling test (2 men) and a prolonged submaximal cycling test using 1 leg at a time (13 men) — were used. While there was no difference in work capacity between the control and nicotinic acid-supplemented trials, there were some metabolic changes. Plasma FFA and plasma glycerol were lower and the RQ higher during both exercise trials after nicotinic acid administration. Glycogen content of the quadriceps femoris was significantly lowered with prolonged submaximal exercise, especially in the nicotinic acid-supplemented trials. Bergstrom and co-workers concluded that nicotinic acid administration significantly reduced the availability of FFA as a source of fuel for the working muscle and increased the utilization of glycogen, without impairing the ability to do work. However, the authors did note a significant increase in heart rate and $\dot{V}O_2$

during exercise in the nicotinic acid-supplemented trials. The subjects also reported that the prolonged exercise appeared heavier and more fatiguing after nicotinic acid administration.

Pernow and Saltin[47] went one step further and looked at work capacity and substrate utilization with a combination of nicotinic acid supplementation and glycogen depletion. Using a one-leg bicycle exercise (performed to exhaustion) on 2 consecutive days and a low carbohydrate diet between the 2 days, they significantly lowered muscle glycogen prior to the start of the second day of exercise. Prior to the testing of the second leg on the second day, intermittent administration of 1.2 g of nicotinic acid significantly reduced work load (kpm/min) and time to exhaustion compared to results from both legs on day 1 and the first leg on day 2. Prolonged work at less than 60 to 70% of $\dot{V}O_2$max can be continued even with lowered muscle glycogen stores so long as FFA is available. Once FFA release is blocked via nicotinic acid, the capacity to perform exercise is significantly reduced.

In a single-blind, randomized design, supplementation with 2 g of nicotinic acid to 10 well-trained runners, performance did not improve or decrease on a 10-mi timed run.[48] The same metabolic response of depressed FFA was observed and, as in other studies, performance was not different from those nonsupplemented subjects. The 10-mi run, with times of 76 ± 3 min and 78 ± 3 min for the placebo and nicotinic acid groups, respectively, was probably not severe enough to deplete muscle glycogen stores and limit performance.[49] However, Galbo et al.[50] showed in subjects run to exhaustion (60% $\dot{V}O_2$max), that total run time was decreased with nicotinic acid administration.

Carbohydrate supplementation during prolonged exercise, like nicotinic acid, attenuates the release of FFA, but also delays fatigue during prolonged exercise.[51] Murray et al.[52] hypothesized that because nicotinic acid increases the reliance on carbohydrate as a fuel source during exercise, supplementation with both nicotinic acid and carbohydrate might be expected to improve performance. A group of 10 subjects in a double-blind, randomized design study completed 5 trials including a baseline trial and beverage supplementation with either water placebo (WP), 6% carbohydrate-electrolyte (CE), water plus nicotinic acid (280 mg/l; WP + NA), and carbohydrate-electrolyte plus nicotinic acid (CE + NA). Subjects ingested 3.5 ml/kg LBM of the beverages every 15 min during exercise. Subjects were asked to cycle at approximately 70% $\dot{V}O_2$max for 120 min and then perform a 3.5-mi time trial. While the addition of nicotinic acid to the carbohydrate beverage (CE + NA) did attenuate FFA rise during exercise and increase carbohydrate oxidation, performance time on the 3.5-mi cycling time trial was not improved. In fact, while the results were not statistically different, trends in the data suggest the possibility that nicotinic acid administration may be detrimental to performance time (CE < CE + NA and WP < WP + NA). However, the authors recommended that further work is needed to ascertain these trends towards impaired performance.

Heath et al.[53] were interested in the possibility of an adaptive response to nicotinic acid administration and investigated the influence of longer-term (3 weeks) administration, in addition to supplementation prior to exercise, on fuel utilization. There were four 30-min submaximal runs conducted by 8 men over the course of a 3-week period and, similar to the results of the earlier studies, they found a depression in plasma FFA and glycerol and an elevated respiratory exchange ratio (RER). Because RER was significantly lower in trials 3 and 4 compared to trial 2, the authors speculate that adaptation to the high intakes of nicotinic acid is possible and that longer-term supplementation trials are needed.

The observations of attenuated FFA utilization and enhanced dependence on carbohydrate during exercise with nicotinic acid is not limited to skeletal muscle. Lassers et al.[54] showed that intravenous infusion of nicotinic acid depressed plasma FFA and resulted in an estimated 42% reduction of lipid substrate for myocardial oxidative metabolism at rest and 56% during exercise. After infusion the estimated contribution from carbohydrate increased 39% at rest and 47% during exercise.

Keith[35] summarized some of the studies investigating the relationship between nicotinamide supplementation and performance[55,56] and found that only Frankau[55] had reported improved performance (agility test) with nicotinamide administration. These were apparently healthy cadets, but Keith points out that the pre-test niacin status was not reported.[35] Hilsendager and Karpovich,[56] in a well-designed, double-blind placebo-controlled study, found no influence of 75 mg of supplemental niacin on endurance performance (bicycle ergometry).

While the available data on niacin status and performance are limited, Jett'e et al.[57] reported niacin intake, NMN excretion, and performance in four male subjects. Aerobic performance was assessed following glycogen supercompensation, achieved through exhaustive exercise and followed by low- and high-carbohydrate diets.[57] Nutrient consumption as well as nutritional biochemical parameters were reported. Aerobic performance, as measured by $\dot{V}O_2$max during a progressive treadmill run, was slightly decreased following the high-carbohydrate diet, compared to the control or baseline $\dot{V}O_2$max test. Niacin intake was lower and NMN excretion lower during the high-carbohydrate diet phase compared to values during the high-protein, low-carbohydrate phase. The authors speculated that the decreased aerobic performance following consumption of the high-carbohydrate diet may have been related to lower intakes of niacin and altered oxidative metabolism. Intakes of niacin, while reduced somewhat, were still adequate. In addition, urinary NMN excretion was not different from baseline values and could be considered clinically normal.

D. SUMMARY AND RECOMMENDATIONS DURING EXERCISE AND SPORT

A large segment of the population uses pharmacological doses of nicotinic acid as treatment for hypercholesterolemia. Supplementation with nicotinic acid alters fuel availability and utilization in skeletal and cardiac muscle during exercise and could possibly impact performance. There is overwhelming evidence that pharmacological administration of nicotinic acid reduces the availability of FFA and potentiates the use of carbohydrate as a fuel for exercise. Performance does not appear to be enhanced or compromised; however, when nicotinic acid administration is combined with limited carbohydrate substrate availability, the ability to perform work is significantly reduced.[47]

Because of the metabolic roles of NAD in glycolysis and respiratory metabolism, a deficiency of the vitamin would be expected to impair performance by limiting substrate oxidation during prolonged exercise. There is no evidence of inadequate niacin status in athletes or active individuals, and based on reported intakes of niacin in the general population, it is unlikely that niacin intakes would be low enough to compromise aerobic performance. The observation of decreased intakes of niacin with high-carbohydrate diets[57] deserves further attention, especially as current dietary guidelines recommend diets higher in carbohydrate.

In summary, the metabolic responses to pharmacological administration of nicotinic acid, including profound reductions in plasma FFA and increased carbohydrate utilization, do not appear to impair performance unless carbohydrate substrate is limited. Based on the current evidence, there is no need or advantage for niacin supplementation in exercise and sport.

REFERENCES

1. **McCormick, D. B.,** Riboflavin, in *Modern Nutrition in Health and Disease,* Shils, M. E., Olson, J. A., and Shike, M., Eds., Lea & Febiger, Malvern, PA, 1994, 366.
2. **Berdanier, C. D.,** *Advanced Nutrition: Macronutrients,* CRC Press, Boca Raton, FL, 1995, 50-177.
3. **Glatzle, D., Körner, Christeller, S., and Wiss, O.,** Method for the detection of a biochemical riboflavin deficiency stimulation of $NADPH_2$-dependent glutathione reductase from human erythrocytes by FAD in vitro investigations on the vitamin B_2 status in healthy people and geriatric patients, *Int. J. Vitam. Res.,* 40, 166, 1970.

4. **National Academy of Sciences,** Water-soluble vitamins, in *Recommended Dietary Allowances,* National Academy Press, Washington, D.C., 1989, 115.

5. **Bro-Rasmussen, F.,** The riboflavin requirement of animals and men and associated metabolic relations. II. Relation of requirement to the metabolism of protein and energy, *Nutr. Abstr. Rev.,* 28, 369, 1958.

6. **Horwitt, M. K.,** Nutritional requirements of man, with special reference to riboflavin, *Am. J. Clin. Nutr.,* 18, 458, 1966.

7. **Russell, R. M.,** Water-soluble vitamins in the elderly: background and overview, in *Nutritional Assessment of Elderly Populations: Measure and Function,* Rosenberg, I. H., Ed., Raven Press, New York, 1995, 215.

8. **Short, S. H.,** Surveys of dietary intake and nutrition knowledge of athletes and their coaches, in *Nutrition in Exercise and Sport,* Wolinsky, I. and Hickson, J. F., Jr., Eds., CRC Press, Boca Raton, FL, 1994, 367.

9. **Bloch, A. S. and Shills, M. E., Eds.,** Vitamin A, vitamin E, α-tocopherol (TOC), vitamin C, thiamin, riboflavin, niacin, vitamin B_6, vitamin B_{12}, and folate content of selected common foods per serving portion, in *Nutrition Facts Manual: A Quick Reference,* Williams & Wilkins, Media, PA, 1996, 148.

10. USPHS, Nutrition Monitoring in the United States: Chartbook I: Selected Findings from the National Nutrition Monitoring and Related Research Program, 29th ed., U.S. Public Health Service, Hyattsville, MD, 1993, 29.

11. **Kirchner, E. M., Lewis, R. D., and O'Connor, P. J.,** Bone mineral density and dietary intake of female college gymnasts, *Med. Sci. Sports Exercise,* 27, 542, 1995.

12. **Sauberlich, H. E., Dowdy, R. P., and Skala, J. H.,** *Laboratory Tests for the Assessment of Nutritional Status,* CRC Press, Boca Raton, FL, 1974, 30.

13. **Belko, A. Z., Obarzanek, E., Kalkwarf, H. J., Rotter, M. A., Bogusz, S., Miller, D., Haas, J. D., and Roe, D. A.,** Effects of exercise on riboflavin requirements of young women, *Am. J. Clin. Nutr.,* 37, 509, 1983.

14. **Campbell, T. C., Brun, T., Junshi, C., Zulin, F., and Parpia, B.,** Questioning riboflavin recommendations on the basis of a survey in China, *Am. J. Clin. Nutr.,* 51, 436, 1990.

15. **Horwitt, M. K.,** Comments on methods for estimating riboflavin requirements, *Am. J. Clin. Nutr.,* 39, 159, 1984.

16. **Gibson, R. S.,** Assessment of the status of thiamin, riboflavin, and niacin, in *Principles of Nutritional Assessment,* Gibson, R. S., Ed., Oxford University Press, New York, 1990, 425.

17. **Tucker, R. G., Mickelsen, D., and Keys, A.,** The influence of sleep, work, diuresis, heat, acute starvation, thiamine intake and bed rest on human riboflavin excretion, *J. Nutr.,* 72, 251, 1960.

18. **Belko, A. Z., Obarzanek, M. P., Rotter, B. S., Urgan, G., Weinberg, S., and Roe, D. A.,** Effects of aerobic exercise and weight loss on riboflavin requirements of moderately obese, marginally deficient young women, *Am. J. Clin. Nutr.,* 40, 553, 1984.

19. **Belko, A. Z., Meredity, M. P., Kalkwarf, H. J., Obarzanek, E., Weinberg, S., Roach, R., McKeon, G., and Roe, D. A.,** Effects of exercise on riboflavin requirements: biological validation in weight reducing women, *Am. J. Clin. Nutr.,* 41, 270, 1985.

20. **Evelo, C. T. A., Palmen, N. G. M., Artur, Y., and Janssen, G. M. E.,** Changes in blood glutathione concentrations, and in erythrocyte glutathione reductase and glutathione S-transferase activity after running training and after participation in contests, *Eur. J. Appl. Physiol.,* 64, 354, 1992.

21. **Fogelholm, M.,** Micronutrient status in females during a 24-week fitness-type exercise program, *Ann. Nutr. Metab.,* 36, 209, 1992.

22. **Lewis, R. D., Yates, C. Y., and Driskell, J. A.,** Riboflavin and thiamin status and birth outcome as a function of maternal aerobic exercise, *Am. J. Clin. Nutr.,* 48, 110, 1988.

23. **Winters, L. R. T., Yoon, J., Kalkwarf, H. J., Davies, J. C., Berkowitz, M. G., Haas, J., and Roe D. A.,** Riboflavin requirements and exercise adaptation in older women, *Am. J. Clin. Nutr.,* 56, 526, 1992.

24. **Soares, M. J., Satyanarayana, K., Bamji, M. S., Jacob, C. M., Venkata Ramana, Y., and Sudhakar Rao, S.,** The effect of exercise on the riboflavin status of adult men, *Br. J. Nutr.,* 69, 541, 1993.

25. **Ohno, H., Yahata, T., Sato, Y., Yamamura, K., and Taniguchi, N.,** Physical training and fasting erythrocyte activities of free radical scavenging enzyme systems in sedentary men, *Eur. J. Appl. Physiol.,* 57, 173, 1988.

26. **Delachaux, A. and Ott, W.,** Quelques observations sur le metabolisme du fer et de vitamines au cours de l'effort physique et de l'entrainement, *Schweiz. Med. Wochenschr.,* 73, 1026, 1943.

27. **Friedemann, T. E., Ivy, A. C., Jung, F. T., and Sheft, B. B.,** Work at high altitudes. IV. Utilization of thiamine and riboflavin at low and high density intakes, *Q. Bull. Northwest. Univ. Med. Sch.,* 23, 177, 1949.

28. **Roe, D. A. and Belko, A. Z.,** Reply to letter by Horwitt, *Am. J. Clin. Nutr.,* 39, 161, 1984.

29. **Hunter, K. E. L. and Turkki, P. R.,** Effect of exercise on riboflavin status of rats, *J. Nutr.,* 117, 298, 1987.

30. **Haralambie, G.,** Vitamin B_2 status in athletes and the influence of riboflavin administration on neuromuscular irritability, *Nutr. Metab.,* 20, 1, 1976.

31. **Keith, R. E. and Alt, L. A.,** Riboflavin status of female athletes consuming normal diets, *Nutr. Res.,* 11, 727, 1991.

32. **Guilland, J., Penaranda, T., Gallet, C., Boggio, V., Fuchs, F., and Klepping, J.,** Vitamin status of young athletes including the effects of supplementation, *Med. Sci. Sports Exercise,* 21, 441, 1989.

33. **Tremblay, A., Boiland, F., Breton, M., Bessette, H., and Roberge, A. G.,** The effects of a riboflavin supplementation on the nutritional status and performance of elite swimmers, *Nutr. Res.,* 4, 201, 1984.

34. **Singh, A., Moses, F. M., and Deuster, P. A.,** Vitamin and mineral status in physically active men: effects of a high-potency supplement, *Am. J. Clin. Nutr.,* 55, 1, 1992.

35. **Keith, R. E.,** Vitamins and physical activity, in *Nutrition in Exercise and Sport,* Wolinsky, I. and Hickson, F. J., Jr., Eds., CRC Press, Boca Raton, FL, 1994, 159.

36. **van Dokkum, W. and van der Beek, E. J.,** Vitamines en prestatievermogen, *Voeding,* 46, 50, 1985.

37. **van der Beek, E. J., van Dokkum, W., Schrijver, J., Wedel, M., Gaillard, A. W. K., Wesstra, A., van de Weerd, H., and Hermus, R. J. J.,** Thiamin, riboflavin, and vitamins B_6 and C: impact of combined restricted intake on functional performance in man, *Am. J. Clin. Nutr.,* 48, 1451, 1988.

38. **Gollnick, P. D., Armstrong, R. B., Saubert, C. W., IV, Piehl, K., and Saltin, B.,** Enzyme activity and fiber composition in skeletal muscle of untrained and trained men, *J. Appl. Physiol.,* 33, 312, 1972.

39. **Swendseid, M. E. and Jacob, R. A.,** Niacin, in: *Modern Nutrition in Health and Disease,* Shils, M. E., Olson, J. A., and Shike, M., Eds., Lea & Febiger, Malvern, PA, 1994, 376.

40. **DiPalma, J. R. and Thayer, W. S.,** Use of niacin as a drug, *Annu. Rev. Nutr.,* 11, 169, 1991.

41. **Ekstrom-Jodal, B., Harthon, L., Haggendal, E., Malmberg, R., and Svedmyr, N.,** Influence of nicotinic acid and pentaerythritol tetraniconate on the cardiac output in man, *Pharmacol. Clin.,* 2, 86, 1970.

42. **Otani, H., Engelman, R. M., Datta, S., Jones, R. M., Cordis, G. A., Rousou, J. A., Breyer, R. H., and Das, D. K.,** Enhanced myocardial preservation by nicotinic acid, an antilipolytic compound, *J. Thorac. Cardiovasc. Surg.,* 96, 81, 1988.

43. **Gollnick, P. D. and Saltin, B.,** Fuel for muscular exercise: role of fat, in *Exercise, Nutrition, and Energy Metabolism,* Horton, E. S. and Terjung, R. L., Eds., Macmillan, New York, NY, 1988, 72.

44. **Carlson, L. A., Havel, R. J., Ekelund, L. G., and Holmgren, A.,** Effect of nicotinic acid on the turnover rate and oxidation of the free fatty acids of plasma in man during exercise, *Metab. Clin. Exp.,* 12, 837, 1963.

45. **Jenkins, D. J. A.,** Effects of nicotinic acid on carbohydrate and fat metabolism during exercise, *Lancet,* 1, 1307, 1965.

46. **Bergstrom, J., Hultman, E., Jorfeldt, L., Pernow, B., and Wahnen, J.,** Effect of nicotinic acid on physical working capacity and on metabolism of muscle, *J. Appl. Physiol.,* 26, 170, 1969.

47. **Pernow, B. and Saltin, B.,** Availability of substrates and capacity for prolonged heavy exercise, *J. Appl. Physiol.,* 31, 416, 1971.

48. **Norris, B., Schade, D. S., and Eaton, R. P.,** Effects of altered free fatty acid mobilization on the metabolic response to exercise, *J. Clin. Endocrinol. Metab.,* 46, 254, 1978.

49. **Williams, M. H.,** The role of vitamins in physical activity, in *Nutritional Aspects of Human Physical and Athletic Performance,* Williams, M. H., Ed., Charles C Thomas, Springfield, IL, 1985, 147.

50. **Galbo, H., Holst, J. J., Christensen, N. J., and Hilsted, J.,** The effect of nicotinic acid and propanolol on glucagon and plasma catecholamine responses to prolonged exercise in man, *Diabetologia,* 11, 343, 1975.

51. **Coggan, A. R. and Coyle, E. F.,** Carbohydrate ingestion during prolonged exercise: effects on metabolism and performance, in *Exercise and Sports Sciences Reviews,* Holloszy, J. O., Ed., Williams & Wilkins, Baltimore, MD, 1991, 1.

52. **Murray, R., Bartoli, W. P., Eddy, D. E., and Horn, M. K.,** Physiological and performance responses to nicotinic-acid ingestion during exercise, *Med. Sci. Sports Exercise,* 1057, 1995.

53. **Heath, E. M., Wilcox, A. R., and Quinn, C. M.,** Effects of nicotinic acid on respiratory exchange ratio and substrate levels during exercise, *Med. Sci. Sports Exercise,* 1018, 1993.

54. **Lassers, B. W., Wahlqvist, M. L., Kaijser, J., and Carlson, L. A.,** Effect of nicotinic acid on myocardial metabolism in man at rest and during exercise, *J. Appl. Physiol.,* 33, 72, 1972.

55. **Frankau, I.,** Acceleration of co-ordinated muscular effort by nicotinamide, *Br. Med. J.,* 2, 60, 1943.

56. **Hilsendager, D. and Karpovich, P. V.,** Ergogenic effect of glycine and niacin separately and in combination, *Res. Q. Am. Assoc. Health Phys. Educ. Recreat.,* 35, 389, 1964.

57. **Jetté, M., Pelletier, O., Parker, L., and Thoden, J.,** The nutritional and metabolic effects of a carbohydrate-rich diet in a glycogen supercompensation training regimen, *Am. J. Clin. Nutr.,* 31, 2140, 1978.

Chapter 5

VITAMIN B$_6$

_____ David A. Sampson

CONTENTS

I. INTRODUCTION

Vitamin B$_6$ functions as a coenzyme in several pathways involved in substrate utilization during exercise (discussed below). Many studies in animals and humans have shown that exercise alters vitamin B$_6$ metabolism, and conversely that poor vitamin B$_6$ nutritional status compromises exercise performance. These observations have led to hypotheses that regular exercise increases the requirement for vitamin B$_6$[1] and that supplements of vitamin B$_6$ may enhance athletic performance.[2] These are important claims, if true, for competitive and recreational athletes. However, current evidence supports neither claim.

Manore[3] has recently reviewed the relation between vitamin B$_6$ and exercise. The reader is referred to this paper for a comprehensive discussion of vitamin B$_6$ requirements, nutritional status measures, effects of exercise on vitamin B$_6$, intake and nutritional status in athletes, and relation to growth hormone. The current review will focus on recent papers and other aspects of this topic that were not emphasized in Manore's review. (The reader may want to peruse other recent reviews that have focused on: vitamin B$_6$ requirements,[4,5] metabolism,[6] nutritional status,[7] steroid interaction,[8-10] methods of analysis,[11-14] seizure disorders,[15] CNS interaction,[16,17] behaviorial aspects,[18] bioavailability,[19] cancer aspects,[20] immune aspects,[21] enzymes,[22] toxicity,[23] and general aspects.[24])

Vitamin B_6 is a coenzyme for over 100 mammalian enzymes including about 60 aminotransferases, about 30 lyases, 16 decarboxylases, and various other transferases and racemases. Most of these enzymes are involved in amino acid metabolism, although there are B_6-dependent enzymes involved in metabolism of carbohydrate (including muscle glycogen) and fat; in the synthesis of nucleic acids, heme, phospho- and sphingolipids, polyamines, and neurotransmitters; and in the action of steroid hormones.[9,25] The term "vitamin B_6" refers to a group of interconvertible and biologically active 3-hydroxy 2-methyl pyridine derivatives, including the alcohol, pyridoxine (PN); the aldehyde, pyridoxal (PL); the amine, pyridoxamine (PM); and the 5'-phosphate esters of these compounds, pyridoxine phosphate (PNP), pyridoxal phosphate (PLP), and pyridoxamine phosphate (PMP).[26,27]

According to intake surveys, many Americans consume marginal amounts of vitamin B_6. Data from NHANES II show average vitamin B_6 intake was 1.8 and 1.1 mg/d for adult males and females, respectively, compared to the 1989 Recommended Dietary Allowances (RDAs) of 2.0 and 1.6 mg/d.[28] These data showed further that 71% and 90% of males and females, respectively, habitually consumed only two thirds of the vitamin B_6 RDA. Pao and Mickle[29] reported that women of all ages and elderly men in this country are at risk for vitamin B_6 nutritional status. Other surveys have documented inadequate vitamin B_6 intake in preschool, adult, and elderly Americans of both sexes.[30-33] In spite of this, there is little clinical evidence of widespread vitamin B_6 deficiency in the U.S.

Methods for evaluation of vitamin B_6 nutritional status have been summarized recently by Leklem.[7] Briefly, vitamin B_6 status is usually inferred from concentration of pyridoxal phosphate in plasma, excretion of 4-pyridoxic acid in urine, activity and stimulation of aspartate or alanine aminotransferase in erythrocytes, or from excretion of urinary catabolites following oral loads of tryptophan or other amino acids. Current thinking holds that accurate vitamin B_6 status assessment requires measuring more than one of these response variables.[7]

II. FUNCTIONS OF VITAMIN B_6 RELATED TO EXERCISE: VITAMIN B_6-DEPENDENT SUBSTRATE UTILIZATION

Several aspects of energy metabolism during exercise require PLP-dependent enzymes. First, amino acid oxidation, which provides 5 to 10% of energy during prolonged exercise,[34] involves as a first step the removal of amino groups by PLP-dependent aminotransferases.[35] Second, alanine released from muscle during exercise is the primary hepatic substrate for gluconeogenesis during exhaustive exercise.[36] Alanine is formed in muscle from pyruvate by the action of PLP-dependent alanine aminotransferase. Third, glycogenolysis in liver and skeletal muscle is catalyzed by glycogen phosphorylase, which requires PLP as a coenzyme.[37] Fourth, 80 to 90% of energy for exercising muscle comes from ß-oxidation of fatty acids, which requires the PLP-dependent synthesis of carnitine from lysine[38] to shuttle long-chain fatty acyl thioesters into the mitochondrion. There is evidence that all four of these paths are impaired by frank deficiency of vitamin B_6.[37-41] However, aminotransferases are equilibrium enzymes and as such are regulated *in vivo* by concentration of substrate rather than concentration of coenzyme. There is no evidence that mild deficiency of vitamin B_6 alters glycogen phosphorylase activity or carnitine synthesis. Thus, data are lacking to support the contention[3] that vitamin B_6 status has a practical effect on energy metabolism in muscle during exercise.

III. EXERCISE AND VITAMIN B$_6$ METABOLISM

It is well established that sustained aerobic exercise (such as running or bicycling) produces short-term alteration of various measures of vitamin B$_6$ nutritional status. Leklem and co-workers,[42,43] as well as other investigators,[44-46] have established that concentrations of plasma vitamin B$_6$ rise significantly (10 to 20% in human subjects[45] and >50% in rats[46]) during various types of exercise in both humans and animals. Excretion of the urinary catabolite of vitamin B$_6$, 4-pyridoxic acid, also increases with exercise.[47] Manore[3] has reviewed this literature through the early 1990s. There appears to be a threshold for this effect, because milder exercise, such as walking, does not alter measures of vitamin B$_6$ status.[48]

Hypotheses have been advanced suggesting that the exercise-induced rise in plasma PLP represents an adaptive aspect of substrate utilization reflecting an interorgan shift in the vitamin that promotes fuel supply to exercising muscle. Two variations of this concept have been advanced: one positing that PLP moves from muscle to liver, where it functions coenzymatically in aminotransferase reactions necessary for gluconeogensis.[47] A second view posits that elevated plasma PLP during exercise is destined for skeletal muscle, where it functions either in aminotransferase or glycogen phosphorylase reactions.[44]

Both of these views have been challenged recently by Sampson and co-workers.[45] These authors reasoned that if elevated plasma PLP relates to substrate utilization during exercise, then the rise in plasma PLP should be proportional to the intensity of exercise. Their results in human subjects at two levels of aerobic exercise (60 or 85% of $\dot{V}O_2$max), using bicycle ergometry, showed no effect of exercise intensity on plasma vitamin B$_6$ concentrations, and thus did not support either hypothesis. Furthermore, data from this group showed that the rise in plasma PLP occurred very early in an exercise bout, before glycogen stores would be depleted by the exercise burden. They suggested that the early rise cast further doubt on hypotheses that elevated PLP during exercise is involved in fuel economy of the athlete.

This group presented an alternate explanation for the rise in plasma PLP during exercise. Exercise causes protein, including albumin, to shift (by an unknown mechanism) from the interstitial space into plasma.[49-51] Sampson and co-workers[45] suggested that if PLP is present in the interstitial space bound to albumin, then movement of albumin into plasma during exercise would drag along PLP, and thus account for the observed change in plasma PLP. Confirmation of this hypothesis requires investigation of interstitial PLP concentration. If correct, the hypothesis suggests that elevated plasma PLP is a consequence of exercise, not a regulatory adaptation.

Hadj-Saad et al.[46] reported recently that swimming for 1 to 2.5 h significantly increased vitamin B$_6$ in skeletal muscle of rats, and tended to decrease vitamin B$_6$ in liver. These results would not appear to support a view that elevated plasma PLP during exercise reflects fuel oxidation. However, these authors did conclude that "... the mechanisms involved in the regulation of vitamin B$_6$ distribution, transport, and storage during exercise ..." may be fruitful areas for future research.

Other recent evidence shows that chronic exercise also produces detectable changes in vitamin B$_6$ nutritional status. Fogelholm[52] reported recently that a 24-week aerobic fitness program, in which human subjects increased the frequency of 30-min training bouts (at 75% heart rate reserve) from 2 to 6 sessions per week, resulted in a small but statistically significant rise (+4%) in the activity coefficient for the vitamin B$_6$-dependent enzyme, aspartate aminotransferase, in the subjects' red cells. This change indicates a negative effect of exercise on a functional measure of vitamin B$_6$ nutritional status, but the author noted that the small magnitude of the change makes its physiological significance uncertain.

IV. INADEQUATE VITAMIN B₆ INTAKE AND EXERCISE PERFORMANCE

Van der Beek et al.[53] reported in 1988 that 8 weeks of combined marginal intake (32% of the Dutch RDA) of thiamin, riboflavin, vitamin C, and vitamin B_6 significantly decreased $\dot{V}O_2$max (–10%) and onset of blood lactate accumulation (–20%) in 23 human subjects. The authors speculated that the effect was mediated by an alteration in the redox state of their deficient subjects. However, the variability in the subjects' performance response to the deficiency and the lack of correlation between the degree of vitamin deficiency and the decrease in performance makes the significance of these observations to sports nutrition unclear.

These investigators[54] recently extended this work in 24 male subjects. They used a factorial treatment design to evaluate main effects and interactions of marginal intake of vitamin B_6, thiamin, and riboflavin on exercise performance measures (aerobic power, blood lactate accumulation, and O_2 consumption). This treatment design is more powerful than that in their 1988 report because effects of each vitamin can be evaluated, as well as interaction between the individual vitamins. Vitamin intakes were <55% of the Dutch RDA, with intake for vitamin B_6 at 0.39 mg/d, or 20% of the U.S. 1989 RDA. The authors observed biochemical vitamin deficiencies for all three vitamins, but no significant main effects or interactions for any of the deficiencies on exercise performance. Because few athletes consume diets providing vitamin B_6 at levels as low as those used in these two studies,[3] it seems rather unlikely, based on present evidence, that impaired athletic performance due to inadequate intake of vitamin B_6 is a common or practical problem in sports nutrition.

V. SUPPLEMENTAL VITAMIN B₆ INTAKE AND EXERCISE PERFORMANCE

Manore[3] concluded in her 1994 review that "… supplemental vitamin B_6 … does not appear to impact fuel substrate use during exercise dramatically enough to alter performance." That review did not cite the work of McMillan et al.,[2] who evaluated in rats whether intake of supplemental vitamin B_6 (about 33 times the level currently recommended for rat maintenance and growth[55]), compared to adequate intake, enhanced skeletal muscle strength. Their data showed no positive effect of supplemental vitamin B_6, and in fact showed a trend toward an impairing effect. The conclusion of these authors that a vitamin B_6 supplement provided "… no positive effect on performance …" and had possibly adverse effects would seem a suitable summary of the literature for both human and animal subjects in this area.

Hu et al.[56] recently reported that pyridoxine and thiamin in high concentrations stimulated lipid peroxidation *in vitro* in rat microsomes. These authors speculated that high intakes of these vitamins may have the undesirable side effect of increasing lipid peroxidation. An extrapolation of this concern is that if exercising individuals, who are subjected to elevated oxidant stress from increased oxygen perfusion of tissues, habitually take vitamin B_6 supplements, they may increase lipid peroxidative damage.

VI. VITAMIN B₆ NUTRITIONAL STATUS IN ATHLETES

Manore[3] thoroughly reviewed recent literature through the early 1990s dealing with intake and nutritional status of vitamin B_6 in athletes. She noted that "… some studies report that athletes have low or marginal diet B_6 intakes … whereas others report mean intakes at or above the RDA …", and that "… recent reports suggest that some athletes may have poor status." The collective dietary data for both male (12 reports) and female (7 reports) athletes discussed in Manore's review[3] suggest clearly that athletes in general consume adequate vitamin B$_6$.

Rokitzki et al.[57] recently have added to this literature. They evaluated dietary intake and nutritional status for vitamin B$_6$ in a group of 57 German athletes that included body builders, wrestlers, and players of handball, soccer, and basketball. These investigators reported that >30% of their subjects consumed vitamin B$_6$ at less than recommended levels. However they found no evidence of vitamin B$_6$ deficiency as measured by plasma concentration of vitamin B$_6$ or activity of red cell aspartate aminotransferase. These data suggest that this diverse group of athletes had no biochemical evidence of vitamin B$_6$ inadequacy, although the authors concluded that the lack of reference values for athletes makes evaluation of their dietary intake difficult.

VII. SPECULATION AND FUTURE DIRECTIONS

Oxidant stress — Exercise increases oxidant stress in muscle and other tissues, due in part due to increased perfusion with oxygen and the concomitant increase in production of reactive oxygen species.[58-60] There has been considerable recent interest in the possible interaction between antioxidant nutrient status and oxidant stress related to exercise.[61] Maxwell et al.[62] reported that antioxidant capacity of plasma increases significantly after 1 h of eccentric exercise, and that supplements of vitamin C and E affected this rise. Although vitamin B$_6$ does not appear on the list of well-documented antioxidant nutrients,[63,64] there is evidence in rats that vitamin B$_6$ deficiency impairs oxidant defense. Selvam and Ravichandran[65] reported that frank vitamin B$_6$ deficiency in rats significantly decreased hepatic glutathione, glutathione peroxidase activity, and concentrations of vitamin C and E, while increasing hepatic hydroperoxide concentrations. These rat data raise the possibility that suboptimal vitamin B$_6$ nutritional status during exercise may impair oxidant defense in muscle. More generally, Ji[66] has noted recently that "… exercise provides an excellent model to study the dynamic balance between oxidative challenge and antioxidant defense …" In particular, evaluating the molecular mechanisms by which exercise elevates expression of antioxidant defense enzymes[66] would appear to be an exciting area for future exercise/nutrition research.

Glutathione — Glutathione (GSH) is a well-documented part of mammalian oxidant defense,[64] and is present at high concentrations (millimolar) in most tissues.[66] GSH, administered either i.p. or per os, affords dose-responsive improvement in exercise endurance in animal models.[67] GSH is synthesized from methionine/homocysteine in the transsulfuration pathway that has two vitamin B$_6$-dependent enzymes (cystathionine ß-synthase and cystathionine γ-lyase).[68] Activity of this synthetic path is high in liver but relatively low in skeletal muscle.[66] The vitamin B$_6$ dependence raises the possibility that vitamin B$_6$ nutritional status may alter GSH synthesis, oxidant defense, and exercise endurance in humans. However, evidence in rats suggests that although vitamin B$_6$ deficiency decreases activity of the enzymes, it does not significantly alter tissue concentration of GSH.[69] Thus a potential link between vitamin B$_6$ status and exercise endurance involving GSH does not appear to have practical effects.

Ischemia/reperfusion — One current hypothesis about muscle damage during exercise posits that muscle ischemia occurs during vigorous contractions and is followed by reperfusion during the subsequent relaxation.[70,71] In this model, superoxide radical formation occurs during reperfusion, which then damages the muscle tissue. The vitamin B$_6$-dependent enzyme ornithine decarboxylase (ODC) and its product, putrescine, as well as other polyamines synthesized from putrescine, have been implicated in ischemia/reperfusion injury in nervous tissue[72] and intestine.[73] In those tissues, ischemia/reperfusion evokes a large spike in expression of this enzyme. The polyamines that result accumulate in high concentrations, and may lead to peroxide production.[74] However, the literature is confusing at present because evidence is available showing both a protective[75] as well as a toxic role[74] for increased ODC expression in ischemia/reperfusion in these tissues. ODC expression in exercising muscle has not been studied. Deficiency of vitamin B_6 elevates activity of ODC significantly in rat liver, kidney, and intestine.[76,77] An explanation for this paradoxical effect has been advanced by Meisler and Thanassi,[78] who postulated that maintenance of ODC activity is so critical to the organism that deficiency of ODC's coenzyme (i.e., vitamin B_6) elicits increased expression of the apoprotein (by an unknown mechanism) which traps the limited vitamin B_6, which in turn assures that flux through the enzyme will be maintained in spite of the deficiency. From this comes the speculation that the status of vitamin B_6 in strenuously exercising muscle may modulate ischemia/reperfusion-related muscle damage, although future work will be necessary to establish this.

Group-specific protease (GSP) — Katunuma and co-workers[80,81] published a series of papers in the 1970s that characterized a serine protease in tissues of rats that is induced by vitamin B_6 deficiency, starvation, and zero-protein diets. This protease is substrate-specific for some pyridoxal phosphate-dependent enzymes, and may function to make limited pyridoxal phosphate available for critical B_6-dependent enzymes. Katunuma et al.[80,81] showed this protease to be highly inducible in skeletal muscle and to attack glycogen phosphorylase in that tissue.[82] These authors did not investigate expression of GSP as affected by exercise, nor did they establish its functional significance in whole-body vitamin B_6 metabolism. However, this may prove a fertile area for future vitamin B_6/exercise research from several perspectives, given that glycogen phosphorylase functions both as a storage pool for vitamin B_6 which is mobilized during starvation,[83] as well as the flux-generating enzyme in oxidation of muscle glycogen, which is critical for ATP production during endurance exercise.[84] This seems particularly relevant for future research in light of Leklem's hypothesis that endurance exercise elicits a biochemical response similar to starvation.[42]

Exercise and homocysteinemia — Elevated plasma homocysteine has been recognized recently as an independent risk factor for cardiovascular disease,[85,86] even when the magnitude of elevation is mild.[87,88] Vitamins B_6, B_{12}, and folate all function as coenzymes or substrates in homocysteine metabolism.[68] Homocysteine is either transmethylated to methionine or transsulfurated to cysteine.[68] Vitamin B_6 is indirectly involved in transmethylation because of its coenzymatic role in serine hydroxymethyltransferase, an upstream enzyme which catalyzes synthesis of 5,10-methylene tetrahydrofolate from tetrahydrofolate. As discussed above, vitamin B_6 is directly involved in transsulfuration because of its coenzymatic function in cystathionine ß-synthetase and cystathionine γ-lyase, which together catalyze conversion of homocysteine to cysteine. Although the current evidence[89] suggests that folate is the primary nutritional regulator of this path, the literature shows clearly that deficits of any of these three vitamins elevates homocysteine.[90,91]

Physical activity is known to lower the risk of cardiovascular disease[82,93] and also to raise blood levels of vitamin B_6 (see discussion above).[45] It is possible that some of exercise's protective effect on cardiovascular disease is mediated through the elevating effect of exercise on plasma vitamin B_6, which could function coenzymatically in these pathways to lower plasma homocysteine. This hypothesis needs verification from exploration of effects of exercise on plasma and tissue homocysteine concentrations.

VIII. CONCLUSIONS

The recent literature reviewed here does not lend support to the contention that vitamin B_6 intake — either inadequate or supplemental — has much practical impact on exercise performance. However, it does appear that several significant research topics in vitamin B_6 nutritional biochemistry as well as sports nutrition can be explored profitably in the future using experimental designs involving interaction between vitamin B$_6$ status and exercise. As discussed in this review, a list of such topics includes: the significance and mechanism of pyridoxal phosphate redistribution into plasma during exercise; a role for group-specific protease in vitamin B$_6$ metabolism of skeletal muscle; possible involvement of vitamin B$_6$ in oxidant stress and ischemia/reperfusion in exercising muscle; and an involvement of vitamin B$_6$ in the protective effect of exercise on cardiovascular disease.

REFERENCES

1. **Guilland, J. C., Penaranda, T., Gallet, C., Boggio, V., Fuchs, F., and Klepping, J.**, Vitamin status of young athletes including the effects of supplementation, *Med. Sci. Sports Exercise*, 21, 441, 1989.
2. **McMillan, J., Keith, R. E., and Stone, M. H.**, The effects of supplemental vitamin B$_6$ and exercise on the contractile properties of rat muscle, *Nutr. Res.*, 8, 73, 1988.
3. **Manore, M. M.**, Vitamin B$_6$ and exercise, *Int. J. Sport Med.*, 4, 89, 1994.
4. **Bender, D. A.**, Vitamin B$_6$ requirement and recommendations, *Eur. J. Clin. Nutr.*, 43, 289, 1989.
5. **Driskell, J. A.**, Vitamin B$_6$ requirements of humans, *Nutr. Res.*, 14, 293, 1994.
6. **Merrill, A. H. and Henderson, J. M.**, Vitamin B-6 metabolism by human liver, *Ann. N.Y. Acad. Sci.*, 585, 110, 1990.
7. **Leklem, J. E.**, Vitamin B$_6$: a status report, *J. Nutr.*, 120, 1503, 1990.
8. **Allgood, V. E., Powell-Oliver, F. E., and Cidlowski, J. A.**, The influence of vitamin B$_6$ on the structure and function of the glucocorticoid receptor, in *Vitamin B$_6$*, Vol. 585, Dakshinamurti, K., Ed., New York Academy of Sciences, New York, 1990, 452.
9. **Allgood, V. E. and Cidlowski, J. A.**, Novel role for vitamin B$_6$ in steroid hormone action. A link between nutrition and the endocrine system, *J. Nutr. Biochem.*, 2, 523, 1991.
10. **Tully, D. B., Allgood, V. E., and Cidlowski, J. A.**, Vitamin B$_6$ modulation of steroid induced gene expression, in *Nutrition and Gene Expression*, Berdanier, C. D. and Hargrove, J. L., Eds., CRC Press, Boca Raton, FL, 1993, 547.
11. **Gregory, J. F.**, Methods for determination of vitamin B$_6$ in foods and other biological materials: a critical review, *J. Food Compos. Anal.*, 1, 105, 1988.
12. **Guilarte, T. R.**, Radiometric microbiological assay of B vitamins. Part 1. Assay procedure, *J. Nutr. Biochem.*, 2, 334, 1991.
13. **Bitsch, R. and Moller, J.**, Analysis of B-6 vitamers in foods using a modified high-performance liquid chromatographic method, *J. Chromatogr.*, 463, 207, 1989.
14. **Guilarte, T. R.**, Radiometric microbiological assay of B vitamins. Part 2. Extraction methods, *J. Nutr. Biochem.*, 2, 399, 1991.
15. **Anon.**, Infant vitamin B$_6$ deficiency and preconvulsant activity in brain, *Nutr. Rev.*, 46, 358, 1988.
16. **Guilarte, T. R.**, Vitamin B$_6$ and cognitive development. Recent research findings from human and animal studies, *Nutr. Rev.*, 51, 193, 1993.
17. **Kirksey, A. and Wasynczuk, A. Z.**, Morphological, biochemical, and functional consequences of vitamin B$_6$ deficits during central nervous system development, *Ann. N.Y. Acad. Sci.*, 678, 62, 1993.
18. **Anon.**, Behavioral consequences of pyridoxine deficiency in mothers and infants, *Nutr. Rev.*, 49, 312, 1991.
19. **Gregory, J. F.**, The bioavailability of vitamin B$_6$ — recent findings, *Ann. N.Y. Acad. Sci.*, 585, 86, 1990.
20. **Gregory, J. F., III**, A novel vitamin B$_6$ metabolite may be a circulating marker of cancer, *Nutr. Rev.*, 50, 295, 1992.
21. **Rall, L. C. and Meydani, S. N.**, Vitamin B$_6$ and immune competence, *Nutr. Rev.*, 51, 217, 1993.
22. **John, R. A.**, Pyridoxal phosphate-dependent enzymes, *Biochim. Biophys. Acta*, 1248, 81, 1995.
23. **Dordain, G. and Deffond, D.**, Pyridoxine neuropathy, *Therapie*, 49, 333, 1994.
24. **Leklem, J. E.**, Vitamin B$_6$: reservoirs, receptors, and red-cell reactions, *Ann. N.Y. Acad. Sci.*, 669, 34, 1992.
25. **Merrill, A. H. and Burnham, F. S.**, Vitamin B$_6$, in *Present Knowledge in Nutrition*, 6th ed., Brown, M. L., Ed., International Life Sciences Institute, Washington, D.C., 1990, 155.
26. **Sauberlich, H. E.**, Vitamin B$_6$, in *The Vitamins*, 2nd ed. Vol. VII, Gyorgy, P. and Pearson, W. N., Eds., Academic Press, New York, 1967, 169.
27. **Snell, E. E.**, Vitamin B$_6$, in *Comprehensive Biochemistry*, Vol. 11, Florkin, M. and Stotz, E. H., Eds., Elsevier, New York, 1963, 48.
28. **Kant, A. K. and Block, G.**, Dietary vitamin B$_6$ intake and food sources in the U.S. population: NHANES II, 1976-1980, *Am. J. Clin. Nutr.*, 52, 707, 1990.
29. **Pao, E. M. and Mickle, S. J.**, Problem nutrients in the United States, *Food Technol.*, 35, 58, 1981.
30. **Fries, M. E., Chrisley, B. M., and Driskell, J. A.**, Vitamin B-6 status of a group of preschool children, *Am. J. Clin. Nutr.*, 34, 2706, 1981.

31. **Chrisley, B. M. and Driskell, J. A.**, Vitamin B-6 Status of adults in Virginia, *Nutr. Rep. Int.*, 19, 553, 1979.
32. **Garry, P. J., Goodwin, J. S., Hunt, W. C., Hooper, E. M., and Leonard, A. G.**, Nutrition status in a healthy elderly population: dietary and supplemental intakes, *Am. J. Clin. Nutr.*, 36, 319, 1982.
33. **Lowik, M. R. H., van den Berg, H., Westenbrink, S., Wedel, M., Schrijver, J., and Ockhuizen, T.**, Dose-response relationships regarding vitamin B-6 in elderly people: a nationwide nutritional survey (Dutch Nutritional Surveillance System), *Am. J. Clin. Nutr.*, 50, 391, 1989.
34. **Poortmans, J. R.**, Protein turnover and amino acid oxidation during and after exercise, *Med. Sports Sci.*, 17, 130, 1984.
35. **Graham, T. E. and MacLean, D. A.**, Ammonia and amino acid metabolism in human skeletal muscle during exercise, *Can. J. Physiol. Pharmacol.*, 70, 132, 1992.
36. **Jahoor, F., Peters, E. J., and Wolfe, R. R.**, The relationship between gluconeogenic substrate supply and glucose production in humans, *Am. J. Physiol.*, 258, E288, 1990.
37. **Helmreich, E. J. M.**, How pyridoxal 5'-phosphate could function in glycogen phosphorylase catalysis, *Biofactors*, 3, 159, 1992.
38. **Feller, A. G. and Rudman, D.**, Role of carnitine in human nutrition, *J. Nutr.*, 118, 541, 1988.
39. **Takami, M., Fujioka, M., Wada, H., and Taguchi, T.**, Studies on pyridoxine deficiency in rats, *Proc. Soc. Exp. Biol. Med.*, 129, 110, 1968.
40. **Okada, M. and Suzuki, K.**, Amino acid metabolism in rats fed a high protein diet without pyridoxine, *J. Nutr.*, 104, 287, 1974.
41. **Cochary, E. F., Gershoff, S. N., and Sadowski, J. A.**, Effects of vitamin B-6 deficiency and aging on pyridoxal 5'-phosphate levels and glycogen phosphorylase activity in rats, *J. Nutr. Biochem.*, 2, 135, 1991.
42. **Leklem, J. E. and Shultz, T. D.**, Increased plasma pyridoxal 5'-phosphate and vitamin B_6 in male adolescents after a 4500-meter run, *Am. J. Clin. Nutr.*, 38, 541, 1983.
43. **Manore, M. M., Leklem, J. E., and Walter, M. C.**, Vitamin B-6 metabolism as affected by exercise in trained and untrained women fed diets differing in carbohydrate and vitamin B-6 content, *Am. J. Clin. Nutr.*, 46, 995, 1987.
44. **Hofmann, A., Reynolds, R. D., Smoak, B. L., Villanueva, V. G., and Deuster, P. A.**, Plasma pyridoxal and pyridoxal 5'-phosphate concentrations in response to ingestion of water or glucose polymer during a 2-h run, *Am. J. Clin. Nutr.*, 53, 84, 1991.
45. **Crozier, P. G., Cordain, L., and Sampson, D. A.**, Exercise-induced changes in plasma vitamin B-6 concentrations do not vary with exercise intensity, *Am. J. Clin. Nutr.*, 60, 552, 1994.
46. **Hadj-Saad, F., Lhuissier, M., and Guilland, J.-C.**, Effects of acute, submaximal exercise on vitamin B_6 metabolism in the rat, *Nutr. Res.*, 15, 1181, 1995.
47. **Leklem, J. E.**, Physical activity and vitamin B-6 metabolism in men and women: interrelationship with fuel needs, in *Vitamin B-6: Its Role in Health and Disease,* Reynolds, R. D. and Leklem, J. E., Eds., Alan R. Liss, New York, 1985, 221.
48. **Yates, C. Y., Boylan, L. M., Lewis, R. D., and Driskell, J. A.**, Maternal aerobic exercise and vitamin B-6 status, *Am. J. Clin. Nutr.*, 48, 117, 1988.
49. **Lanne, R., Barnes, J. R., and Brouha, L.**, Changes in concentration of plasma protein fractions during muscular work and recovery, *J. Appl. Physiol.*, 13, 97, 1958.
50. **Van Beaumont, W., Greenleaf, J. E., and Juhos, L.**, Disproportional changes in hematocrit, plasma volume, and proteins during exercise and bed rest, *J. Appl. Physiol.*, 33, 55, 1972.
51. **Harrison, M. H.**, Effects of thermal stress and exercise on blood volume in humans, *Physiol. Rev.*, 65, 149, 1985.
52. **Fogelholm, M.**, Micronutrient status in females during a 24-week fitness-type exercise program, *Ann. Nutr. Metab.*, 36, 209, 1992.
53. **Van der Beek, E. J., Van Dokkum, W., Schrijver, J., Wedel, M., Gaillard, A. W. K., Wesstra, A., Van de Weerd, H., and Hermus, R. J. J.**, Thiamin, riboflavin, and vitamins B_6 and C: impact of combined restricted intake on functional performance in man, *Am. J. Clin. Nutr.*, 48, 1451, 1988.
54. **Van der Beek, E. J., Van Dokkum, W., Wedel, M., Schrijver, J., and Van den Berg, H.**, Thiamin, riboflavin and vitamin B_6: impact of restricted intake on physical performance in man, *J. Am. Coll. Nutr.*, 13, 629, 1994.
55. **Reeves, P. G., Nielsen, F. H., and Fahey, G. C.**, AIN-93 purified diets for laboratory rodents: final report of the American Institute of Nutrition ad hoc writing committee on the reformulation of the AIN-76A rodent diet, *J. Nutr.*, 123, 1939, 1993.
56. **Hu, M.-L., Chen, Y.-K., and Lin, Y.-F.**, The antioxidant and prooxidant activity of some B vitamins and vitamin-like compounds, *Chem. Biol. Interact.*, 97, 63, 1995.
57. **Rokitzki, L., Sagredos, A. N., Reuss, F., Cufi, D., and Keul, J.**, Assessment of vitamin B_6 status of strength and speedpower athletes, *J. Am. Coll. Nutr.*, 13, 87, 1994.
58. **Davies, K. J. A., Quintanilha, A. T., Brooks, G. A., and Packer, L.**, Free radicals and tissue damage produced by exercise, *Biochem. Biophys. Res. Commun.*, 107, 1198, 1982.
59. **Jenkins, R. R.**, Free radical chemistry: relationship to exercise, *Sports Med.*, 5, 156, 1988.

60. **Sjodin, B., Westing, Y. H., and Apple, F. S.**, Biochemical mechanisms for oxygen free radical formation during exercise, *Sports Med.*, 10, 236, 1990.

61. **Robertson, J. D., Maughan, R. J., Duthie, G. G., and Morrice, P. C.**, Increased blood antioxidant systems of runners in response to training load, *Clin. Sci.*, 80, 611, 1991.

62. **Maxwell, S. R. J., Jakeman, P., Thomason, H., Leguen, C., and Thorpe, G. H. G.**, Changes in plasma antioxidant status during eccentric exercise and the effect of vitamin supplementation, *Free Rad. Res. Commun.*, 19, 191, 1993.

63. **Bendich, A.**, Exercise and free radicals. Effects of antioxidant vitamins, *Med. Sports Sci.*, 32, 59, 1991.

64. **Frei, B.**, Reactive oxygen species and antioxidant vitamins. Mechanisms of action, *Am. J. Med.*, 97 (Suppl. 3A), 5S, 1994.

65. **Selvam, R. and Ravichandran, V.**, Lipid peroxidation in liver of vitamin B$_6$ deficient rats, *J. Nutr. Biochem.*, 2, 245, 1991.

66. **Ji, L.**, Oxidative stress during exercise: implication of antioxidant nutrients, *Free Rad. Biol. Med.*, 18, 1079, 1995.

67. **Cazzulani, P., Cassin, M., and Ceserani, R.**, Increased endurance to physical exercise in mice given oral reduced glutathione (GSH), *Med. Sci. Res.*, 19, 543, 1991.

68. **Selhub, J. and Miller, J. W.**, The pathogenesis of homocysteinemia: interruption of the coordinate regulation by S-adenosylmethionine of the remethylation and transsulfuration of homocysteine, *Am. J. Clin. Nutr.*, 55, 131, 1992.

69. **Takeuchi, F., Izuta, S., Tsubouchi, R., and Shibata, Y.**, Glutathione levels and related enzyme activities in vitamin B$_6$-deficient rats fed a high methionine and low cystine diet, *J. Nutr.*, 121, 1366, 1991.

70. **Stainby, W. N., Brechere, W. F., O'Drobnack, D. N., and Barclay, J. K.**, Oxidation/reduction state of cytochrome oxidase during repetitive contractions, *J. Appl. Physiol.*, 67, 2158, 1989.

71. **McCord, J. M.**, Oxygen-derived free radicals in post-ischaemic tissue injury, *N. Engl. J. Med.*, 312, 159, 1985.

72. **Packianathan, S., Cain, C. D., Stagg, R. B., and Longo, L. D.**, Ornithine decarboxylase activity in fetal and newborn rat brain. Responses to hypoxic and carbon monoxide hypoxia, *Dev. Brain Res.*, 76, 131, 1993.

73. **Kummerlen, C., Seiler, N., Galluser, M., Gosse, F., Knodgen, B., Hasselmann, M., and Raul, F.**, Polyamines and the recovery of intestinal morphology and function after ischemic damage in rats, *Digestion*, 55, 168, 1994.

74. **Muszynski, C. A., Robertson, C. S., Goodman, J. C., and Henley, C. M.**, DFMO reduces cortical infarct volume after middle cerebral artery occlusion in the rat, *J. Cereb. Blood Flow Metab.*, 13, 1033, 1993.

75. **Sauer, D., Martin, P., Allegrini, P. R., Bernasconi, R., Amacker, H., and Fagg, G. E.**, Differing effects of alpha-difluoromethylornithine and CGP 40116 on polyamine levels and infarct volume in a rat model of focal cerebral ischaemia, *Neurosci. Lett.*, 141, 131, 1992.

76. **Sturman, J. A. and Kremzner, L. T.**, Regulation of ornithine decarboxylase synthesis. Effect of a nutritional deficiency of vitamin B$_6$, *Life Sci.*, 14, 977, 1974.

77. **Sampson, D. A., Harrison, S. C., Clarke, S. D., and Yan, X.**, Dietary protein quality alters ornithine decarboxylase activity but not vitamin B$_6$ nutritional status in rats, *J. Nutr.*, 125, 2199, 1995.

78. **Meisler, N. T. and Thanassi, J. W.**, Vitamin B$_6$ metabolism and its relation to ornithine decarboxylase activity in regenerating rat liver, *J. Nutr.*, 112, 314, 1982.

79. **Anon.**, Control of enzyme levels in vitamin deficiency, *Nutr. Rev.*, 30, 232, 1972.

80. **Kominami, E., Kobayashi, K., Kominami, S., and Katunuma, N.**, Properties of a specific protease for pyridoxal enzymes and its biological role, *J. Biol. Chem.*, 247, 6848, 1972.

81. **Banno, Y., Shiotani, T., Towatari, T., Yoshikawa, D., Katunuma, T., Afting, E. G., and Katunuma, N.**, Studies on new intracellular proteases in various organs of rat. 3. Control of group-specific protease under physiological conditions, *Eur. J. Biochem.*, 52, 59, 1975.

82. **Katunuma, N.**, Enzyme degradation and its regulation by group-specific proteases in various organs of rats, in *Current Topics in Cellular Regulation,* Vol. 7, Horecker, B. L. and Stadtman, E. R., Eds., Academic Press, New York, 1973, 175.

83. **Black, A. L., Guirard, B. M., and Snell, E. E.**, The behavior of muscle phosphorylase as a reservoir for vitamin B$_6$ in the rat, *J. Nutr.*, 108, 670, 1978.

84. **Newsholme, E. A. and Leech, A. R.**, *Biochemistry for the Medical Sciences,* John Wiley & Sons, New York, 1983.

85. **Malinow, M. R.**, Plasma homocysteine and arterial occlusive diseases: a mini-review, *Clin. Chem.*, 40, 173, 1994.

86. **Kang, S. S., Wong, P. W. K., and Malinow, M. R.**, Hyperhomocysteinemia as a risk factor for occlusive vascular disease, *Annu. Rev. Nutr.*, 12, 279, 1992.

87. **Stampfer, M. J., Malinow, R., Willet, W. C., Newcomer, L. M., Upson, B., Ullmann, D., Tishler, P. V., and Hennekens, C. H.**, A prospective study of plasma homocyst(e)ine and risk of myocardial infarction in U.S. physicians, *J. Am. Med. Assoc.*, 268, 877, 1992.

88. **Mason, J. B. and Miller, J. W.**, The effects of vitamins B_{12}, B_6 and folate on blood homocysteine levels, *Ann. N.Y. Acad. Sci.*, 669, 197, 1992.
89. **Ubbink, J. B., Vermaak, W. J. H., Van der Merwe, A., Becker, P. J., Delport, R., and Potgieter, H. C.**, Vitamin requirement for the treatment of hyperhomocysteinemia in humans, *J. Nutr.*, 124, 1927, 1994.
90. **Malinow, M. R.**, Hyperhomocyst(e)inemia — a common and easily reversible risk factor for occlusive atherosclerosis, *Circulation*, 81, 2004, 1990.
91. **Ubbink, J. B.**, Vitamin nutrition status and homocysteine: an atherogenic risk factor, *Nutr. Rev.*, 52, 383, 1994.
92. **Blair, S. N., Kohl, H. W., Paffenbarger, R. S., Clark, D. G., Cooper, K. H., and Gibbons, L. W.**, Physical fitness and all-cause mortality: a prospective study of healthy men and women, *J. Am. Med. Assoc.*, 262, 2395, 1989.
93. **Lee, I. M., Hsieh, C., and Paffenbarger, R. S.**, Exercise intensity and longevity in men: the Harvard Alumni Health Study, *J. Am. Med. Assoc.*, 273, 1179, 1995.

Chapter **6**

FOLATE AND VITAMIN B$_{12}$

———— Kenneth McMartin

CONTENTS

I. INTRODUCTION

The roles of folate and vitamin B$_{12}$ (cobalamin) in sport and exercise are poorly defined today. Both are B vitamins that are crucial for DNA synthesis, hence are involved in cell division and growth. These vitamins are required for proper erythrocyte production, so could theoretically be important for endurance athletes. Folate and cobalamin are also involved in other enzymatic steps that regulate amino acid and other cellular metabolic pathways. This chapter presents information on the intake and status of these vitamins in the general population as well as in athletic populations. In addition, evidence for their role in affecting exercise performance is discussed.

0-8493-8192-4/97/$0.00+$.50

A. CHEMISTRY

Folate is a general term used to include the many forms that have the biologic activity of the commercial vitamin form, folic acid. The chemical structure, pteroylmonoglutamic acid (PteGlu), consists of a pteridine ring structure linked to paraaminobenzoic acid and L-glutamic acid residues. The commercial vitamin does not exist naturally in the body, but is rapidly converted to the physiologic forms in tissues (derivatives of tetrahydrofolate, $H_4PteGlu$).[1] Tissue folates exist mainly as polyglutamyl folates, where additional glutamates are attached to the base structure through peptide bonds.

Vitamin B_{12} in the commercial form is generally cyanocobalamin. The chemical structure of cyanocobalamin consists of a planar coordination complex of four conjoined pyrrole rings surrounding a central cobalt atom. This structure is similar to the iron porphyrins as found in heme. The CN group is attached to one of the available Co sites, while attached to the other site is a ribonucleotide, which is additionally attached to the pyrrole ring structure by an aminopropanol linkage. There are three main physiologic cobalamins, in which the CN group is replaced with an OH group (hydroxocobalamin, which is sometimes available commercially), a methyl group (methylcobalamin), or a 5'-deoxyadenosyl group (adenosyl-cobalamin). The latter two are the coenzyme forms of the vitamin in humans. Cyanocobalamin is used commercially and in most research studies because of its greater stability.[2] In addition to the cobalamins, human plasma often contains cobalamin analogues, which are generally inactive as coenzymes.[2]

B. METABOLIC FUNCTIONS

Folate coenzymes mainly function in one-carbon transfer reactions that involve amino acid metabolism and the synthesis of pyrimidine and purine nucleotides.[3] The latter are the bases of DNA and RNA, so clinical folate deficiency is primarily linked with defects in DNA biosynthesis. Hence, rapidly proliferating tissues such as the hematopoietic system, the gastrointestinal epithelium, and the developing fetus have the greatest requirement for DNA synthesis and are the major tissues affected in clinical folate deficiency. Recently, folate deficiency has been linked with an elevation in plasma homocysteine concentration, which has been recognized as an important risk factor for the development of atherosclerosis.[4]

For athletes, the primary importance of folates would be in providing for proper synthesis of erythrocytes to maintain the normal oxygen-carrying capacity of the blood. There may also be as-yet unrecognized consequences of malfunctions in the folate-dependent interconversions of amino acids, such as glycine *N*-methyltransferase or serine hydroxymethyltransferase.

Cobalamins act as coenzymes in humans in only two reactions, methylcobalamin in methionine synthase and adenosylcobalamin in methyl malonyl CoA mutase. The former reaction involves the remethylation of homocysteine using 5-methyltetrahydrofolate as the methyl donor. Through this reaction, vitamin B_{12} is linked with the folate system.[3] In the absence of B_{12}, the methyl group cannot be transferred from the folate, leading to increased levels of 5-methyltetrahydrofolate. The latter cannot be converted to tetrahydrofolate by reversal of its formation, so the folate pool becomes "trapped" in the methyl form. Then tetrahydrofolate is not available to transfer one-carbon groups, especially in the thymidylate synthetase reaction, which leads to diminished DNA synthesis. The second reaction, i.e., mutase, converts methyl malonyl CoA to succinyl CoA and is involved in metabolism of propionate groups generated in fatty acid oxidation.

Because of the link with the folate system, vitamin B_{12}'s importance for athletes also lies in proper erythropoiesis to maintain oxygen transport in the blood. In addition, cobalamin deficiency is associated with development of nervous system damage leading to neurologic and mental symptoms, through as-yet undetermined mechanisms. Hence, vitamin B_{12} may be needed for proper functioning of the nervous system. Athletes, who depend on central coordination of movement, timing, strength, etc., would probably be dependent on sufficient cobalamin to maintain proper CNS function.

C. INDICATORS OF STATUS

Folate and vitamin B$_{12}$ status can be assessed by biochemical measurements and by clinical indications, although the latter generally appear in severe deficiency conditions so are of little use in diagnosing the initial development of deficiency.[5] The diagnosis of sub-clinical deficiency depends on the demonstration of lower than normal tissue vitamin levels by biochemical measurements. The development of folate deficiency has been classified by Herbert[6] in stages. Stage 1, or initial negative balance occurs when the intake of folate is not as great as that being lost. This stage is indicated by a decrease in the serum folate level, measured biochemically, below 6.5 nmol/l (3 ng/ml). Since tissue stores are not initially affected, a decrease in serum folate does not, by itself, indicate folate deficiency. Stage 2 of negative folate balance is tissue folate depletion, as indicated by a decrease in the red cell folate level below 300 nmol/l (140 ng/ml). Erythrocyte folate levels generally parallel those in the liver, so are considered a reliable indication of the status of the body folate pool. Stage 3 is characterized as severe folate deficiency and is correlated with the development of abnormal intracellular folate-dependent metabolism. This stage is indicated biochemically by an abnormal deoxyuridine suppression test (in bone marrow or peripheral lymphocytes) and morphologically by the presence of hypersegmented neutrophils, both suggesting alterations in DNA synthesis. Stage 4 deficiency is the presence of macrocytic anemia (increased mean cell volume [MCV] and decreased hemoglobin levels) and clinical symptomatology.

The most common biochemical indicator of B$_{12}$ status is the demonstration of low serum or plasma cobalamin concentrations, which are associated with decreased tissue body content of the vitamin. The lower levels of the normal range are about 200 to 250 pg/ml.[7] Serum B$_{12}$ levels can be determined by microbiological or radioisotope dilution assay. Although the latter procedures are used most often and are generally quite accurate, the presence of cobalamin analogues in the plasma can sometimes obfuscate the binding of cobalamin,[8] leading to erroneous results. Since the most common cause of cobalamin deficiency is an abnormal intestinal absorption of B$_{12}$, a clinical procedure for diagnosing cobalamin malabsorption is the urinary excretion or Schilling test.[9] Diminished excretion of a radiolabeled oral dose of cobalamin after a flushing parenteral dose indicates gastrointestinal malabsorption. A specific indicator of diminished vitamin B$_{12}$ status is an increased plasma or urinary level of methylmalonate (because of the block in methylmalonate conversion to succinate). Recent studies have shown the value of urinary or plasma methylmalonate determinations for diagnosis of cobalamin deficiency,[10] but these tests are not yet widely available.

Many of the hematologic changes in folate and B$_{12}$ deficiency are identical, so are not true indicators of status of the individual vitamins. Megaloblastic changes in the bone marrow plus macroovalocytes and neutrophilic hypersegmentation in the peripheral blood are indicators of megaloblastic anemia resulting from either folate or B$_{12}$ deficiency. Hence, laboratory methods are needed to distinguish the two types of deficiency — measurements of serum and red cell folate and of serum vitamin B$_{12}$ are needed to ascertain the cause of the macrocytic anemias. A wide range of neurologic signs and symptoms can indicate diminished cobalamin status. These include paresthesias of the extremities, loss of sensation, confusion, loss of memory and, even in severe cases, delusional psychosis. It is critically important to identify the cause of the hematologic abnormality because folate therapy for a cobalamin deficiency can reverse the megaloblastic symptomatology, but exacerbate the neurologic damage.[11]

There is no evidence that exercise has any direct effects on the biochemical or clinical indicators of folate and vitamin B$_{12}$ status per se. Nevertheless, exercise could change the optimal vitamin status by a decrease in availability or an increase in requirement. Availability of folate or B$_{12}$ is decreased when there is reduced dietary supply or reduced absorption of ingested vitamin. Dietary supply would primarily be determined by socioeconomic factors; exercise, if anything, should increase dietary intake by stimulating the overall intake of food and the general concern of the exercising individual for health. Because polyglutamyl folates are not directly absorbed across the intestinal mucosa, the bioavailability of dietary folates will depend on food composition, i.e., on the relative amounts of polyglutamylation in the ingested food.[12] The bioavailability of supplements and of fortified foods such as cereals would be greatest because the folate is present in the monoglutamate form. Hence, athletes who consume fortified cereals or supplements should have no problems with bioavailability.

Because recent studies have demonstrated that folate has an ameliorating effect on neural tube defects, fortification of grains with folic acid has been recommended as a means of increasing the intake of folate by potentially affected females.[13] Such fortification should diminish the frequency of marginal folate deficiency in females, including those who exercise regularly. Food preparation techniques can influence dietary folate supply in that folates are readily destroyed by lengthy boiling of food such as vegetables.[12] Malabsorption of food folate and B_{12} occurs in disorders of the intestinal tract such as in tropical sprue. Lack of intrinsic factor secretion (see below) is the most common cause of diminished vitamin B_{12} status. Gastric mucosal atrophy, such as in pernicious anemia, and loss of gastric function through surgical resection, are the major causes of loss of intrinsic factor secretion.

Folate and vitamin B_{12} requirements are increased in persons who need increased amounts because of rapid growth (infants, pregnant and lactating women), presence of disease (malignancy, inflammation), and use of certain drugs (antifolates used in cancer chemotherapy or as antimicrobials, oral contraceptives, alcohol, and certain anticonvulsants). Functional B_{12} deficiency can be produced by chronic exposure (24 h) to high levels of the anesthetic gas nitrous oxide.[14] Nitrous oxide combines with the Co atom in cobalamin, hence specifically and irreversibly inhibiting the enzyme methionine synthase. Except for persons affected by such categories, there is no reason to expect exercise or sporting activities to increase the requirements for folate or B_{12}. However, malabsorption of vitamin B_{12} increases in frequency with age, so that masters athletes are more likely to have an increased requirement for B_{12}.

D. CONTENT OF FOODS

Folate is not produced by mammals so it must be ingested by humans as an essential vitamin. Food sources that contain the highest concentration of folate include liver, green leafy vegetables, certain fruits (and juices), legumes (especially pinto and navy beans), and fortified products like cereals.[5,15] The folate molecule is sensitive to oxidation so it can be destroyed by excessive exposure to heat and light, and is water soluble so it can be readily leached by cooking in water. Hence, food preparation styles greatly influence the amount of unchanged folates that are presented to the intestine. Although the above foods may contain high concentrations of folate, they do not necessarily represent the foods that provide for the highest intake by the general population. Liver, for example, is not consumed to a great extent by most people today. McNulty[5] has noted that beer, which contains less than 5% of the amount of folate as liver on a per gram basis, provides for about 10% of the total folate intake in a British population, while liver contributes essentially nothing. The highest contribution to dietary folate intake appears to come from breads, orange juice, cereals, and vegetables including beans.[5,15]

The ultimate sources of vitamin B_{12} are cobalamin-synthesizing microorganisms that are found in soil, water, or the intestinal lumen of animals. Vegetable products do not contain cobalamins unless they are contaminated with such microorganisms. Hence, the primary source of vitamin B_{12} is the consumption of animal products such as meat, eggs, and milk containing B_{12}. Small amounts of B_{12} are available from legumes, due to contamination with soil bacteria. Hence, because the daily requirement is only 2 to 3 µg, strict vegetarians often have marginal B_{12} status, but rarely become overtly deficient by dietary insufficiency alone.

However, infants breast-fed by strictly vegetarian mothers are susceptible to B_{12} deficiency because of the very low concentration of cobalamin in milk of mothers with diminished B_{12} intake.[16]

E. ABSORPTION, DISTRIBUTION, AND ELIMINATION

Dietary sources of folates are primarily polyglutamyl forms, which cannot cross cell membranes. Polyglutamate folates must be cleaved to the monoglutamate forms to be absorbed by the intestinal mucosa. Hydrolysis of the glutamate moieties is catalyzed by the enzyme pteroylpolyglutamate hydrolase (conjugase), which is found in pancreatic secretions as well as in the brush-border membranes of the jejunal mucosa.[12] The monoglutamate folates are then transported across the mucosa by a specific carrier-mediated uptake system, although significant amounts can also be transported by passive diffusion down an electrochemical gradient.[17] The bioavailability of folates from different food sources is extremely inconsistent because of the presence or absence of factors which can interfere with polyglutamate hydrolysis or bind with folates.[12] The primary folate in the plasma is 5-methyl-H_4PteGlu,[18] which is then transported to the liver and peripheral tissues, where it is taken up. In cells, the 5-methyl-H_4PteGlu is converted eventually to the polyglutamyl derivatives, which act as physiologic substrates for the folate-dependent enzymes, as physiologic regulators of one-carbon metabolism, and as storage forms of folates. The liver contains the majority of the total body folate pool; folates can be secreted into the bile, then reabsorbed in the intestine to establish an active enterohepatic circulation. Folates are eliminated from the body in small amounts through fecal excretion, but mostly through urinary excretion of unchanged folates and of folate catabolites.[19] Because of loss of body stores via these latter processes, folate deficiency can occur relatively rapidly (i.e., in 2 to 3 months) whenever dietary sources are restricted.

The absorption of B_{12} is a highly regulated process and defects in it are the primary cause of deficiency.[8] Dietary B_{12} is cleaved from dietary and salivary proteins by acid in the stomach and by pancreatic proteases. B_{12} is then bound to intrinsic factor, a glycoprotein secreted by the gastric parietal cells.[8] Binding to intrinsic factor protects B_{12} from enzymatic digestion in the gastrointestinal tract. The cobalamin-intrinsic factor complex traverses the intestinal tract to the ileum where it binds to specific receptors on ileal mucosal cells.[2] Absorption through the mucosa occurs via intracellular cleavage from intrinsic factor and transport into the portal circulation by binding to a specific protein, transcobalamin II. Some absorption of pharmacologic levels of B_{12} can be mediated by a separate, diffusion-type mechanism.[2] Vitamin B_{12} is carried in the circulation by binding to transcobalamin II. Uptake into tissues, primarily by the liver, occurs by binding of transcobalamin II to specific receptors, followed by receptor-mediated endocytosis.[2] About 90% of the total body stores of cobalamin is found in the liver. Excretion via the urine and the feces is minor, accounting for the minimal daily requirement of 2 to 3 μg. Biliary secretion of cobalamin occurs, but most of the vitamin is reabsorbed in the ileum after binding to the intrinsic factor. Efficient conservation of vitamin B_{12} can explain why a deficiency takes years to develop, even in cases of strict vegetarians who consume almost no B_{12}.[7]

II. INTAKE

A. GENERAL POPULATION

Folate deficiency is a major problem in societies where there is poverty and general malnutrition. It is often second only to iron deficiency as a cause of anemia. In our current society in the U.S., overt folate deficiency occurs infrequently because of poor dietary intake. In fact because of a recent reduction in the recommended daily intake from 400 to 180–200 μg (see below), the general population is considered in most surveys to be taking in sufficient amounts of folate. New studies that relate folate status with development of neural tube defects or elevated homocysteine levels (and atherosclerosis) suggest that the definitions of sufficient intake may need to be refined. Surveys of populations in the U.S., Canada, and the U.K. have shown mean folate intakes of 185 to 305 μg/day.[5,15] Not surprisingly, dietary supplements contribute substantially to the daily folate intakes at the high end of the intake distribution curve, while contributing little at the low end of the curve. There are several reasons that dietary folate intake is probably underestimated in such surveys: (1) general underestimation of total food intake; or (2) inexact food composition data due to variabilities in food sample preparation (loss during cooking) and in analytical methodologies used to measure food folate content (variations in extraction from food matrices and in deconjugation of polyglutamates).[15]

Vitamin B_{12} deficiency is most often associated with absorption defects, so intake per se may not be as relevant as for folate. Even so, population studies indicate that most humans in Western societies consume more than adequate amounts of B_{12}. People at most risk for B_{12} deficiency would be the elderly, especially post 60 years, when increasing gastric atrophy contributes to malabsorption. Population studies of intake in the U.S. and U.K., reported 20 to 30 years ago (cited by Herbert[7]), suggest that vitamin B_{12} intakes range from 3 to 15 μg/day. A recent study of the Framingham heart study cohort of elderly subjects (>67 years old) showed B_{12} intakes averaging 5 to 6 μg/day.[20] A study of the vitamin B_{12} and folate status of a group of 132 Thai vegetarians (ingesting no animal products except milk) and a control group, reported B_{12} intakes of 0.4 μg/day in the vegetarians, confirming the reduced levels of B_{12} in vegetarian diets.[21] As expected, the vegetarian group was relatively B_{12} deficient (mean serum levels of 117 and 152 pg/ml in males and females, respectively, compared to about 500 pg/ml in controls). However, serum folate levels in the vegetarians were about twice those in controls.

B. ATHLETES

Total folate and B_{12} intakes by athletes do not seem to be much different from those of other groups that are active consumers of balanced diets and vitamin supplements, although such intakes would be above those of the general population. Barry et al.[22] surveyed the reported intakes of 108 international (I) class athletes and of 35 club (C) class athletes (involving both endurance and strength sports) using weighed inventories over 3 alternative days. Both I- and C-class males consumed about 315 μg of folate per day (similar to the RDA of 300 present at the time), while females consumed only 180 to 200 μg/day. I- and C-class males consumed 19 and 13 μg of B_{12} per day (much higher than the RDA of 3 μg, probably due to a high meat consumption), while I- and C-class females consumed 3 and 6 μg/day, respectively. About 50% of both groups of athletes were active consumers of some type of vitamin supplement. Singh et al.[23] recorded the 4-day dietary records of ultramarathoners who averaged 67 mi/week in training. The estimated vitamin intake from food alone was 320 to 400 μg of folate per day and 4.5 to 6 μg of B_{12} per day (compared to the existing RDAs of 200 and 2, respectively). Since 70% of this population used vitamin supplements, the total daily intakes were estimated at 510 to 630 μg folate and 50 to 55 μg B_{12}, well above the RDAs.

In a separate study of the effects of vitamin supplements on physically active men, Singh et al.[24] reported baseline 4-day diet records (no subjects on supplements for 3 weeks prior to baseline data). Folate and B_{12} intakes were about 400 and 5.5 μg/day, respectively. Worme et al.[25] surveyed male and female participants in a forthcoming triathlon (about a 17% response). Subjects completed a 3-day dietary record during normal training periods within 6 weeks after the event, including no competition during the 3 days. From food alone, daily folate intakes for males and females were 380 ± 20 and 300 ± 245 μg, respectively, while B_{12} intakes for both genders were about 5 μg/day. About 40% of the population consumed vitamin supplements on a regular basis and the total folate intakes for both genders increased to about 500 μg/day, the total B$_{12}$ intake for males increased to 10 μg/day, but that for females remained the same as for food alone. The RDAs cited at the time of this study were 400 and 3 μg/day for folate and B$_{12}$, respectively. Hence, it would appear that total intake of both vitamins from this population was greater than the RDA. However, when the data were shown for individuals, it was noted that about 45% of the females and about 30% of the males consumed less than the RDA, including both food and supplements. The population means cited above were apparently inflated by the presence of a few excess consumers of food and supplements such that these populations included a significant number of active athletes with less than the recommended vitamin consumptions.

A special concern should be noted since there are subsets of athletes who follow vegetarian diets for reasons of health or otherwise. As discussed above, the vitamin B$_{12}$ intake of strict vegetarians can be very low (0.4 μg/day), and well below the RDA for B$_{12}$ (2 μg/day).[21]

III. BIOCHEMICAL STATUS IN ATHLETES

Several studies have examined the folate and vitamin B$_{12}$ status of humans and animals during training as well as the effects of vitamin supplements on such status. Brotherhood et al.[26] compared the status of numerous hematologic parameters in 40 male long-distance runners with 12 matched controls. They reported no differences between these groups in serum or red cell folate levels, nor in serum B$_{12}$ levels. Runners showed a 20% increase in blood volume and total hemoglobin. Matter et al.,[27] in a study of 85 female marathoners, described a subgroup of 23 (27%) that showed low serum folate levels (<4.5 ng/ml, group mean of 3 ng/mL, which was half that of the other subgroups). The folate-deficient group showed an increased MCV, but no other indications of anemia; vitamin B$_{12}$ levels were normal in these subjects, as in the folate-normal subgroups. Daily supplementation with 5 mg of folate for 1 week returned the folate status to normal in the deficient group. The biochemical status of 17 of the I-class athletes was characterized by Barry et al.[22] Serum B$_{12}$ and folate levels were in the normal range for all athletes, although there were several females at the low end of the reference range for folate. Red cell folates were normal for all males, and the mean value was low, but normal for the females. However, some individual females had below normal red cell folate levels, so would be considered folate deficient. None of these athletes was an active consumer of vitamin supplements. Since the dietary intakes of folates by some females in this study were less than the RDA, the low red cell folate levels probably resulted from the low dietary intake, rather than from the intensity of training.

Singh et al.[23] reported on a group of ultramarathoners whose total folate and B$_{12}$ intakes from foods and supplements were found to be significantly above the RDAs. The serum folate levels averaged 56 nmol/l, above the reference range, while the blood B$_{12}$ levels averaged 226 pmol/l, in the middle of the reference range. Singh et al.[24] also reported on the status of physically active men before and during daily ingestion of a commercially available, high potency multivitamin and mineral supplement (400 μg folate, 200 μg B$_{12}$) for 12 weeks. Plasma folate levels before supplementation averaged 23 nmol/l, in the middle of the reference range, and did not increase with supplementation. Blood B$_{12}$ levels averaged about 200 pmol/l before supplementation, in the middle of the reference range, and significantly increased to 300 pmol/l by 6 weeks of supplementation, with no further increase at 12 weeks. The rise in B$_{12}$ levels, with no such increase in folate levels, can readily be explained by the fact that the folate concentration in the supplements was limited to 400 μg, in the range of the RDA, while the B$_{12}$ content was orders of magnitude greater than the RDA. Weight et al.[28] conducted a similar double-blind, placebo-controlled trial of multivitamin and mineral supplementation (500 μg folate and 60 μg B$_{12}$) in a group of male runners who averaged more than 40 mi/week. Background (presupplementation) folate and B$_{12}$ statuses were normal in these endurance athletes — serum folate averaged 11 nmol/l, red cell folate was 630 nmol/l, and serum B_{12} was 340 pmol/l — all in the middle of the normal ranges. Supplementation for up to 3 months did not affect folate or B_{12} status significantly; similarly, administration of a placebo did not affect these vitamins, suggesting that the control subjects maintained a well-balanced diet throughout the study.

These studies of populations of heavy-endurance exercisers show that folate and B_{12} statuses seem to be closely related to the diets consumed, i.e., those who consume a well-balanced diet or supplements have normal or elevated status, while those who consume a marginal diet without supplements tend to have lowered serum folate levels, although B_{12} status was normal in all studies. Supplements may raise folate or B_{12} levels to above normal status, but only if the supplement contains a grossly elevated content of the vitamin. In a direct study of the effect of intensive exercise, Allen[29] reported that the serum folate levels of thoroughbred horses significantly decreased from 4.6 to 3.5 µg/l during a 6-month period of intense training. There was no mention about whether any dietary changes were made due to training, but this could confound the interpretation that training lowered folate levels.

IV. STUDIES RELATED TO EXERCISE PERFORMANCE

A. ANIMAL

Apparently there have not been any studies conducted in animals that relate folate or B_{12} status or consumption of excess folate or B_{12} with changes in exercise performance.

B. HUMAN

Numerous studies have examined the effects of folate or vitamin B_{12} on exercise performance. Most of these have been conducted in conjunction with intake of other vitamins, especially other B vitamins (reviewed by Van der Beek[30]). Such studies are complicated in their interpretation as to the effects of folate or B_{12} per se. None of the studies of these vitamins individually have shown significant effects of folate or B_{12} on exercise performance, with the exception of one study in which the subjects were already anemic, i.e., they were already suffering from deficiency symptoms.

Matter et al.[27] studied the effects of folate supplementation (5 mg/day for 10 weeks) on a subgroup of 23 female marathoners with low serum folate levels (<4.5 ng/ml) compared to a group with normal folate status given placebo similarly. The subjects underwent treadmill exercise testing before, and at 1 and 10 weeks of supplementation. Also, various physiological parameters relevant to exercise were measured, including heart and respiratory rate, minute ventilation, forced expiratory CO_2 and O_2, and rise in blood lactate. None of these parameters were affected by folate supplementation, although serum folate levels more than doubled. The author concluded that neither low nor normal serum folate status affected treadmill performance nor biochemical or physiological parameters linked with maximal exercise. Tin-May-Tan et al.[31] studied the effects of parenteral vitamin B_{12} supplementation (1 mg, 3 times per week for 6 weeks) on physical performance in a double-blind placebo-controlled study in male students. B_{12} supplementation had no effect on resting heart rate, nor on recovery heart rate after maximal exercise, on oxygen uptake ($\dot{V}O_2max$), nor on measures of strength and coordination.

Rodger et al.[32] reported on a mass screening study of a university population in which serum folate and B_{12} levels in 300 subjects were compared to an assessment of exercise habits by questionnaire. The authors observed no significant relation between folate or B_{12} levels and levels of exercise in hours per week in either men or women. Read and McGuffin[33] reported a double-blind placebo-controlled study of B vitamin supplementation in age-matched male college students. Subjects received 0.5 µg B_{12} per day for 6 weeks in a multivitamin complex containing near or above RDA levels of B$_1$, B$_2$, B$_6$, niacin, and pantothenic acid. No significant effects of supplementation were noted in three tests of endurance capacity (treadmill) during the 6-week period.

In contrast to these negative reports, Seshadri and Malhotra[34] showed significant effects of folate supplementation on physical performance in a placebo-controlled study. Subjects were age- and income-matched pairs of boys (5 to 6 years old) with mild anemia (hemoglobin of 8 to 10.5 g/dl). Supplements included 0.2 mg folate and 40 mg iron per day for 2 months. Physical performance was assessed by running and jumping tests. The increase in performance in the treated group was significantly greater than that in the placebo group.

Although most sports require physical athletic exercise, there are other sports requiring mental conditioning and proper sensory-motor control, such as marksmanship. Bonke and Nickel[35] studied the effects of megadoses of B$_{12}$ in combination with B$_1$ (thiamin) and B$_6$ (pyridoxine) on performance by experienced marksmen in two studies: one of open design with 120 µg B$_{12}$ per day for 8 weeks and one of double-blind design with 600 µg/day for 8 weeks. In the latter study, the vitamin-treated group showed an increase in performance during the treatment period, with no such effect in the placebo group, suggesting minimal effects of training per se on the increased performance. These results are intriguing, although a crossover study in the same subjects might have eliminated some bias. Also, the doses of all the B vitamins were 60 to 300 times the respective RDAs.

V. REQUIREMENTS

A. RECOMMENDED DIETARY ALLOWANCES

The Recommended Dietary Allowance (RDA) is the term used to describe the amount of intake of a necessary nutrient considered to be sufficient to meet the needs of most healthy persons, i.e., what is needed to prevent a deficiency. These allowances utilize certain margins of safety (mean requirement plus two standard deviations) to cover the degree of variability in requirements among people and in bioavailability from most food sources. The RDAs undergo changes, depending on the presence of new scientific data. For instance, the RDAs promulgated in 1989 (Table 1) represent a marked reduction from those established in 1980.[36,37] Ironically, these reductions were controversial and stimulated a number of new scientific studies, especially of the folate status. Further impetus for reevaluation of the folate RDAs has come from studies linking neural tube defects with folate intake and from studies showing a relationship between poor folate status and elevated homocysteine levels, which is an acknowledged risk factor for various cardiovascular diseases. In fact, plasma homocysteine concentrations are often used as a functional measure of folate and B$_{12}$ status. O'Keefe et al.[38] have recently shown that daily consumption of 200 µg of folate (provided by supplementing low-folate food with folic acid) by a group of healthy nonpregnant women is not sufficient to maintain serum and red cell folate levels. They suggest that the current RDA for nonpregnant women is not adequate to meet their dietary needs.

B. SPECIFIC FOR ATHLETES

The popular or lay recommendation for intakes of folate and B$_{12}$ by athletes appears to be to take as much as one can. This is especially true for vitamin B$_{12}$, which is often hyped as an ergonomic aid or as a tonic for tiredness and poor mental status. The reasons behind the hype are probably derived from the known rapid improvement in mental status that occurs when a person with the neurologic symptoms of B$_{12}$ deficiency is injected with B$_{12}$. Hence, it is "logically" derived that if B$_{12}$ works in such a situation, then B$_{12}$ should be good for other situations where a person feels the need to be stimulated by something healthy.

**TABLE 1   Current Dietary Folate and
Vitamin B$_{12}$ Recommendations**

Age/gender	Folate (µg/day)	B$_{12}$ (µg/day)
Children		
0–0.5 years	25	0.3
0.5–1 years	35	0.5
1–3 years	50	0.7
4–6 years	75	1.0
7–10 years	100	1.4
Males		
11–14 years	150	2.0
15+ years	200	2.0
Females		
11–14 years	150	2.0
15+ years	180	2.0
Pregnant	400	2.2
Lactating	280	2.6

Note: Recommended Dietary Allowance (RDA)
determined by the Food and Nutrition Board
of the National Academy of Sciences, 1989.

The intake studies that have been conducted in athletes show that a substantial portion of lay and highly trained athletes consume high-potency vitamin supplements on a regular basis.[22-24] Such consumption brings the folate and B$_{12}$ status of these populations up to or above the recommended normal. In particular, B$_{12}$ levels are often elevated, since supplements are often superfortified in B$_{12}$. Despite the fact that supplements have decreased the frequency of marginal or deficient status in exercising populations, the studies of performance have indicated that the added amounts of folate and B$_{12}$ offer little if any improvement in endurance or athletic ability. Hence, there appears to be no need to recommend a different requirement of folate or B$_{12}$ intake for athletes as compared to the general population. However, the 1989 RDAs may be inadequate to meet the needs of a substantial portion of the population, based on more subtle measures such as homocysteine status. Thus, an increase in folate and B$_{12}$ intake by exercising populations (through well-balanced diets or via supplements) may have an unintended benefit of diminishing the occurrence of neural tube defects or of elevated homocysteine concentrations and the adverse effects thereof.

VI. CONCLUSIONS

Folate and vitamin B$_{12}$ are B vitamins that are primarily needed to maintain proper growth and development of cells through DNA synthesis. Deficiency of either vitamin leads to hematopoietic defects and possibly to anemia. In persons that have reached such morbidity, the administration of folate or B$_{12}$ in diets or supplements will have marked effects, including increasing endurance and athletic performance. In the athlete with normal or marginal folate or B$_{12}$ status, with no accompanying signs of deficiency, there is no scientific evidence that increased amounts of folate or B$_{12}$ will provide any benefits in terms of athletic performance or exercise physiology. Hence, athletes and physically active persons should consume a well-balanced diet to obtain sufficient folate and B$_{12}$. Supplements may be added to such a diet to ensure that the person does not suffer some of the subtle effects of marginal folate or B$_{12}$ status. But there is no reason to recommend consumption of added amounts of folate or B$_{12}$ to increase one's ability to exercise or perform athletically. Although vitamin B$_{12}$ is often given to patients complaining of tiredness, there is no evidence from controlled studies that B$_{12}$ improves alertness or well-being in nondeficient subjects.

REFERENCES

1. McMartin, K. E., Virayotha, V., and Tephly, T. R., High-pressure liquid chromatography separation and determination of rat liver folates, *Arch. Biochem. Biophys.*, 209, 127, 1981.
2. Ellenbogen, L. and Cooper, B. A., Vitamin B$_{12}$, *Handbook of Vitamins,* 2nd ed., Machlin, L. J., Ed., Marcel Dekker, New York, 1991, 491.
3. Shane, B. and Stokstad, E. L. R., Vitamin B$_{12}$-folate relationships, *Annu. Rev. Nutr.,* 5, 115, 1985.
4. Ueland, P. M. and Refsum, H., Plasma homocysteine, a risk factor for vascular disease: plasma levels in health, disease, and drug therapy, *J. Lab. Clin. Med.*, 114, 473, 1989.
5. McNulty, H., Folate requirements for health in different population groups, *Br. J. Biomed. Sci.*, 52, 110, 1995.
6. Herbert, V., Development of human folate deficiency, *Folic Acid Metabolism in Health and Disease,* Picciano, M. F., Stokstad, E. L. R., and Gregory, J. F., Eds., Wiley-Liss, New York, 1990, 195.
7. Herbert, V., Recommended dietary intakes (RDI) of vitamin B-12 in humans, *Am. J. Clin. Nutr.*, 45, 671, 1987.
8. Nexø, E., Hansen, M., Rasmussen, K., Lindgren, A., and Gräsbeck, R., How to diagnose cobalamin deficiency, *Scand. J. Clin. Lab. Invest.*, 54, 61, 1994.
9. Schilling, R. F., Intrinsic factor studies. II. The effect of gastric juice on the urinary excretion of radioactivity after the oral administration of radioactive vitamin B$_{12}$, *J. Lab. Clin. Med.,* 42, 860, 1953.
10. Marcell, P. D., Stabler, S. P., Podell, E. R., and Allen, R. H., Quantitation of methylmalonic acid and other dicarboxylic acids in normal serum and urine using capillary gas chromatography-mass spectrometry, *Anal. Biochem.,* 150, 55, 1985.
11. Savage, D. G. and Lindenbaum, J., Folate-cobalamin interactions, *Folate in Health and Disease,* Bailey, L. B., Ed., Marcel Dekker, New York, 1995, 237.
12. Gregory, J. F., III, The bioavailability of folate, *Folate in Health and Disease,* Bailey, L. B., Ed., Marcel Dekker, New York, 1995, 195.
13. Crane, N. T., Wilson, D. B., Cook, D. A., Lewis, C. J., Yetley, E. A., and Rader, J. I., Evaluating food fortification options: General principles revisited with folic acid, *Am. J. Public Health*, 85, 660, 1995.
14. Amess, J. A. L., Burman, J. F., Rees, G. M., Nancekievill, D. G., and Mollin, D. L., Megaloblastic haemopoiesis in patients receiving nitrous oxide, *Lancet*, 2, 339, 1978.
15. Bailey, L. B., Folate requirements and dietary recommendations, *Folate in Health and Disease,* Bailey, L. B., Ed., Marcel Dekker, New York, 1995, 123.
16. Schneede, J., Dagnelie, P. C., Van Staveren, W. A., Vollset, S. E., Refsum, H., and Ueland, P. M., Methylmalonic acid and homocysteine in plasma as indicators of functional cobalamin deficiency in infants on macrobiotic diets, *Pediatr. Res.*, 36, 194, 1994.
17. Selhub, J., Dhar, G. J., and Rosenberg, I. H., Gastrointestinal absorption of folates and antifolates, *Pharm. Ther.,* 20, 397, 1983.
18. Eisenga, B. H., Collins, T. D., and McMartin, K. E., Differential effects of acute ethanol on urinary excretion of folate derivatives in the rat, *J. Pharmacol. Exp. Ther.*, 248, 916, 1988.
19. Geoghegan, F. L., McPartlin, J. M., Weir, D. G., and Scott, J. M., *para*-Acetamidobenzoylglutamate is a suitable indicator of folate catabolism in rats, *J. Nutr.*, 125, 2563, 1995.
20. Selhub, J., Jacques, P. F., Wilson, P. W. F., Rush, D., and Rosenberg, I. H., Vitamin status and intake as primary determinants of homocysteinemia in an elderly population, *J. Am. Med. Assoc.*, 270, 2693, 1993.
21. Tungtrongchitr, R., Pongpaew, P., Prayurahong, B., Changbumrung, S., Vudhivai, N., Migasena, P., and Schelp F. P., Vitamin B$_{12}$, folic acid and haematological status of 132 Thai vegetarians, *Int. J. Vitam. Nutr. Res.,* 63, 201, 1993.
22. Barry, A., Cantwell, T., Doherty, F., Folan, J. C., Ingoldsby, M., Kevany, J. P., O'Broin, J. D., O'Connor, H., O'Shea, B., Ryan, B. A., and Vaughan, J., A nutritional study of Irish athletes, *Br. J. Sports Med.*, 15, 99, 1981.
23. Singh, A., Evans, P., Gallagher, K. L., and Deuster, P. A., Dietary intakes and biochemical profiles of nutritional status of ultramarathoners, *Med. Sci. Sports Exercise*, 25, 328, 1993.
24. Singh, A., Moses, F. M., and Deuster, P. A., Vitamin and mineral status in physically active men: effects of a high-potency supplement, *Am. J. Clin. Nutr.*, 55, 1, 1992.
25. Worme, J. D., Doubt, T. J., Singh, A., Ryan, C. J., Moses, F. M., and Deuster, P. A., Dietary patterns, gastrointestinal complaints, and nutrition knowledge of recreational triathletes, *Am. J. Clin. Nutr.*, 51, 690, 1990.
26. Brotherhood, J., Brozovic, B., and Pugh, L. G. C., Haematological status of middle-and long-distance runners, *Clin. Sci. Mol. Med.*, 48, 139, 1975.
27. Matter, M., Stittfall, T., Graves, J., Myburgh, K., Adams, B., Jacobs, P., and Noakes, T. D., The effect of iron and folate therapy on maximal exercise performance in female marathon runners with iron and folate deficiency, *Clin. Sci.*, 72, 415, 1987.
28. Weight, L. M., Noakes, T. D., Labadarios, D., Graves, J., Jacobs, P., and Berman, P. A., Vitamin and mineral status of trained athletes including the effects of supplementation, *Am. J. Clin. Nutr.*, 47, 186, 1988.
29. Allen, B. V., Serum folate levels in horses, with particular reference to the English thoroughbred, *Vet. Rec.*, 103, 257, 1978.

30. Van der Beek, E. J., Vitamins and endurance training, Food for running or faddish claims?, *Sports Med.*, 2, 175, 1985.
31. Tin-May-Tan, Ma-Win-May, Khin-Sann-Aung, and Mya-Tu, M., The effect of vitamin B_{12} on physical performance capacity, *Br. J. Nutr.*, 40, 269, 1978.
32. Rodger, R. S. C., Fletcher, K., Fail, B. J., Rahman, H., Sviland, L., and Hamilton, P. J., Factors influencing haematological measurements in healthy adults, *J. Chronic Dis.*, 40, 943, 1987.
33. Read, M. H. and McGuffin L., The effect of B-complex supplementation on endurance performance, *J. Sports Med.*, 23, 178, 1983.
34. Seshadri, S. and Malhotra, S., The effect of hematinics on the physical work capacity in anemics, *Indian Pediatr.*, 21, 529, 1984.
35. Bonke, D. and Nickel, B., Improvement of fine motoric movement control by elevated dosages of vitamin B_1, B_6, and B_{12} in target shooting, *Int. J. Vitam. Nutr. Res.*, Suppl. 30, 198, 1989.
36. Food and Nutrition Board, *Recommended Dietary Allowances*, 10th ed., National Academy of Sciences, Washington, D.C., 1989.
37. Food and Nutrition Board, *Recommended Dietary Allowances*, 9th ed., National Academy of Sciences, Washington, D.C., 1980.
38. O'Keefe, C. A., Bailey, L. B., Thomas, E. A., Hofler, S. A., Davis, B. A., Cerda, J. J., and Gregory, J. F., Controlled dietary folate affects folate status in nonpregnant women, *J. Nutr.*, 125, 2717, 1995.

Chapter 7

PANTOTHENIC ACID AND BIOTIN

———— Elizabeth A. Thomas

CONTENTS

I. INTRODUCTION

Pantothenic acid and biotin are essential water-soluble vitamins that serve as regulators for several metabolic processes, many of which are important for exercise performance. Pantothenic acid was recognized as a growth cofactor for yeast in 1933,[1] and was identified as an essential nutrient in humans in 1939.[2] The biologically active forms of pantothenic acid, coenzyme A (CoA) and acyl carrier protein, are cofactors for acetylation reactions which are essential in many biosynthetic pathways, as well as in energy production. Pantothenic acid-containing coenzymes are involved in acylation of alcohols, amines, and amino acids; oxidation of pyruvate and α-ketoglutarate; β-oxidation of fatty acids; and synthesis of fatty acids, cholesterol, citrate, acetoacetate, and porphyrins.[3] Acetyl-CoA is a central intermediate in the degradation of fats, carbohydrates, and some proteins.

Biotin was identified as the factor that protected rats against hair loss and skin lesions induced by raw egg white feeding in the 1930s.[4] However, the critical role of biotin in human nutrition was not recognized until the 1960s and 1970s.[5] Biotin is an essential cofactor for four carboxylation reactions in intermediary metabolism. Acetyl-CoA carboxylase catalyzes the incorporation of bicarbonate into acetyl-CoA to form the fatty acid substrate malonyl-CoA. Pyruvate carboxylase and propionyl-CoA carboxylase function in the synthesis of TCA cycle intermediates. Oxalacetate, the product of the reaction catalyzed by pyruvate carboxylase, also serves as a glucose precursor in the gluconeogenic pathway. Methyl crotonyl-CoA carboxylase catalyzes an essential step in the degradation of the branched-chain amino acid leucine.[5]

This chapter will present a summary of available data related to pantothenic acid and biotin status in athletes. Dietary and supplemental intake, as well as biochemical and functional indicators of status will be discussed. Studies of the relationship between pantothenic acid or biotin intake and exercise performance will be presented.

II. DIETARY AND SUPPLEMENTAL INTAKE

Pantothenic acid is widely distributed among foods. Animal tissues, whole grain cereal, and legumes provide the greatest concentrations, while milk, vegetables, and fruits contribute lesser amounts. The usual intake of pantothenic acid in the U.S. has been reported to range from 5 to 10 mg/day.[6] The best sources of biotin are liver, egg yolk, soy flour, cereals, and yeast. Fruits and meats are poor sources of biotin.[7] Dietary intake of biotin in the U.S. has been reported to be between 28 and 42 µg/day.[8] Additionally, biotin synthesized by intestinal microorganisms is apparently available for absorption. On average, about one half of the pantothenic acid and biotin in food is biologically available. Avidin, a glycoprotein found in raw egg whites, binds biotin, making it unavailable for absorption. Avidin is stable over a wide pH range but is degraded by heat. Chronic consumption of large amounts of raw egg whites may induce a biotin deficency, but this is an unlikely occurrence. The recently published nutrient intake data from the Third National Health and Nutrition Examination Survey did not include information on dietary intake of pantothenic acid or biotin in the U.S.[9]

Analysis of pantothenic acid and biotin intake has not been included in published studies of nutrient intake of athletes. A review of the vitamin/mineral supplement use among athletes found the overall mean prevalence of athletes' supplement use was 46%.[10] While pantothenic acid and biotin are not traditionally supplemented as single nutrients, studies of the prevalence of types of vitamin/mineral supplement use by athletes indicate that B-complex supplements, which include pantothenic acid and biotin, are the most frequently consumed.

III. BIOCHEMICAL STATUS

In the healthy adult, normal pantothenic acid levels are 1120 to 1960 ng/ml in whole blood and 211 to 1096 ng/ml in serum.[11] Whole-blood pantothenic acid levels were studied in 96 high-performance athletes participating in various sports.[12] Compared to the reference values, the marathon runners and soccer players had suboptimal circulating pantothenic acid levels. According to relative frequencies, more than 30% of the athletes studied had pantothenic acid concentration below the lower limit of normal. Dietary intake information was not provided for the athletes studied.

Established normal biotin values are 215 to 750 pg/ml in whole blood, and 200 to 700 pg/ml in serum.[13] Singh et al.[14] found blood pantothenic acid and biotin levels within normal ranges in a group of highly trained athletes. Changes in the biochemical status of a number of nutrients following supplementation with a high-potency multivitamin/mineral supplement were examined in 22 physically active men randomly assigned to take a supplement or placebo for 12 weeks.[14] The supplement contained 100 mg of pantothenic acid and 200 mg of biotin. Baseline mean blood concentrations of pantothenic acid and biotin were within normal ranges. Concentrations rose significantly in the blood of the supplemented group by 6 weeks, and the higher concentrations were maintained at 12 weeks. Values returned to baseline levels following cessation of supplementation. These findings indicated that supplementation with high levels of pantothenic acid and biotin raised blood concentrations in healthy physically active men. Unfortunately, measures of the effect of these increased vitamins level on exercise performance were not assessed.

IV. EFFECTS ON EXERCISE PERFORMANCE

A double-blind exercise protocol was followed to compare the effects of a pantothenic acid supplement with a placebo on the exercise capacity of male distance runners.[15] A group of 18 highly conditioned men (age 30 to 35 years) were randomly assigned to consume either 1 g of pantothenic acid or a placebo daily for 2 weeks. While diet and training were kept constant, each subject completed two runs to exhaustion; one before and one after the supplementation period. Venous blood samples were taken throughout each run. Run times to exhaustion for each trial as well as mean individual run time changes were similar between the pantothenic acid-supplemented and placebo groups. No significant differences in pulse rate or blood biochemical parameters were seen between groups.

Preliminary data of a study that examined the effects of pantothenic acid supplementation on human exercise reported a decrease in blood lactate and decreased oxygen consumption during exercise to exhaustion.[16] Highly trained male runners took a 2-g supplement of pantothenic acid or placebo for 14 days. However, details of the exercise and analytical protocols and results have not been published. At this time, no clear evidence of a beneficial effect of pharmacological dosages of pantothenic acid on exercise capacity is available.

Smith et al.[17] studied the changes in fuel metabolism during a fast and exercise in mice maintained on pantothenate-deficient and pantothenate-supplemented diets. Compared to trained mice on pantothenate-supplemented diets, the trained pantothenate-deficient mice had lower running times until exhaustion, lower body weights, lower liver and muscle glycogen content (even after rest), and elevated liver ketone bodies both during rest and after running. No studies of the effect of physiological doses of pantothenic acid on athletes in suboptimal pantothenic acid status have been reported.

No controlled research has been carried out on the role of biotin alone on physical performance. Pantothenic acid and biotin were components of a vitamin/mineral supplement studied in athletes over 7 to 8 months of training and competition.[18] Participants in basketball, gymnastics, rowing, and swimming were included. All participants were monitored to ensure the recommended daily intakes of vitamins and minerals were provided by diet alone; 82 athletes were randomly assigned to take the supplement or a placebo daily. Groups were matched for sex, age, weight, height, place of residence, and specific sport and/or position played. No evidence of an effect of supplementation to athletic performance for athletes consuming adequate diets was found.

V. REQUIREMENTS AND RECOMMENDATIONS

To date, no Recommended Dietary Allowances have been established for pantothenic acid or biotin.[6,7] However, Estimated Safe and Adequate Daily Dietary Intakes have been determined. Daily intakes of 4 to 7 mg pantothenic acid and 30 to 100 μg biotin have been recommended for healthy adults.[6,7] Like many other individual nutrients, it is not uncommon to find much higher intake levels recommended in nonscientific literature. Daily intakes as high as 20 to 200 mg pantothenic acid and 300 to 5000 μg biotin have been suggested for athletes.[19] Although available evidence suggests that pantothenic acid and biotin are relatively nontoxic, effects of chronic ingestion of megadoses of these vitamins have not been documented.

VI. CONCLUSIONS

Pantothenic acid and biotin are two of the several micronutrients involved in energy metabolism. Based on their metabolic functions, it can be assumed that these vitamins would be of particular importance to an athlete. To date, minimal controlled research has been conducted to evaluate the direct effect of either of these vitamins on exercise performance. Vitamin supplements are often used by athletes in an attempt to improve performance. Although pantothenic acid and biotin are rarely taken as individual supplements, many athletes include them in B-complex supplements. Provided the biochemical status of pantothenic acid and biotin is adequate, supplementation does not appear beneficial to an athlete. Considering the many and varied dietary sources of pantothenic acid, and the availability of biotin synthesized by intestinal microorganisms, it is not surprising that deficiencies of these vitamins are rarely seen in humans. Biochemical status of pantothenic acid and biotin in athletes, however, deserves further investigation.

REFERENCES

1. Williams, R. J., Lyman, C. M., Goodyear, G.H., Truesdail, J.H., and Holaday, D., "Pantothenic acid," a growth determinant of universal biological occurrence, *J. Am. Chem. Soc.*, 55, 2912, 1933.
2. Williams, R. J., Pantothenic acid — a vitamin, *Science*, 89, 486, 1939.
3. Olson, R. E., Pantothenic acid, in *Present Knowledge in Nutrition*, 6th ed., Brown, M. L. Ed., International Life Sciences Institute, Washington, D.C., 1990, 208.
4. Combs, G. F., Discovery of the vitamins, in *The Vitamins, Fundamental Aspects in Nutrition and Health*, Academic Press, San Diego, CA, 1992, 9.
5. Mock, D. M., Biotin, in *Present Knowledge in Nutrition*, 6th ed., Brown, M. L., Ed., International Life Sciences Institute, Washington, D.C., 1990, 189.
6. National Research Council, *Recommended Dietary Allowances*, 10th ed., National Academy Press, Washington, D.C., 1989, 169.
7. National Research Council, *Recommended Dietary Allowances*, 10th ed., National Academy Press, Washington, D.C., 1989, 165.
8. Marshall, M. W., Judd, J. T., and Baker, H., Effects of low- and high-fat diets varying in ratio of polyunsaturated to saturated fatty acids on biotin intakes and biotin in serum, red cells and urine of adult men, *Nutr. Res.*, 5, 801, 1985.
9. Alaimo, K., McDowell, M. A., Briefel, R. R., Bischof, A. M., Caughman, C. R., Loria, C. M., and Johnson, C. L., Dietary Intake of Vitamins, Minerals, and Fiber of Persons Ages 2 Months and Over in the United States: Third National Health and Nutrition Examination Survey, Phase 1, 1988-91. Advance Data, U.S. Department of Health and Human Services, Washington, D.C., Number 258, 1994.
10. Sobal, J. and Marquart, L. F., Vitamin/mineral supplement use among athletes: a review of the literature, *Int. J. Sports Nutr.*, 4, 320, 1994.
11. Combs, G. F., Pantothenic acid, in *The Vitamins, Fundamental Aspects in Nutrition and Health*, Academic Press, San Diego, CA, 1992, 345.
12. Tokitzki, L., Sagredos, A., Reuss, F., Petersen, G., and Keul, L., Pantothenic acid levels in blood of athletes at rest and after aerobic exercise, *Z. Ernaehrungswiss.*, 32, 282, 1993.
13. Baker, H., Assessment of biotin status: clinical implications, in *Biotin*, Dakshinamurti, K. and Bhagavan, H. N., Eds., New York Academy of Sciences, New York, 1985, 129.
14. Singh, A., Moses, F. M., and Deugler, P. A., Vitamin and mineral status in physically active men: effects of a high-potency supplement, *Am. J. Clin. Nutr.*, 55, 1, 1992.
15. Nice, C., Reeves, A. G., Brink-Johnson, T., and Noll, W., The effects of pantothenic acid on human exercise capacity, *J. Sports Med.*, 24, 26, 1984.
16. Litoff, D., Scherzertt, H., and Harrison, J., Effects of pantothenic acid supplementation on human exercise, *Med. Sci. Sports Exercise*, 17, 287 (abstract), 1985.
17. Smith, C. M., Narrow, C. M., Kendrick, Z. V., and Steffen, C., The effect of pantothenate deficiency in mice on their metabolic response to fast and exercise, *Metabolism*, 36, 115, 1987.
18. Telford, R. D., Catchpole, E. A., Deakin, V., Hahn, A. G., and Plank, A. W., The effect of 7 to 8 months of vitamin/mineral supplementation on athletic performance, *Int. J. Sports Nutr.*, 2, 135, 1992.
19. Colgan, M., Vitamins are nuts and bolts, in *Optimum Sports Nutrition*, Advanced Research Press, New York, 1993, 167.

Chapter 8

VITAMIN A AND CAROTENOIDS

Maria Stacewicz-Sapuntzakis

CONTENTS

I. INTRODUCTION

Fat-soluble vitamin A, an essential factor for vision, growth, and reproduction of animals, is derived from certain carotenoids, polyene hydrocarbon compounds synthesized by plants. Humans are unique among mammals in their ability to absorb a wide range of carotenoids.[1] About 40 carotenoids are regularly consumed in our diet, but only a few of them have provitamin A activity. β-Carotene, the orange-red pigment of carrots, theoretically can produce two molecules of vitamin A aldehyde (retinal) by central cleavage. An asymmetric cleavage, producing one molecule of retinal from β-carotene, is also postulated.[2] Other carotenoids, like α-carotene and β-cryptoxanthin, may yield only one molecule of vitamin A because they possess only one required cyclical structure of the β-ionone ring. Carotenoids which do not possess this structure, like the tomato pigment lycopene, do not exhibit vitamin A activity. If the β-ionone ring is substituted with hydroxyl groups, as in xanthophylls, lutein, and zeaxanthin, vitamin A activity also disappears. A carotenoid cleavage enzyme (15,15′-dioxygenase) has been found in intestinal mucosa of many animals and is believed to exist in human intestine and liver.[3] Retinal is reduced to retinol (vitamin A alcohol), which in turn is esterified by long-chain fatty acids, and transported by the lymphatic system to the liver in the form of chylomicrons. The liver is a main site of vitamin A reserves in the body, where retinol is stored in esterified form and repackaged for circulation in plasma as retinol binding protein (RBP) complex. RBP carries retinol to other tissues, where it can be reversibly oxidized to retinal and to retinoic acid (irreversibly). The steady-state level of circulating retinol is governed by liver stores, which appear to buffer any changes in dietary supply or tissue utilization. Besides liver, significant amount of retinyl esters are deposited in milk and

0-8493-8192-4/97/$0.00+$.50

101

egg yolks, which constitute a rich source of preformed vitamin A in the human diet. In the upper intestine, dietary retinyl esters are hydrolyzed by pancreatic ester hydrolase to retinol, which is absorbed into enterocytes, and transported as described above.

The absorption of carotenoids from dietary sources requires sufficient digestion of food to release carotenoids and the formation of lipid micelles in the small intestine, which is aided by the presence of dietary fat and secretion of bile from the gall bladder.[4] In most species of laboratory animals, absorbed provitamin A carotenoids are immediately converted to retinol in the intestinal mucosa and do not appear in circulation and tissues. In humans carotenoids are stored primarily in adipose tissue, but they are also found in liver, adrenals, testes, ovaries, and macula of the eye. Levels of various carotenoids in serum reflect recent dietary intake, while tissue levels are slower in response to dietary changes.

Calculations of the nutritional value of carotenoids are based solely on their perceived conversion to vitamin A. There is a great deal of confusion in conversion factors, and even recent publications often contain errors, sometimes amended later by authors or readers. The food labels still list total vitamin A content in international units (IU), without specifying the contribution of preformed vitamin A and carotenoids. It is estimated that, on average, preformed vitamin A contributes half of the recommended dietary allowance (RDA) in the U.S. diet. The RDA is 1000 RE for an adult man and 800 RE for a woman.[5]
Retinol equivalents (RE) are defined as follows:

    1 RE = 1 µg retinol
         = 6 µg β-carotene
         = 12 µg other carotenoid vitamin A precursors
         = 3.33 IU vitamin A activity from retinol
         = 10 IU vitamin A activity from β-carotene
         = 20 IU vitamin A activity from other carotenoid vitamin A precursors

The conversion factors were derived from studies with young, vitamin A-deficient rats, and assume that in humans one sixth of the dietary provitamin A carotenoids are converted to retinol.[6] However, a recent study with an oral dose of deuterated β-carotene in a well-nourished human subject indicates that only 22% of β-carotene was absorbed and only 1.2% converted to retinol.[7] Of the total retinol produced from the ingested β-carotene, 57% was formed in the liver and 43% in the intestinal mucosa. These preliminary results are in better agreement with observed data of normal vitamin A and carotenoid metabolism in healthy subjects.

II. FUNCTIONS OF VITAMIN A AND CAROTENOIDS

Vitamin A constitutes a vital part of our visual system. Photoreceptors of retina in the eye contain a photosensitive pigment composed of retinal, as a chromophore, and a protein, opsin.[8] Visual impulse is produced when 11-*cis* retinal absorbs a photon, changes to all-*trans* retinal, and disengages from the protein. In the dark, retinal is converted by a specific isomerase back to 11-*cis* retinal, which combines with opsin to regenerate rhodopsin. The first symptom of vitamin A deficiency is an impaired dark adaptation, eventually noticed by subjects as night blindness.

Vitamin A (retinoic acid) is also required for differentiation of epithelial tissues.[6] However, in deficiency, the epithelium becomes hyperkeratinized — thickened, dry, and scaly. It may lead to total blindness when the changes occur in conjunctiva of the eye (xerophthalmia) and progresses to destruction of the cornea. Other epithelial tissues (of the skin, the respiratory, and the urogenital tract) also respond to vitamin A deficiency with histological changes which prevent their normal functions and facilitate infections.

Normal reproduction, fetal development, and growth of young animals require vitamin A for their sustained function. Vitamin A takes part in regulation of bone formation, spermatogenesis, and gestation. On the cellular level it probably functions in regulating stability of the biological membrane structure, possibly through participation in biosynthesis of glycopeptides. Wide-ranging effects of retinoids may be connected with their postulated role in control of gene expression.

Vitamin A is extremely toxic when consumed in excess.[9] The acute poisoning causes an increase in cerebrospinal fluid pressure with resulting headache, nausea, and disorientation. The chronic hypervitaminosis A may occur when doses of retinol exceeding RDA by a factor of five (5000 RE for humans) are taken for prolonged periods. The symptoms include bone and joint pain, skin redness and desquamation, disturbed hair growth, headache, nausea, and anorexia. It is of great importance that comparatively mild hypervitaminosis A may produce teratogenic effect in the offspring. More than 70 types of anomalies affecting every organ were produced in all kinds of mammals, including monkeys, by doses which do not cause overt toxicity in the pregnant female.

Large doses of provitamin A carotenoids do not cause hypervitaminosis A or exert any toxic effects. Apparently, vitamin A is produced from carotenoids to a limited extent, with the remaining precursors eliminated by excretion or absorbed intact and deposited in various tissues. Humans can develop carotenemia,[10] characterized by yellowing of the skin and high circulating plasma levels of carotenoids. The high content of carotenoids in skin has a photoprotective effect used in the therapy of human photosensitivity diseases. In cases of erythropoietic protoporphyria, large doses of β-carotene (300 mg) are taken daily to develop limited tolerance to sunlight.[11] *In vitro* evidence suggests that carotenoids may exert their protective function by quenching singlet oxygen ($^1O_2$) and perhaps also free radicals produced on illumination of protoporphyrin. Another example of the photoprotective function of carotenoids is provided by specific accumulation of two dihydroxycarotenes, zeaxanthin and lutein, in human macula.[12] The same carotenoids protect chlorophyll in green plant tissues against light damage, and may guard the human retina against macular degeneration, a leading cause of blindness in the older U.S. population.

Carotenoids have many biological functions independent of any provitamin A activity. Their antioxidant capacity possibly protects cell membranes from singlet oxygen and chain-reaction lipid peroxidation. There is even a hypothesis that humans owe their unusual longevity in part to the presence of carotenoids in their tissues and blood.[13] Carotenoids appear to enhance many indicators of immune functions both in laboratory animals and, more importantly in humans, also in HIV-infected patients.[14] Carotenoids seem to inhibit neoplastic transformations in cell cultures, and high intake of carotenoid-containing vegetables and fruits was associated with decreased risk of cancer in many epidemiological trials.[15] β-Carotene supplementation decreased the size and recurrence of leukoplakia, an oral precancerous lesion.[16] It may be connected with the possible role of carotenoids in cell to cell communication. Carotenoids can activate the expression of genes which encode the production of connexin 43, a protein forming the structure of intercellular gap junctions.[17]

However, it is possible that carotenoids are merely markers of high intake of fruits and vegetables, which may be beneficial to human health due to vitamin C, fiber, and other substances in plants. Recently publicized intervention trials among smokers in the U.S. and Finland failed to show any benefit of supplementation with pure β-carotene.[18,19] Unexpectedly, higher incidence of lung cancer and heart disease was found among the supplemented groups of subjects, who were at high risk for these diseases due to the history of smoking, drinking alcohol, or working with asbestos.

It is difficult to discuss the concept of carotenoid deficiency because the nutritional requirement for this compound has not been established; there are indigenous populations, like the Eskimo of the Far North, who traditionally consume negligible amounts of carotenoids. However, in a study of 9 premenopausal women, maintained for 68 days on a carotenoid-deficient diet, 7 developed skin problems (rash, acne, and eczema), and 6 experienced disturbances of menstrual patterns (delayed ovulation and prolonged cycles).[20]

III. VITAMIN A AND CAROTENOID STATUS IN PHYSICALLY ACTIVE SUBJECTS

A great majority of the available studies report total vitamin A intake without specifying the proportion obtained from animal and plant sources. Therefore, it is difficult to estimate the carotenoid intake in reported subjects. Adult athletes are usually well nourished with respect to the total vitamin A content of their diet. The cyclists of the Tour de France were estimated to consume an adequate amount of vitamin A (1.3 ± 0.4 mg daily) during the race.[21] However, individual variations can be quite large. Two elite U.S. male cyclists participating in an endurance ride (10 days, 2050 mi, 3300 km) showed very different results.[22] One consumed 87% and the other 163% of the RDA, when the food intake was measured and recorded by trained dietitians. In a study of female collegiate heavyweight rowers the women met 100% of the RDA for vitamin A.[23] Male cross-country runners had an average intake of twice the RDA for vitamin A.[24]

The prevalence of adequate vitamin A nutrition is not as universal as it may seem from the above-mentioned studies. When 32 young college women took part in a 40-week planned exercise program (30 min daily on a bicycle ergometer), their self-reported dietary records indicated a decrease in vitamin A intake (to 70% RDA), unrelated to any decrease in total energy intake.[25] This group of young women seemed to have a relatively high fat intake (40% energy) and very low fruit and vegetable consumption. In a study of Finnish children in early puberty, the average intake of total vitamin A was significantly higher than the RDA only for physically active boys, but a large proportion of children, both active and controls, had inadequate intakes (60% control boys, 30% active boys, 50% control girls, 45% active girls).[26] The authors stress the availability of fruits and vegetables in Finland and think that the food choices of children resemble those of middle class white children in the U.S.

Many athletes and their coaches consider the supplementation of vitamins necessary at doses greatly exceeding the RDA. Body builders take 60,000 IU vitamin A over a period of 4 to 6 weeks before a competition.[27] Although there are many cases of vitamin A abuse among athletes, there is not much documentation of toxic effects, except one case of hypervitaminosis A in an adolescent soccer player who experienced a strong leg pain after consuming at least 100,000 IU vitamin A for 2 months.[28] Among U.S. high school students, greater knowledge about supplements was associated with less use.[29] Nevertheless, 42% of all students used multivitamins and 13% used vitamin A supplements (weekly to daily); 34% did not know that taking high doses of vitamin A can be harmful.

More accurate assessment of vitamin A and carotenoid status emerges from studies which include the analysis of serum or plasma in addition to the estimates of dietary intake. At present, it is possible to obtain accurate measurements of vitamin A and carotenoids in serum by high performance liquid chromatography (HPLC).[30] Older studies used less accurate colorimetric methods with crude estimate of total carotene, without separation of individual carotenoids.[31]

When serum levels of retinol and β-carotene were tested in West German national teams, none of the athletes exhibited low value of retinol (range 49.5 to 93.1 µg/dl), while β-carotene varied considerably (14.0 to 122.5 µg/dl).[27] The results for 24 athletes from 4 disciplines were reported individually (marathon runners, weight lifters, swimmers, and cyclists) and compared with average retinol and β-carotene levels of 150 blood donors (59.8 ± 14.1 and 37.6 ± 25.2 µg/dl, respectively). These data indicate an adequate intake of vitamin A among the athletes and a varied, but not extremely low, intake of β-carotene.

Among physically active older women in the Netherlands (n = 25, 60 to 80 years) the total intake of vitamin A was similar to that of sedentary (n = 23) controls (1.0 mg vs. 1.1 mg per day).[32] Active women consumed more vegetables, fruits, and nonalcoholic drinks, while sedentary women had a higher consumption of milk and meat. Consequently, physically active older women had significantly higher serum β-carotene levels (0.99 ± 0.59 vs 0.67 ± 0.22 mmol/l, p <.05), while their retinol levels were practically identical (1.99 ± 0.41 vs. 2.02 ± 0.39 mmol/l). Similar results were obtained from a U.S. study of physically active older male veterans (n = 26, 69 ± 7 years) participating in Golden Age Games.[33],[34] Their level of activity was calculated to be three times higher than their sedentary controls (n = 17), matched in age and height. Their dietary intake of β-carotene significantly exceeded that of their sedentary peers, although their consumption of β-carotene from supplements was not significantly higher. Serum levels of retinol were nearly identical (65.7 ± 22.6 vs. 63.3 ± 19.7 μg/dl), but β-carotene levels were significantly higher in the active group (23.4 ± 15.0 vs. 12.4 ± 8.0 μg/dl, p <.01). Other carotenoids were also higher in serum of active veterans, but the differences did not reach statistical significance.

Seeming discrepancy between the high intake of carotenoid-rich food in physically active older adults and low intake in young people, even those physically active, found confirmation in an analysis of a large Heidelberg-Michelstadt-Berlin study.[35] Active older men had higher carotene intake than sedentary older men. Younger active women had lower absolute intakes of vitamin A than less active younger women. It may simply reflect the fact that younger people are less concerned with healthy lifestyle, which includes attention to diet containing a high proportion of fruits and vegetables, than the health-conscious elderly people.

However, among young people, primarily women, there are some who are extremely weight obsessed and likely to consume excessive amounts of raw vegetables, with resulting carotenemia. If their diet is severely limited in total energy, the weight loss may put them in the category of anorexia and/or they may also exhibit amenorrhea (cessation of menses). There was some concern among clinicians that amenorrhea may be associated with high carotenoid intake, which causes "golden ovary" syndrome,[36] but it is more likely due to the low body fat content caused by anorexia and/or excessive exercise. In sports where dieting is used to reduce body weight (gymnastics and ballet), there may be a higher incidence of carotenemia (if a high-calorie diet is replaced with carotenoid-containing fruits and vegetables) and amenorrhea (if a severe reduction of body fat content occurs). Total serum carotene levels were studied among female long-distance runners (>25 mi/week) compared with sedentary controls.[37] Eumenorrheic runners (n = 7) had similar intake of calories and dietary carotenoids as sedentary controls (n = 5), while anovulatory runners (n = 8) had a slightly higher carotenoid and lower energy intake than the controls. The anovulatory group had higher serum carotene than the other two groups (all within normal range), but the differences in carotenoid status and intake were not significant. It was concluded that anovulatory dysfunction in long-distance runners did not correlate with hypercarotenemia, which was absent in this group of subjects. When a group of 20 clearly hypercarotenemic Swiss women was studied in respect to ovarian function, the subjects could be divided into three groups: two groups with amenorrhea and low estrogen levels, and one with normal menses and estrogen levels.[38] Amenorrheic patients included those with low weight (below 85% ideal) and nearly normal weight (90 to 99% of ideal). Most were on vegetarian diets, engaged in strenuous sport activity, and had a history of large weight changes. The high levels of carotene in serum were not considered to be responsible for the amenorrhea, but indicative of vegetarian diet or a biological marker of fat mobilization occurring during weight loss.[39]

IV. VITAMIN A, CAROTENOIDS, AND EXERCISE PHYSIOLOGY

Strenuous exercise may raise oxygen comsumption with an increase in free radical production, leading to lipid peroxidation and possible tissue damage.[40] Carotenoids, as antioxidants, may be expected to protect tissues against oxidative damage, but themselves could undergo oxidation and destruction in the process. Vitamin A, although not a strong antioxidant, is probably required for tissue repair and one can expect an increased metabolism of vitamin A under conditions of increased physical activity. Can we observe changes in serum or tissue concentration of vitamin A or carotenoids following controlled exercise? Does supplementation with vitamin A or carotenoids improve physical performance or any indicators of oxidative stress?

There is a paucity of studies of the effect of vitamin A supplementation on physical performance. No decrease of ability to perform hard muscular exercise was noted in men maintained on vitamin A-deficient diets for 6 months, nor did it improve after 6 weeks of high supplementation.[41] This is not surprising, considering that before starting the deficient diet the subjects consumed a daily dose of 75,000 IU vitamin A for 1 month and probably had large liver stores.

A few studies observed transient changes in serum vitamin A and carotenoid levels immediately after exercise. In one study, a group of young athletes (n = 12) exhibited a striking increase of serum vitamin A following strenuous physical activity consisting of a 15-min warm-up and 5 or 6 220-yd (201 m) dashes at full speed at intervals of 5 min.[42] The average blood vitamin A increased 43%, while average total carotene levels decreased 10%. The fact that a simple absorbance assay, followed by irradiation to remove vitamin A,[43] was used on minute samples obtained from finger pricks may have generated some of the great variability in the the response. Similar results were found in another study of 14 males performing a step-up test.[44] The same method was used to estimate vitamin A and β-carotene levels in plasma, but on larger samples of venous blood. Vitamin A levels rose significantly after the exercise period, while β-carotene levels were on the average decreased, with considerable variability between subjects and even between repeated tests of the same individual. It is interesting to note that vitamin A was found to rise by 18% ($p < .05$) after completing a half-marathon, in a recent study of 7 trained athletes.[45] Dehydration, which caused a 6% decrease in plasma volume, could not explain this significant increase of retinol concentration, measured by HPLC assay in samples obtained from venipuncture. However, the researchers cautiously state that it is uncertain whether the 18% increase in plasma vitamin A reflected mobilization of the vitamin to the circulation.

Studies with laboratory rats indicated a significant decrease in liver vitamin A content after 12 days of daily 90-min exercise on a moving track at 20 m/min.[46] Shorter sessions of exercise elicited proportionately smaller effect. Kidney levels of vitamin A remained stable, as did plasma levels.

The above-described studies indicate that there could be a significant mobilization of vitamin A stores from the liver during strenuous exercise if the athlete remains on a vitamin A-deficient diet. Assessment of plasma retinol levels will not reveal any deficiency until liver stores are severely depleted; indeed, they may even be elevated by exercise.

The effect of β-carotene on stress-related hormone production was investigated in young, healthy males who took a single dose of β-carotene 2-h before ergometric bicycling to complete exhaustion.[47] The control group experienced a large rise in corticotropin-releasing hormone, adrenocorticotropic hormone, noradrenaline, and adrenaline. This stress reaction was progressively reduced with increasing doses of β-carotene and completely suppressed in subjects who took 30 mg. This rapid response to a single dose of β-carotene is quite surprising, and should be confirmed on a group of subjects serving as their own control in a double-blind experiment including a placebo.

As an antioxidant, β-carotene was used in a few studies to investigate if it could ameliorate exercise-induced lipid peroxidation and skeletal muscle damage. Unfortunately, because β-carotene was supplied in a mixture containing other antioxidants, vitamins C and E, it is difficult to decide if any positive result can be ascribed to β-carotene or the other components. In one study, supplementation of 10 mg β-carotene, 800 mg vitamin E, and 1000 mg vitamin C daily for 2 months increased the antioxidant potential of the blood glutathione system, counteracting exercise-induced GSSG (oxidized glutathione) elevation and significantly diminishing the indicators of muscle damage (plasma lactate dehydrogenase and creatine phosphokinase).[48] A similar study with a higher dose of 1000 mg vitamin E, 1250 mg vitamin C, and 37.5 mg β-carotene failed to demonstrate any positive effect on muscle damage or lipid peroxidation indicators.[49] The authors speculated that their exercise regimen of downhill running at 65% of maximal heart rate did not present enough metabolic challenge. Another study with the same vitamin mixture consumed daily for 5 weeks decreased lipid peroxidation (measured by serum malondialdehyde and breath pentane) at rest and following exercise at 60 and 90% $\dot{V}O_2$max on a level treadmill.[50] Trying to assess oxidative damage to nucleic acids, the urinary output of 8-hydroxyguanosine was studied before and during 3 consecutive days of submaximal exercise, with and without supplementation (553 mg of α-tocopherol, 1000 mg vitamin C, 10 mg β-carotene).[51] No significant differences were noted due to exercise or supplementation. In elderly women, β-carotene supplementation at 90 mg/day for 3 weeks increased plasma antioxidant capacity measured *in vitro* by induction of phosphatidylcholine hydroperoxides production in presence of a free radical generator.[52]

The equivocal results of the above-described intervention studies stem from differences in methodology. The researchers used different tests, different levels of supplementation, and different intensities and durations of exercise. Nevertheless, there is a promise in the antioxidant capacity of β-carotene and other carotenoids, which should be assessed as single supplements with a whole battery of oxidative damage tests. The treatments should include both athletes and sedentary subjects, and compare the effects of training, of exercise duration, and severity of metabolic challenge. Although carotenoids have to be investigated preferably in human subjects, vitamin A experiments may be performed on laboratory animals. The assessment of liver stores after long-term strenuous exercise should be given priority, in view of increasingly poor nutrition choices in adolescent athletes and some young women on calorie-restricted diets. Modern methods of analysis would lend more credibility to a distinct possibility that sustained physical labor increases utilization of vitamin A.

V. SUGGESTED INTAKE OF VITAMIN A AND CAROTENOIDS

Although review of existing literature indicates that vitamin A intake in developed countries, and especially in athletes, is usually adequate and often exceeds recommended daily allowance, we still have to be vigilant and pay attention to each athlete's diet. The intake should be estimated separately for the preformed vitamin A from animal sources, fortified foods, and supplements; and separately for β-carotene and other carotenoids from plant, animal, and supplemental sources. It would be useful to confirm the dietary interview with serum analysis by using modern chromatographic (HPLC) methods which measure retinol, retinyl esters, individual carotenoids, and tocopherol status. If serum retinol values are found to be below 30 μg/dl, it would be helpful to perform a noninvasive test of liver stores of vitamin A using the relative dose-response procedure.[53] Serum retinol levels below 20 μg/dl are considered to be deficient and a dark adaptation test may be employed for further evaluation. In general, no supplements of preformed vitamin A should be used to avoid possible toxicity. However, an intake of 1000 RE of preformed vitamin A daily from animal food sources or fortified food products should probably be recommended to all strenuously exercising athletes, since it is uncertain how much (if any) vitamin A is produced by conversion from carotenoids.

Carotenoids, in the form of a variety of fruits and vegetables, should be consumed in their own right for antioxidant protection and not as means to obtain necessary vitamin A. The current recommendation of 3 to 5 daily servings of vegetables and 2 to 4 servings of fruits, preferably red, orange, and dark green, should be followed to provide maximum benefit of increased carotenoid consumption together with other healthful phytochemicals contained in such a diet.[54] As recent intervention trials failed to show benefits of β-carotene supplementation,[18,19] large doses of β-carotene in the form of pills are not recommended, especially among heavy smokers and frequent users of alcoholic beverages.

REFERENCES

1. Klaui, H. and Bauerfeind, J. C., Carotenoids as food colors, in *Carotenoids as Colorants and Vitamin A Precursors*, Bauerfeind, J. C., Ed., Academic Press, New York, 1981, 186.
2. Krinsky, N. I., Wang, X.-D., Tang, G., and Russell, R. M., Mechanism of carotenoid cleavage to retinoids, *Ann. N.Y. Acad. Sci.*, 691, 167, 1993.
3. Goodman, D. S. and Blaner, W. S., Biosynthesis, absorption and hepatic metabolism of retinol, in *The Retinoids*, Vol. 2, Sporn, M. B., Roberts, A. B., and Goodman, D. S., Eds., Academic Press, New York, 1984, 4.
4. Erdman, J. W., Jr., Bierer, T. L., and Gugger, E. T., Absorption and transport of carotenoids, *Ann. N.Y. Acad. Sci.*, 691, 76, 1993.
5. National Research Council, *Recommended Dietary Allowances*, National Academy Press, Washington, D.C., 1989, 78.
6. Underwood, B., Vitamin A in animal and human nutrition, in *The Retinoids*, Vol. 1, Sporn, M. B., Roberts, A. B., and Goodman, D. S., Eds., Academic Press, New York, 1984, 281.
7. Novotny, J. A., Dueker S. R., Zech, L. A., and Clifford, A. J., Compartmental analysis of the dynamics of β-carotene metabolism in an adult volunteer, *J. Lipid Res.*, 36, 1825, 1995.
8. Bridges, C. D. B., Retinoids in photosensitive systems, in *The Retinoids*, Vol. 2, Sporn, M. B., Roberts, A. B., and Goodman, D. S., Eds., Academic Press, New York, 125, 1984.
9. Kamm, J. J., Ashenfelter, K. O., and Ehmann, C. W., Preclinical and clinical toxicology of selected retinoids, in *The Retinoids*, Vol. 2, Sporn, M. B., Roberts, A. B., and Goodman, D. S., Eds., Academic Press, New York, 1984, 288.
10. Leung, A. K. C., Carotenemia, *Adv. Pediatr.*, 34, 223, 1987.
11. Mathews-Roth, M. M., Carotenoids in medical applications, in *Carotenoids as Colorants and Vitamin A Precursors*, Bauerfeind, J. C., Ed., Academic Press, New York, 1981, 755.
12. Handelman, G. J., Dratz, E. A., Reay, C. C., and van Kuijk, F. J. G. M., Carotenoids in human macula and whole retina, *Invest. Ophthalmol. Visual Sci.*, 29, 850, 1988.
13. Cutler, R. G., Antioxidants and aging, *Am. J. Clin. Nutr.*, 53, 373S, 1991.
14. Coodley, G. O., Nelson, H. D., Loveless, M. O., and Folk, C., Beta carotene in HIV Infection, *J. Acquired Immune Deficiency Syndr.*, 6, 272, 1993.
15. Ziegler, R. G., Vegetables, fruits, and carotenoids and the risk of cancer, *Am. J. Clin. Nutr.*, 53, 2525, 1991.
16. Gareval, H. S., Carotenoids in Oral Cancer Prevention, *Ann. N.Y. Acad. Sci.*, 691, 139, 1993.
17. Bertram, J. S., Cancer prevention by carotenoids, *Ann. N.Y. Acad. Sci.*, 691, 177, 1993.
18. Omenn, G. S., Goodman, G. E., Thornquist, M. D., Balmes, J., Cullen, M. R., Glass, A., Keogh, J. R., Meyskens, F. L., Valanis, B., Williams, J. H., Barnhart, S., and Hammar, S., Effects of a combination of beta carotene and vitamin A on lung cancer and cardiovascular disease, *N. Engl. J. Med.*, 334, 1150, 1996.
19. The α–Tocopherol, β–Carotene Cancer Prevention Study Group, The effect of vitamin E and β–carotene on the incidence of lung cancer and other cancers in male smokers, *N. Engl. J. Med.*, 330, 1029, 1994.
20. Burri, B. J., Dixon, Z. R., Fong, A. K. H., Kretsch, M. J., Clifford, A. J., and Erdman, J. W., Jr., Possible association of skin lesions with low-carotene diet in premenopausal women, *Ann. N.Y. Acad. Sci.*, 691, 279, 1993.
21. Saris, W. H. M., Schrijver, J. V., Erp Baart, M. A., and Brouns, F., Adequacy of vitamin supply under maximal sustained workloads: The Tour de France, in *Elevated Dosages of Vitamins*, Walter, P., Brubacher, G., and Stahelin, H., Eds., Hans Huber Publishers, Lewiston, NY, 1989, 205.
22. Gabel, K. A., Aldous, A., and Edgington, C., Dietary intake of two elite male cyclists during 10-day, 2050-mile ride, *Int. J. Sport Nutr.*, 5, 56, 1995.
23. Nelson Steen, S., Mayer, K., Brownell, K. D., and Wadden, T. A., Dietary intake of female collegiate heavyweight rowers, *Int. J. Sport Nutr.*, 5, 225, 1995.
24. Niekamp, R. A. and Baer, J. T., In-season dietary adequacy of trained male cross-country runners, *Int. J. Sport Nutr.*, 5, 45, 1995.
25. Johnson., R. E., Mastropaolo, J. A., and Wharton, M. A., Exercise, dietary intake and body composition, *J. Am. Diet. Assoc.*, 61, 399, 1972.

26. Rankinen, T., Fogelholm, M., Kujala, U., Rauramaa, R., and Uusitupa, M., Dietary intake and nutritional status of athletic and nonathletic children in early puberty, *Int. J. Sport Nutr.*, 5, 136, 1995.

27. Rokitzki, L., Berg, A., and Keul, J., Blood and serum status of water and fat soluble vitamins in athletes and non-athletes, in *Elevated Dosages of Vitamins*, Walter, P., Brubacher, G. and Stahelin, H., Eds., Hans Huber Publishers, Lewiston, NY, 1989, 192.

28. Fumich, R. and Essig, G., Hypervitaminosis A case report in an adolescent soccer player, *Am. J. Sports Med.*, 11, 37, 1983.

29. Massad, S. J., Shier, N. W., Koceja, D. M., and Elliss, N. T., High school athletes and nutritional supplements: a study of knowledge and use, *Int. J. Sport Nutr.*, 5, 232, 1995.

30. Barua, A. B. and Furr, H. C., Extraction and analysis by high performance liquid chromatography of carotenoids in human serum, *Methods Enzymol.*, 213, 273, 1992.

31. Frolik, C. A. and Olson, J. A., Extraction, separation and chemical analysis of retinoids, in *The Retinoids*, Vol. 1, Sporn, M. B., Roberts, A. B., and Goodman, D. S., Eds., Academic Press, New York, 1984, 182.

32. Voorrips, L. E., van Staveren, W. A., and Hautvast, J. G. A. J., Are physically active elderly women in a better nutritional condition than their sedentary peers?, *Eur. J. Clin. Nutr.*, 45, 545, 1991.

33. Connor-Bote, E., Murphy, P. A., Orloff, S. B., Ottosen, W., Rothschild, R. L., Sullivan, J. M., and Iber, F. L., Dietary intake in active veterans participating in the Golden Age Games compared with healthy sedentary veterans, in *National Veterans Golden Age Games Research Monograph*, Langbein, W. E., Wyman, D. J., and Osis, A., Eds., Edward Hines, Jr.,VA Hospital, Hines, IL, 1995, 11.

34. Kazi, N., Murphy, P. A., Connor, E. S., Bowen, P. E., Stacewicz-Sapuntzakis, M., and Iber, F. L., Serum antioxidant and retinol levels in physically active vs. physically inactive elderly veterans, in *National Veterans Golden Age Games Research Monograph*, Langbein, W. E., Wyman, D. J., and Osis, A., Eds., Edward Hines, Jr., VA Hospital, Hines, IL, 1995, 50.

35. Mensink, G. B. and Arab, L., Relationship between nutrient intake, nutritional status and activity levels in an elderly and in a young population; a comparison of physically more active and more inactive people, *Z. Gerontol.*, 22, 16, 1989.

36. Page, S. W., Golden ovaries, *Austr. N.Z. J. Obstet. Gynaecol.*, 11, 32, 1971.

37. Richards, S. R., Chang, F. E., Bossetti, B., Malarkey, W. B., and Kim, M. H., Serum carotene levels in female long distance runners, *Fertil. Steril.*, 43, 79, 1985.

38. Martin-Du Pan, R. C., Hermann, W., and Chardon, F., Hypercarotinemia, amenorrhea and vegetarian diet, (in French), *J. Gynecol. Obstet. Biol. Reprod.*, 19. 290, 1990.

39. Mordasini, R., Klose, G., and Greten, H., Secondary Type II hyperlipoproteinemia in patients with anorexia nervosa, *Metabolism*, 27, 71, 1978.

40. Kanter, M. M., Free radicals, exercise, and antioxidant supplementation, *Int. J. Sport Nutr.*, 4, 205, 1994.

41. Wald, G., Brouha, L., and Johnson., R., Experimental human vitamin A deficiency and ability to perform muscular exercise, *Am. J. Physiol.*, 137, 551, 1942.

42. James, W. H. and El Gindi, I. M., Effect of strenuous physical activity on blood vitamin A and carotene in young men, *Science*, 118, 629, 1953.

43. Bessey, O. A., Lowry, O. H., Brock, M. J., and Lopez, J. A., The determination of vitamin A and carotene in small quantities of blood serum, *J. Biol. Chem.*, 166, 177, 1946.

44. Hillman, R. W. and Rosner, M. C., Effects of exercise on blood (plasma) concentrations of vitamin A, carotene and tocopherols, *J. Nutr.*, 64, 605, 1958.

45. Duthie, G. G., Robertson, J. D., Maughan, R. J., and Morrice, P. C., Blood antioxidant status and erythrocyte lipid peroxidation following distance running, *Arch. Biochem. Biophys.*, 282, 78, 1990.

46. Kobylinski, Z., Gronowska-Senger, A., and Swarbula, D., Effect of exercise on vitamin A utilization by rat organism (in Polish), *Rocz. Panstw. Zakl. Hig.*, 41, 247, 1990.

47. Hosegawa, T., Anti-stress effect of β–carotene, *Ann. N.Y. Acad. Sci.*, 691, 281, 1993.

48. Viguie, C. A., Packer, L., and Brooks., G. A., Antioxidant supplementation affects indices of muscle trauma and oxidant stress in human blood during exercise, *Med. Sci. Sports Exercise*, 21, S16, 1989.

49. Kanter, M. M. and Eddy, D. E., Effect of antioxidant supplementation on serum markers of lipid peroxidation and skeletal muscle damage following eccentric exercise, *Med. Sci. Sports Exercise*, 24, S17, 1992.

50. Kanter, M. M., Nolte, L. A., and Holloszy, J. O., Effects of an antioxidant vitamin mixture on lipid peroxidation at rest and postexercise, *J. Appl. Physiol.*, 74, 965, 1993.

51. Witt, E. H., Reznick, A. Z., Viguie, C. A., and Starke-Reed, P., Packer, L., Exercise, oxidative damage and effects of antioxidant manipulation, *J. Nutr.*, 122, 766, 1992.

52. Meydani, M., Martin, A., Ribaya-Mercado, J., Gong, J., Blumberg, J. B., and Russel, R. M., β–Carotene supplementation increases antioxidant capacity of plasma in older women, *J. Nutr.*, 124, 2397, 1994.

53. Underwood, B. A. and Olson, J. A., A brief guide to current methods of assessing vitamin A status, International Vitamin A Consultative Group, ILSI-NF, Washington, D.C., 1993.

54. Anon., The Food Guide Pyramid, Home and Garden Bulletin, Department of Agriculture, Human Nutrition Information Service, Washington, D.C., 1992, 252.

Chapter 9

VITAMINS D AND K

Nancy M. Lewis
Andrea M. Frederick

CONTENTS

I. VITAMIN D

A. INTRODUCTION

Because vitamin D has been clearly associated with specific deficiency diseases, rickets and osteomalacia, it has been classified as a vitamin. However, vitamin D actually is a series of sterol compounds called a prohormone, and it performs hormone-like functions.[1-3]

B. METABOLISM

Vitamin D is a fat-soluble vitamin and its dietary form is metabolized similarly to other fat-soluble molecules, beginning with absorption through the small intestine. When absorbed, the vitamin is first incorporated into chylomicrons and then it is transported through the lymphatic system.[4] Once it reaches the circulation it binds with vitamin D binding proteins and eventually reaches the liver. In the liver it is hydroxylated and becomes 25-hydroxyvitamin D_3 (25-OH-D_3), also called 25-hydroxycholecalciferol. Although 25-OH-D_3 is the major circulating form of vitamin D, this form is not active under physiological conditions. To become physiologically active another hydroxylation reaction must occur on carbon 1. This occurs in the kidney with the assistance of the enzyme 25-OH-D-1α-hydroxylase, producing 1α, 25 dihydroxyvitamin D_3, or 1α,25 dihydroxycholecalciferol ($1,25(OH)_2D_3$). The $1,25(OH)_2D_3$ form is the form which carries out the metabolic functions of vitamin D.[5]

$1,25(OH)_2D_3$ can also be formed from compounds in the skin. The cholesterol precursor 7-dehydrocholesterol, which is made in the liver and stored in the skin, is converted to previtamin D_3 by the ultraviolet rays of the sun or by an artificial source of ultraviolet light. The previtamin D_3 is then converted to vitamin D_3. Finally, vitamin D_3 is converted to $1,25(OH)_2D_3$ through hydroxylation reactions in the liver and kidney, just as the dietary form of vitamin D is hydroxylated.[6,7]

C. FUNCTIONS

The primary role of vitamin D is to maintain homeostasis of calcium (Ca) and phosphorus (Pi) in order to maintain bone formation and maintenance, neuromuscular function, and cellular processes. Vitamin D accomplishes this role through a tightly controlled system involving three organs of the body. This system serves to assure the exact amount of Pi and Ca available to properly carry out their specific functions in the body.

When blood levels of Ca and Pi are low and the minerals are needed somewhere in the body, the first response of vitamin D is to begin the production of the hormone, calcitrol. Calcitrol is formed from vitamin D in the kidneys by an enzyme, dipeptide parathyroid hormone, secreted by the parathyroid. Calcitrol circulates through the body to the intestines, and stimulates the synthesis of Ca and Pi binding proteins. These binding proteins then cause an increase in the intestinal absorption of dietary Ca and Pi. Calcitrol also works together with parathyroid hormone to stimulate the release of Ca and Pi from the surface of the bones into the bloodstream. Finally, calcitrol stimulates the kidneys to reabsorb Ca and Pi that would otherwise be excreted from the body in urine.[6,7] These three metabolic functions of calcitrol all work together to increase the levels of Ca and Pi in the blood. When an adequate amount of Pi and Ca are made available to tissues, calcitrol formation is shut down, and vitamin D is stored in the adipose tissue and muscles to be used later.[8]

After gaining an understanding of the mechanisms surrounding the role of vitamin D and bone mineralization, researchers shifted the focus of vitamin D research to identification of other actions of vitamin D. Following is a summary of possible functions of vitamin D that relate to exercise and sport.

One possible relationship involves vitamin D having an influence in the metabolism of citrate, one of the intermediates of the aerobic energy production pathway. No definitive explanation of the influence of vitamin D has been identified, and the practical implications of this relationship to athletes has not been adequately explored.[9]

Recent animal research has also shown that $1,25 (OH)_2D_3$ can increase the Ca uptake of skeletal muscle through high-voltage-gated calcium channels. It is essential that Ca be present in the muscle sarcoplasmic reticulum in order for the muscle to contract.[10]

Suggested functions of vitamin D in exercise and sport are few and the basis of these functions is not completely understood. This can be attributed mainly to the paucity of research on the topic of vitamin D and exercise.

D. EXERCISE-RELATED RESEARCH

Much of the early research in the area of vitamin D and exercise did not yield interesting or highly significant results. This may partially explain the lack of current literature on this topic; however, the past research is notable. In 1957 German scientists reported on six subjects that were observed for a period of two years. Seidel and Hettinger[11] administered oral doses of vitamin D to the subjects and periodically recorded bicycle ergometer performance. No improvements in performance were seen throughout the study.

Another early study reported by Berven[12] in 1963 assessed the effects of daily vitamin D supplementation on the physical working capacity of 60 children aged 10 to 11 years in Stockholm. The PWC-170 test, a submaximal performance test, was used to measure physical working capacity. Berven first supplemented some of the children with 1500 IU of vitamin D daily, while others received placebo pills. He also administered large single doses of 400,000 IU vitamin D to some participants during a different phase of the study. No indication of significant beneficial effects on physical performance due to either daily supplementation or large single doses of vitamin D were seen.[12] Unfortunately, there has been no subsequent research on the effects of vitamin D supplementation on exercise performance. Therefore, data available at this time indicate that vitamin D does not appear to be effective as an ergogenic aid.

A more recent study was designed to assess the effect of endurance training on plasma levels of vitamin D and physiologically related compounds, such as parathyroid hormone, calcitonin, and Ca.[13] Plasma levels were measured on nine male marathon runners during training, after three weeks of a training break, and two and four weeks after retraining. Results revealed that plasma $1,25(OH)_2D_3$ was nonsignificantly elevated after the training break, and then significantly decreased at two and four weeks of retraining. Plasma $25\text{-}OH\text{-}D_3$ showed no significant changes, nor did the ratio of $1,25(OH)_2D_3$ to $25\text{-}OH\text{-}D_3$. After controlling for related factors, these researchers attributed the decrease of $1,25(OH)_2D_3$ during retraining to the inhibition of 1-hydroxylation of $25(OH)D_3$ during periods of intense training. Other factors also indicated a possibility of lower intakes of vitamin D during the training period. The authors proposed that the effects of training on vitamin D levels remain to be verified through further research.[13]

E. DEFICIENCY

Adequate exposure to sunlight and ingestion of dietary sources of vitamin D is often enough to ward off deficiencies; however, they can occur and some segments of the population may be at risk.

One deficiency disease associated with vitamin D is known as rickets, and despite fortification of foods with vitamin D, this disease still affects a large number of children worldwide.[7] Similarly, the vitamin D deficiency of adulthood is called osteomalacia. Some of the common signs of rickets include poor calcification of bones, resulting in bow legs, retarded growth, enlargement of long bone ends, rib deformities, delayed fontanel closing, and poorly formed teeth. Other deficiency signs may include lax muscles which cause protrusion of the abdomen, muscle spasms, or involuntary twitching.[7] Osteomalacia as a result of vitamin D deficiency results in a softening effect of the bones which causes deformities and pain in the back, pelvis, and limbs. Involuntary twitching and muscle spasms may also accompany these symptoms.[7]

Although vitamin D deficiencies in athletes have not been reported, such a deficiency could potentially result in fractures of the bones and problems of muscle control. In nonathletes, researchers have observed skeletal muscle weakness with vitamin D deficiency.[14]

F. TOXICITY

Because it is a fat-soluble vitamin, vitamin D can be stored by the body, and therefore can be potentially toxic. Symptoms of toxicity are generally not observed until consumption of vitamin D reaches 50,000 IU/day for several months.[15] Toxicity generally is not a result of overexposure to sunlight or excessive dietary intake, but rather from the use of vitamin D supplements.[8]

Toxicity of vitamin D, also called hypervitaminosis D, can result in kidney stones, irreversible kidney damage, and calcification of soft tissues such as blood vessels, kidney, heart, lungs, and tissues surrounding joints — all of which could lead to death.[7] Other reported vitamin D toxicity symptoms include weight loss, vomiting, nausea, lethargy, and loss of muscle tone.[16] Excess metabolites of vitamin D have also been shown to decrease collagen synthesis and cross-linking,[17,18] resulting in increased susceptibility of musculoskeletal injuries in athletes.[14]

G. SUPPLEMENTATION

Vitamin D supplements are available and may be warranted for individuals with medical problems interfering with vitamin D absorption or metabolism, or for those with a low intake of vitamin D sources and limited sun exposure.[14] Individuals most at risk for developing a deficiency include those who suffer from chronic intestinal malabsorption caused by cystic fibrosis, Crohn's disease, chronic liver disease, Whipple's disease, and the elderly. Because vitamin D can be toxic, caution must be taken when considering frequency and dosage of vitamin D supplements. Research on vitamin D supplementation and exercise is limited, and does not support its use for athletes.[14,19]

H. RECOMMENDATIONS

The Recommended Dietary Allowance (RDA) for vitamin D, which is intended for the general healthy population, is 10 µg for males and females up to age 24, and 5 µg after age 24 for both males and females.[20] The RDA can be met through dietary sources of vitamin D such as fish, eggs, liver, and vitamin D-fortified milk, and also through exposure to the ultraviolet rays of the sun.

Athletes, like the general healthy population, require an adequate intake of vitamin D as well as all other essential vitamins and minerals in order to perform effectively. However, no separate recommendation has been given for athletes. Some athletes, for example wrestlers[21] and dancers,[22] may be at risk of low vitamin D intakes due to consumption of low-calorie diets. Currently there is no supporting evidence that increased intakes of vitamin D will enhance performance in athletes.[19]

II. VITAMIN K

A. INTRODUCTION

Vitamin K was discovered in 1929 as a result of investigations into a hemorrhagic disease of cattle feeding on sweetclover silage and of chickens eating a fat-free diet.[23,24] Currently, three biologically active forms of vitamin K have been identified. They are phylloquinone, which is the normal dietary form; menaquinone, which is synthesized by the flora of the intestines; and menadione, which is a synthetic form of the vitamin that the body can metabolize to yield active phylloquinone.[24]

B. METABOLISM

Vitamin K absorption and metabolism is similar to other fat-soluble compounds, beginning with its absorption through the small intestines. The vitamin is first incorporated into chylomicrons and travels through the lymphatic system until it reaches the bloodstream. Within 72 h after absorption, the vitamin K bound by chylomicrons is transferred to the ß-lipoproteins in the liver. Currently, no vitamin K-specific binding protein has been identified.[23]

C. FUNCTIONS

The most common function of vitamin K is its involvement in blood clot formation. The series of reactions involved in the formation of fibrin for blood clots is tightly regulated by substances that depend on vitamin K.[23] In fact, there are four vitamin K-dependent proteins involved in blood clotting.[25]

Another primary function of vitamin K is to serve as a cofactor in the conversion of protein-bound glutamyl residues to γ-carboxyglutamyl residues. Prothrombin activity is dependent upon this conversion.[25,26]

Other vitamin K-dependent proteins not related to blood clot formation exist including osteocalcin (Gla protein, BGP) which osteoblasts secrete,[27,28] and bone matrix GLA protein (MGP) found in the cartilage, dentin, and bone.[29] The synthesis of the BGP and MGP molecules have also been shown to be dependent on vitamin D $(1,25 (OH)_2D_3)$,[30] indicating that some of the functions of vitamin D may be influenced by these vitamin K-dependent compounds, BGP and MGP.[23] The role of the vitamin K-dependent osteocalcin is not completely understood, but is believed to be more related to bone formation than to bone maintenance.[25] This may be important for young athletes who are building their bones so that they can have strong bones to sustain their activities in the future.

D. EXERCISE-RELATED RESEARCH

There is no clear rationale for exercise-related benefits[31] or musculoskeletal healing in humans[14] with supplementation of vitamin K, consequently no studies have been done. Therefore, it is not likely that any will be done until a potential relationship becomes clear.

E. DEFICIENCY

It is unlikely that vitamin K deficiency could by produced by lack of dietary intake alone. This is difficult due to the numerous sources of vitamin K in plants and animals, the recycling of vitamin K by the body to conserve its stores, and the presence of vitamin K-producing microbiologic flora in the intestinal tract of normal humans. However, low intake along with antibiotic therapy affecting the flora of the small intestines could result in symptoms of deficiency.[23] In addition, malabsorption of fats and fat-soluble compounds such as vitamin K could potentially lead to a deficiency of vitamin K.[32]

Symptoms of deficiency include bruising[31] and hemorrhaging.[33] Synthesis of osteocalcin may also be impaired, but the effects on bone mineralization as a result of vitamin K deficiency have only been shown in animals transfused with preformed blood clotting factors.[25] Vitamin K deficiencies have not been documented in the exercising population.[2]

F. TOXICITY

Vitamin K toxicity is uncommon and highly unlikely, however, it has occurred when water-soluble substitutes of vitamin K are prescribed. Symptoms associated with toxicity of vitamin K include hemolysis of red blood cells, jaundice, and brain damage.[33]

G. SUPPLEMENTATION

Although no studies have been conducted, there seems to be no basis for ergogenic benefits from supplementation of vitamin K.[2] Its role in osteocalcin synthesis may indicate that supplemental vitamin K may be helpful in healing of bone fractures.[25]

H. RECOMMENDATIONS

The amount of vitamin K needed by individuals has been difficult to determine because of the difficulties in measuring vitamin K in foods and tissues and to the insensitivity of prothrombin time as the primary method used to determine sufficiency.[34] Recommended Dietary Allowances (RDA) have been established for vitamin K. The current recommendations range from 45 to 80 µg for men and 45 to 60 µg for women. These recommendations increase throughout the life span and during pregnancy and lactation.[20] Again, there is no reason to believe that increased amounts of vitamin K will give ergogenic benefits, therefore, there is no increase in the recommendation for athletes.

Since there is no clear association with vitamin K and exercise, future research is unlikely unless a connection can be seen. The recently discovered relationship between vitamin K and bone, and a possible impact of exercise on this relationship, may be an area of possible research.

REFERENCES

1. Gaby, S. K. and Singh, V. N., Vitamin D, in *Vitamin Intake and Health: A Scientific Review,* Gaby, S. K., Ed., Marcel Dekker, New York, 1991, chap. 4.
2. Bucci, L. R., Micronutrient supplementation and ergogenesis-vitamins, in *Nutrients as Ergogenic Aids for Sports and Exercise,* Bucci, L., Ed., CRC Press, Boca Raton, FL, 1993, chap. 3.
3. DeLuca, H. F., New concepts of vitamin D functions, in *Beyond Deficiency: New Views on the Function and Health Effects of Vitamins,* Vol. 669, Sauberlich, H. E. and Machlin, L. J., Eds., New York Academy of Sciences, New York, 1993, pp. 59-68.
4. Holick, M. F., Vitamin D: biosynthesis, metabolism, and mode of action, in *Endocrinolgy,* Vol. 2, DeGroot, L. J., Ed., Grune & Stratton, New York, 1989, pp. 902-926.
5. Holick, M. F., Vitamin D, in *Modern Nutrition in Health and Disease,* 8th ed., Shils, M. E., Olsen, J. A., and Shike, M., Eds., Lea & Febiger, Philadelphia, 1994, chap. 17.
6. Williams, S. R., Fat-soluble vitamins, in *Nutrition and Diet Therapy,* 7th ed., Smith, J. M., Malinee, V., Stevenson, L. M., and Fannin, S. C., Eds., Mosby-Year Book, St. Louis, 1993, chap. 8.
7. Whitney, E. N., Cataldo, C. B., and Rolfes, S. R., *Understanding Normal and Clinical Nutrition,* 3rd ed., West Publishing, St. Paul, MN, 1991, pp. 251-257.
8. Miller, B. E. and Norman, A. W., Vitamin D, in *Handbook of Vitamins,* Machlin, L. J., Ed., Marcel Dekker, New York, 1984, pp. 45-97.
9. DeLuca, H. F., Vitamin D, in *Modern Nutrition in Health and Disease,* 6th ed., Goodhart, R. and Shils, M. E., Eds., Lea & Febiger, Philadelphia, 1980, chap. 6.
10. de Boland, A. R. and Boland, R. L., Rapid changes in skeletal muscle calcium uptake induced in vitro by 1,25-dihydroxyvitamin D_3 are suppressed by calcium channel blockers, *Endocrinology,* 120, 1858, 1987.
11. Seidl, E. and Hettinger, T., Der Einfluss von Vitamin D_3 auf Kraft und Leistungsfahigkeit des Gesunden Erwachsenen, *Int. Z. Angew. Physiol.,* 16, 365, 1957.
12. Berven, H., The physical working capacity of healthy children: seasonal variation and effects of ultraviolet irradiation and vitamin D supply, *Acta Pediatr.,* Suppl. 148, 1, 1963.
13. Klausen, T., Breum, L., Sorensen, H. A., Schifter, S., and Sonne, B., Plasma levels of parathyroid hormone, vitamin D, calcitonin, and calcium in association with endurance exercise, *Calcif. Tissue Int.,* 52, 205, 1993.
14. Bucci, L. R., *Nutrition Applied to Injury Rehabilitation and Sports Medicine,* CRC Press, Boca Raton, FL, 1995, chap. 5.
15. DeLuca, H. F., Vitamin D and its metabolites, in *Modern Nutrition in Health and Disease,* 7th ed., Shils, M. E. and Young, V. R., Eds., Lea & Febiger, Philadelphia, 1988, p. 313.
16. Tatkon, M., *The Great Vitamin Hoax,* Macmillan, New York, 1968.
17. Tinker, D. and Rucker, R. B., Role of selected nutrients in synthesis, accumulation, and chemical modification of connective tissue proteins, *Physiol. Rev.,* 65, 607, 1985.
18. Berg, R. A. and Kerr, J. S., Nutritional aspects of collagen metabolism, *Annu. Rev. Nutr.,* 12, 369, 1992.
19. Bucci, L.R., Nutritional ergogenic aids, in *Nutrition in Exercise and Sport,* Wolinsky, I. and Hickson, J. F., Jr., Eds., CRC Press, Boca Raton, FL, 1994, chap. 14.
20. National Research Council, *Recommended Dietary Allowances,* 10th ed., National Academy Press, Washington, D.C., 1989.
21. Williams, M. H., *Nutritional Aspects of Human Physical and Athletic Performance,* 2nd ed., Charles C Thomas, Springfield, IL, 1985, chap. 6.
22. Cohen, J. L., Potosnak, L., Frank, O., and Baker, H., A nutritional and hematological assessment of elite ballet dancers, *Phys. Sportsmed.,* 13, 43, 1985.
23. Olson, R. E., Vitamin K, in *Modern Nutrition in Health and Disease,* 8th ed., Shils, M. E., Olson, J. A., and Shike, M., Eds., Lea & Febiger, Philadelphia, 1994, chap. 19.

24. Bender, D. A., *Introduction to Nutrition and Metabolism,* UCL Press, London, 1993.
25. Bender, D. A., Vitamin K, in *Nutritional Biochemistry of the Vitamins,* Bender, D. A., Ed., Cambridge University Press, New York, 1992, chap. 5.
26. Olson, R. E., Vitamin K, in *Modern Nutrition in Health and Disease,* 7th ed., Shils, M. E. and Young, V. R., Eds., Lea & Febiger, Philadelphia, 1988, p. 328.
27. Hauschka, P. V., Lian, J. B., and Gallop, P. M., Direct identification of the calcium-binding amino acid γ-carboxyglutamate in mineralized tissue, *Proc. Natl. Acad. Sci. U.S.A.,* 72, 3925, 1975.
28. Price, P. A., Otsuka, A. S., Poser, J. W., Kristaponis, J., and Raman, N., Characterization of γ-carboxyglutamic acid-containing protein from bone, *Proc. Natl. Acad. Sci. U.S.A.,* 73, 1447, 1976.
29. Price, P. A., Urist, M. R., and Otawara, Y., Matrix Gla protein, a new γ-carboxyglutamic acid-containing protein which is associated with the organic matrix of bone, *Biochem. Biophy. Res. Commun.,* 117, 765, 1983.
30. Price, P. A., The effects of 1,25 dihydroxyvitamin D_3 on the synthesis of the vitamin K-dependent protein of bone, in *Vitamin D: Basic and Clinical Aspects,* Kumar, R., Ed., Martinus Nijhoff, Boston, 1984, chap. 16.
31. Bucci, L. R., Nutritional ergogenic aids, in *Nutrition in Exercise and Sport,* Wolinsky, I. and Hickson, J. F., Jr., Eds., CRC Press, Boca Raton, FL, 1994, chap. 14.
32. van der Meer, J., Hemker, H. C., and Loeliger, E. A., *Pharmacological Aspects of Vitamin K: A Clinical and Experimental Study in Man,* F.K. Schattauer-verlag, Stuttgart, 1968, chap. 6.
33. Whitney, E. N., Cataldo, C. B., and Rolfes, S. R., *Understanding Normal and Clinical Nutrition,* 3rd ed. West Publishing Company, St. Paul, MN, 1991, pp. 261-263.
34. Suttie, J. W., Vitamin K and human nutrition, *J. Am. Diet. Assoc.,* 92, 585, 1992.

Chapter 10

VITAMIN E

Mohsen Meydani
Roger A. Fielding
Nader Fotouhi

CONTENTS

I. INTRODUCTION

Physical activity has been recognized as an important lifestyle factor which contributes to good health and delays the onset of many diseases later in life. Individuals who adopt a regular program of physical activity or exercise training are also more conscious of other environmental factors such as diet and nutrition, alcohol consumption, and smoking, which are also known have a great impact on health and disease. Among these and other factors, nutrition and the components of daily foods of athletes and individuals with regular physical regimens have received great attention not only for maintaining energy balance, but also for improving performance among elite athletes. In recent decades, due to the emerging scientific evidence on the importance of diet and the consumption of fruits and vegetables in the prevention of degenerative diseases such as cancer and cardiovascular disease, public aware-ness and interest in this area of knowledge has increased substantially. Recently, the concept of oxidant/antioxidant balance as a key to the maintenance of health and the prevention of degenerative disease has been introduced to the public.[1]

Exercise influences oxidative metabolism and produces reactive oxygen species (ROS) which elicit a series of metabolic events that lead to muscle fiber degradation and repair processes. Vitamin E, the most effective natural antioxidant in the biological system, has been found to play an important role in preventing cardiovascular disease and certain types of cancer, as well as improving the immune system. It has also been suggested that vitamin E may have an important role in lowering oxidative stress associated with exercise and improving the oxidant/antioxidant balance. Vitamin E deficiency is rarely observed; it is mainly associated with fat malabsorption syndromes. Clinical symptoms such as neuropathy and red blood cell (RBC) hemolysis are only manifested at the point of extreme deficiency of this vitamin. However, marginal deficiency without apparent clinical symptoms may occur — especially among the elderly and individuals engaged in strenuous physical activity or training and consuming a high-carbohydrate, low-fat diet without paying attention to their dietary intake of antioxidants, such as vitamins E, C, and carotenoids. Increased intake of vitamin C may spare vitamin E utilization in the body. *In vitro* studies and some animal studies have shown that vitamin C may recycle the vitamin E radical back to the reduced form during oxidative reactions.[2]

An increase in physical activity without providing an adequate supply of vitamin E and other antioxidant nutrients may predispose skeletal muscle and other organs to oxidative stress and its associated pathology. Evidence from epidemiological and clinical trials indicates that intake of vitamin E above the Recommended Dietary Allowance (RDA) or higher vitamin E status is associated with decreased cardiovascular disease, cancer, and enhancement of the immune system.[3] However, even though a higher intake of vitamin E is associated with decreased production of exercise-induced oxidative stress, a few human studies have shown no improvement in physical performance due to vitamin E supplementation. This chapter briefly reviews the current knowledge about the nature of dietary vitamin E, its relation to other antioxidant defense systems in maintaining the oxidant/antioxidant balance, and muscle fiber function in skeletal muscle.

II. STRUCTURE AND BIOLOGICAL FUNCTION OF VITAMIN E

Vitamin E is an essential fat-soluble vitamin which includes a group of eight naturally occurring compounds in two classes designated as tocopherols and tocotrienols with different biological activities (Figure 1). *RRR*-α-tocopherol (formerly *d*-α-tocopherol) has the highest biological activity and is the most widely available form of vitamin E in food. The other isomers (β, γ, δ), some of which are more abundant in a typical Western diet, are less biologically active than *d*-α-tocopherol.

Commercially available vitamin E supplement pills contain either the natural or synthetic form of α-tocopherol. The synthetic forms of vitamin E are comprised of an approximately equal mixture of eight stereoisomeric forms of α-tocopherol, whereas the natural form contains only *RRR*-α-tocopherol or its esterified form with acetate or succinate. Deuterium-labeled tocopherol studies have suggested that the natural form of vitamin E is more bio-available than synthetic forms.[4] The body's discrimination for the natural vs. the synthetic form is thought to be related to the higher binding capacity of the natural form to liver vitamin E-binding protein.[5]

For practical purposes, one International Unit (IU) of vitamin E is referred to as 1 mg of the synthetic form, *all-rac*-α-tocopheryl acetate (formerly *dl*-α-tocopheryl acetate), and the natural form of *RRR*-α-tocopherol has a biopotency of vitamin E equal to 1.49 IU. In order to easily estimate vitamin E activity in food, 1 mg of *RRR*-α-tocopherol is termed as α-tocopherol equivalent (a-TE). Therefore, in a mixed diet containing either the natural or

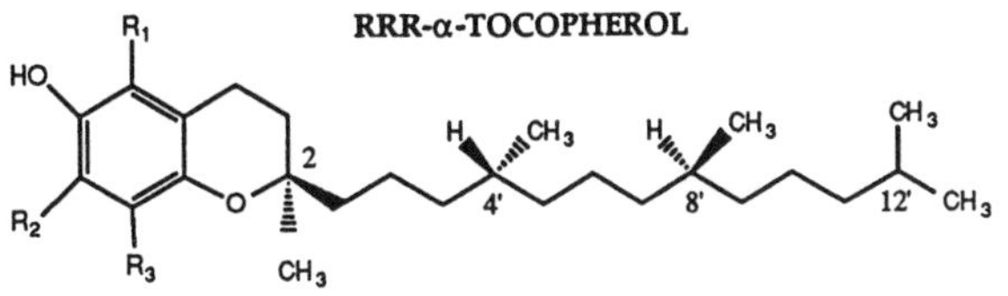

RRR-α-TOCOPHEROL

The eight compounds found in nature that have vitamin E activity:

Compound	R1	R2	R3	Double bound on 4′, 8′ 12′	Biological activity IU/mg compared to d-α-T	
d-α-tocopherol	CH_3	CH_3	CH_3	none	1.49	100%
d-β-tocopherol	CH_3	H	CH_3	none	0.75	50%
d-γ-tocopherol	H	CH_3	CH_3	none	0.15	10%
d-δ-tocopherol	H	H	CH_3	none	0.05	3%
d-α-tocotrienol	CH_3	CH_3	CH_3	yes	0.75	30%
d-β-tocotrienol	CH_3	H	CH_3	yes	0.08	5%
d-γ-tocotrienol	H	CH_3	CH_3	yes	not known	
d-δ-tocotrienol	H	H	CH_3	yes	not known	

FIGURE 1 The eight compounds found in nature that have vitamin E activity.

the synthetic form of vitamin E, the α-TE can be estimated by multiplying the weight concentration of each isomer by the respective isomeric index (relative activity) as shown in Figure 1.

Vegetables; seed oils including soybean, safflower, and corn; sunflower seeds; nuts; whole grains; and wheat germ contain a relatively higher concentration of tocopherols, while animal products are generally poor sources of this vitamin. Data from the Second National Health and Nutrition Examination Survey (NHANES II) study have indicated that while fats and oils are the major contributors of vitamin E to average American diets, fruits and vegetables as well as meat products and breakfast cereals also contribute a substantial amount of vitamin E to the average diet of the U.S. population (Table 1).[6]

Absorption of vitamin E is dependent upon the digestion and absorption of fat. Approximately 45% of a dose is absorbed into the lymph, while metabolites and a small amount of the intact form of vitamin E are absorbed through the portal vein.[7] In the blood, it is principally carried in low-density lipoprotein (LDL) and high-density lipoprotein (HDL).[8] Newly absorbed vitamin E accumulates largely in adipose tissue, liver, and muscle.

The RDAs of vitamin E for men and women are 10 and 8 mg, respectively.[9] The present RDA for vitamin E is based primarily on the customary intake of this vitamin from U.S. food sources and appears to be adequate to maintain normal physiological functions and protect the polyunsaturated fatty acids (PUFA) of tissue from lipid peroxidation. The daily requirement for this vitamin increases with a high intake of PUFA and increasing degree of

TABLE 1   Percent Contribution of Food
Categories to Vitamin E in the
Average American Diet

Food Category	% Total Vitamin E
Fats and oils	20.2
Vegetables	15.1
Meat, poultry, and fish	12.6
Breakfast cereals	9.9
Fruit	5.3
Breads and grain products	5.3
Dairy products	4.5
Mixed main dishes	4.0
Nuts and seeds	3.8
Eggs	3.2
Salty snacks	3.0
Legumes	2.1
Soups, sauces, and gravies	1.7

Data from NHANES II Study, adapted from Murphy,
S.P., Subar, A.F., and Block, G., *Am. J. Clin. Nutr.*,
52, 361, 1990.

unsaturation of fatty acids in the diet. Even though foods that are high in PUFA often contain high levels of vitamin E, this may not always be the case. Vegetable oils and margarine are relatively rich in γ-tocopherol, which has 1/10 the biological activity of α-tocopherol (Figure 1), therefore increasing the PUFA in the diet from these sources may not provide enough α-TE to maintain a proper balance. A ratio of >0.4 mg *RRR*-α-tocopherol per gram of PUFA is desirable to maintain the oxidant/antioxidant balance.[10] This ratio may vary significantly depending on the type of food; for example, it is 0.07 for walnuts whereas it is 1.42 for olive oil.

Several surveys and recent clinical studies have indicated that intake of vitamin E more than several times the RDA is necessary to reduce the risk of cardiovascular disease, certain cancers, as well as to increase immune function, especially among the elderly.[3] Animal studies and a few human studies also point to similar conclusions for the beneficial effect of vitamin E in the prevention of exercise-related disorders. However, according to the NHANES II, the vitamin E content of diets of the majority of the U.S. population is slightly below the RDA (69% of men and 80% of women), and the diets of 20% of men and 32% of women contain less than 50% of the RDA.[6] Murphy et al.[6] also reported that 23% of men and 15% of women in that survey showed a ratio of vitamin E to PUFA of <0.4, which is believed to be critical for the maintenance of antioxidant/oxidant balance.

Vitamin E, relative to other fat-soluble vitamins, is a safe vitamin. Few side effects have been reported, even at doses as high as 3 g/day. Individuals who consume anticoagulant drugs or have a coagulation defect due to vitamin K deficiency should avoid supplemental intake of vitamin E.[11]

Antioxidant properties and prevention of PUFA from lipid peroxidation are the most widely accepted biological function of vitamin E. It is the most effective chain-breaking, lipid-soluble antioxidant in the biological membrane where it contributes to membrane, stability, regulates fluidity, and protects critical cellular structures against damage from ROS and other free radicals (containing an unpaired electron). In normal cellular metabolism, most of the oxygen consumed is utilized in the mitochondrial electron transport system for substrate metabolism and ATP production. However, a small fraction of molecular oxygen (<2%) escapes this process and produces a highly reactive superoxide radical ($O_2 \cdot^-$), hydroxyl radical ($OH\cdot$), and hydrogen peroxide (H_2O_2). These products can cause membrane lipid peroxidation and the loss of membrane integrity. The continuous and increased production of free radicals and their reaction with other critical cellular components such as DNA have been suggested to contribute to the aging process and the pathogenesis of chronic diseases.[12]

Exercise increases oxygen consumption of the whole body dramatically, particularly the skeletal muscles, thus increasing production of ROS. In mitochondria, ROS are produced from ubiquinone oxidation in the respiratory electron transport system located in the inner mitochondrial membrane.[13] Evidence demonstrating mitochondrial involvement in the production of superoxide radicals during exercise has arisen from the work of Davies et al.,[14] who showed that exhaustive exercise in rats resulted in a marked reduction in respiratory control indices of mitochondrial enzymes, suggesting an increasing inner membrane leakiness to proton and decreasing energy coupling efficiency due to exercise. ROS are also produced by the immune inflammatory cells within the muscle tissue where they clear debris from injured fibers following strenuous exercise. Activation of chemotactic factors by superoxide radicals, similar to the early manifestation of the acute phase response in infection, has been suggested to occur following exercise.[15] Following exercise, immune complements are also activated as an initial event in the inflammatory response,[16] then followed by the mobilization and activation of neutrophils,[17] the production of acute phase proteins, and the accumulation of monocytes and macrophages at the site of injury. Neutrophils produce degradative enzymes such as elastase[18] and lysozyme[19] that further break down muscle to be phagocytized by macrophages and monocytes,[16] generating radicals such as $NO\cdot$, $HO\cdot$, and H_2O_2 and hypochlorous acid.[20] Thus, both enzymatic and nonenzymatic antioxidants and particularly vitamin E, which is more abundant in the inner mitochondrial membrane, may play an important role in modulating oxidative stress induced by exercise.

In addition to its antioxidant function, vitamin E has recently been shown to influence cellular response to oxidative stress through modulation of signal transduction pathways.[21] This mechanism of vitamin E has been suggested to contribute to its anticancer and immunostimulatory effects.

The necessity of vitamin E for neurological function, genetic disorders, prevention of RBC hemolysis, and other disorders in premature infants and adults is well established. Current evidence indicates that vitamin E protects tissues from the harmful effects of ROS and, without doubt, it is an essential antioxidant for normal cell function during exercise.

The concentration of vitamin E in plasma is approximately 27 µmol/l; in liver and heart it is about 23 nmol/g wet weight, and in adipose tissue its concentration amounts to 230 nmol/g wet weight. Even though protein is the major constituent of skeletal muscle, it contains approximately 30 to 40 nmol vitamin per gram of wet tissue with considerable differences between muscle fiber types. Concentration of vitamin E can be significantly increased within a relatively short period of time through high intakes of vitamin E.[22] The magnitude of the increase of vitamin E in the muscle may be attributed to the tissue's high oxidative metabolic activity, lipoprotein lipase, and low-density lipoprotein receptor activities, as well as to the nonspecific exchange with plasma vitamin E.[5] We have found that intake of 800 IU of vitamin E for 4 weeks increased α-tocopherol in the *vastus lateralis* muscle from 37 to 57 nmol/g wet tissue.[22] Even though the magnitude of the increase in plasma was much higher than in the muscle (from 21 to 64 µmol/l, ≈300% increase), the increase in skeletal muscle vitamin E, which correlated well with the increase in plasma vitamin E, suggests a close metabolic equilibrium between plasma and muscle vitamin E.

Vitamin E may have a differential role in the oxidative metabolism of different muscle fibers. Human skeletal muscle consists of two main fibers, Type I (red, slow-twitch) and Type II (white, fast-twitch) fibers. Type I fibers are rich in myoglobin and mitochondrial enzymes and replenish their phosphocreatine more efficiently via oxidative phosphorylation than Type II fibers.[23] Relative to Type II fibers, Type I fibers also contain a higher catalase (CAT) activity[24] which may be necessary to eliminate the harmful effects of ROS produced from a higher oxidative metabolism associated with a large number of mitochondria.[25,26] Thus, Type I fibers, which produce energy primarily via aerobic processes, may also utilize more vitamin E than Type II fibers. Muscle composed mainly of Type I fiber has been reported to contain a higher α-tocopherol concentration than muscle composed mainly of Type II fiber.[27] Similar observations have been made in rabbits injected with radiolabelled α-tocopherol;[28] however, a high dietary intake of vitamin E or supplementation may have no effect on the increase of muscle fiber types. We found no effect of 800 IU of vitamin E supplementation for 1 month on the distribution of muscle fiber types in the *vastus lateralis* muscle of young volunteers.

III. VITAMIN E DEFICIENCY AND SKELETAL MUSCLE

Vitamin E deficiency can lead to the degeneration of muscular tissue (nutritional muscular dystrophy, NMD) in animals[29-32] and humans.[33,34] Given the antioxidant function of vitamin E, it is believed that free radical damage is responsible for NMD. It has been shown that a diet containing a high level of PUFA and deficient in vitamin E exasperates NMD.[35] Vitamin E deficiency in rats swimming to exhaustion further increased muscle lipid peroxidation.[36]

Increased *in vitro* muscle lipid peroxidation has also been demonstrated in sheep fed a vitamin E-deficient diet for 12 weeks.[27] Earlier, Dillard and co-workers[37] reported that the production of ethane and pentane, the volatile end products of lipid peroxidation of PUFA in exhaled breath samples, was higher in rats with low vitamin E status compared with vitamin E-sufficient animals. Feeding a vitamin E-deficient diet to mice for 5 or 12 weeks reduced skeletal muscle vitamin E concentrations by 36 and 61%, respectively, and increased susceptibility of muscle to lipid peroxidation.[38]

Vitamin E deficiency in humans has been observed in patients with chronic fat malabsorption syndromes.[34,39] The pathology of vitamin E deficiency in humans is similar to that found in animals.[30,31,33,34] One report showed severe fiber loss with almost complete disappearance of large-diameter fibers.[39] Large-dose vitamin E therapy appears to reverse some of the damages, including 2 shift of fibers from Type I to Type II and reduction in the number of fibers containing lipid and ceroid granules.[33]

Since the Type I fibers are more oxidatively active than Type II fibers, they may be affected more by vitamin E deficiency than Type II fibers. Pillar et al.[40] reported that vitamin E deficiency appears to affect predominantly Type I muscle fibers in rats. However, Smith et al. reported that NMD is primarily associated with Type II muscle fiber in weaned sheep.[41] Neville et al.[34] observed Type I fiber predominance in one patient and fiber type grouping in another patient, with no excessive Type II fiber production. Thus, it appears that vitamin E deficiency alters fiber type population; however, vitamin E supplementation beyond the deficiency does not increase Type I fiber numbers above the normal level.

The exact mechanism by which vitamin E deficiency induces muscle degradation is not known. Muscle from vitamin E-deficient animals appears susceptible to oxidation and free-radical attack, and the deficit may be responsible for the etiology of NMD. Shih et al.[42] reported increased muscle proteolysis and a higher ratio of cystine:cysteine as an index of oxidative degradation of the muscle protein in dystrophic muscle. Vitamin E may be involved in regulation of the synthesis of specific proteins required for normal muscle function.[43]

Loss of calcium homeostasis seems to be a key event in the damaging process. Depletion of cellular thiols and increase of intracellular calcium may potentiate free-radical generation. Vitamin E-deficient muscle appears to be more susceptible to intercellular calcium overload due to leakiness of membranes for the influx of calcium, which activates protease leading to muscle protein degradation.[44] It is also important to note that mitochondria are also very sensitive to increased intracellular calcium concentration, which interferes with production of ATP. The increased protease activity due to the increase of intracellular calcium in vitamin E deficiency may contribute to the thin filament degradation in the Z disk.

In conclusion, severe deficiency of vitamin E increases oxidative stress in skeletal muscles, alters muscle fiber types, and causes degradation and inflammatory processes leading to dystrophic conditions.

IV. EXERCISE, OXIDATIVE STRESS, AND VITAMIN E SUPPLEMENTATION

Skeletal muscle has one of the highest oxygen requirements of all tissues. Exercise increases total oxygen consumption by 10 to 15-fold. Therefore, the rate of production of ROS during exercise is also greatly increased. The exercise-induced increase in free-radical production has been documented both directly and indirectly in muscle tissue. Davies et al.[14] monitored free-radical signals in exercised and control rats by electron paramagnetic resonance. The free-radical signals in homogenates of muscle from exercised rats were more than double those of unexercised muscle. Jackson and co-workers[45] found that excess contractile activity resulted in a 70% increase in the electron spin resonance signal. Injection of spin-trappers or vitamin E to rats prior to swimming to exhaustion significantly increased time to exhaustion, an indirect evidence for the induction of free radicals by exercising and their elimination with antioxidants. The fatty acid oxidation product, pentane, has also been measured as a product of exercise-induced lipid peroxidation in humans.[46] There was a significant increase in expired pentane during exercise at 75% maximum oxygen consumption compared with pentane production before exercise.

It has also been demonstrated that more vitamin E is needed when an exercise regimen is adopted in experimental animals. Endurance-trained rats had lower muscle vitamin E concentration than sedentary animals.[47] After 6 months of exercise training in rats, cytochrome oxidase in skeletal muscles of 12- and 24-month-old rats increased, but vitamin E concentration in muscle tissue decreased and was more pronounced in the older animals.[48] In contrast, Packer et al.[49] found that there was no differences in vitamin E content of muscles between the sedentary and trained animals. However, they found a higher cytochrome C reductase in red quadriceps, plantaris, and soleus muscles of trained rats compared with sedentary animals, resulting in a lower ratio of antioxidant to oxidative capacity in the trained animals. Rats supplemented with a 10,000 IU vitamin E per kilogram diet following exercising to exhaustion had lower vitamin E levels in the gastrocnemius, but not in the white or red quadriceps muscles compared with unexercised controls given the same diet.[50] On the other hand, Tiidues and Houston[51] found that rats performing acute submaximal exercise did not have lower muscle vitamin E levels than the unexercised controls. However, the accumulated evidence indicates that without adequate dietary vitamin E, training decreases vitamin E concentration in tissues which could lead to increased vulnerability to oxidative stress.

A few studies indicate either no increased oxidative stress due to exercise or a protective effect against lipid peroxidation from endurance training. Salminen and Vihko[52] reported a lower peroxidation rate *in vitro* in the red and white skeletal muscle of trained mice compared with controls. The red muscle in both groups contained higher vitamin E and CAT than the white muscle. Red muscle is mainly composed of Type I fibers, whereas Type II fiber is the major constituent of the white muscle. Submaximal exercise for 3 consecutive days had no effect on plasma vitamin E or urinary 8-hydroxyguanosine (an index of DNA oxidative damage) of moderately trained men.[53] There was a short-term reduction in blood glutathione (GSH) and an increase in oxidized glutathione (GSSG) as well as total and reduced ascorbate during exercise, which returned to baseline during recovery. These authors[52] concluded that in healthy young men submaximal exercise has no long-term effect on blood antioxidants, and does not result in damage to DNA.

Several animal and human studies have pointed out that dietary vitamin E might play a significant role in the prevention of injury from oxidative stress. Supplemental vitamin E has been shown to prevent exercise-induced free radical formation in cardiac muscle.[54] Young males receiving 300 mg of α-tocopherol acetate per day for 4 weeks had reduced leakage of enzymes and a lower blood malondialdehyde (MDA) level pre- and postexercise compared to controls.[55] Vitamin E-supplemented exercised rats had lower protein carbonyl content in the gastrocnemius and white quadriceps muscle compared with unsupplemented exercised rats. Rats supplemented with a 250 IU vitamin E per kilogram diet prior to exercise had lower thiobarbituric acid reactive substances (TBARS) in red slow-twitch and white fast-twitch muscles compared to controls.[56] Cannon et al.[57] found that following an eccentric bout of exercise, young subjects (<30 years) had a higher plasma creatine kinase (CK) concentration and a greater number of neutrophils in circulating blood than older subjects (>55 years). Supplementation with 800 IU vitamin E per day in older subjects for 7 weeks tended to eliminate these differences from young subjects. Plasma lipid peroxides were not affected by exercise or vitamin E supplementation in either of the two age groups. This was probably due to rapid clearance of lipid peroxides from plasma.

A variety of factors may contribute to the elimination or neutralization of lipid peroxides following exercise. These include the induction of enzymatic antioxidants, the mobilization of antioxidants from other tissues, and the elimination of end products from breath and urine. From the above study, we found that the excretion of lipid peroxides in urine increased in both age groups following exercise.[22] We also found that the excretion of these products in urine was greatest in the placebo groups at 12 days postexercise and that vitamin E-supplemented subjects excreted a lower level of these compounds, indicating that vitamin E supplementation may have suppressed oxidative damage induced by eccentric exercise. Further, we observed that the protective effect of vitamin E was more prominent in older subjects.

The delayed increase in urinary lipid peroxides coincided with an increased protein breakdown as indicated by urinary excretion of 3-methylhistidine.[58] Davies et al.[14] have suggested that oxidatively modified proteins are more rapidly and selectively degraded by intracellular proteolytic systems. This process may be further accelerated by ROS produced by mononuclear cells and neutrophils infiltrating damaged muscle tissue to clear debris.[14,59] The catabolic breakdown of protein and the anabolic utilization of amino acid products for remodeling and the generation of new fibers is a continuous process that may last several weeks after initial muscle injury.[16] Therefore, the increased excretion of urinary TBARS, which are, in part, derived from lipid peroxidation, appear to parallel the proteolytic process which was also elevated 12 days postexercise.[58]

In a recent study, a significant increase of DNA strand breakage was demonstrated in individuals 24 h after exhaustive exercise.[60] Intake of 1200 mg vitamin E per day for 14 days showed no increase in DNA damage following the exercise bout in 4 out of 5 subjects.

It is important to note that a few studies have found no protective effect of vitamin E supplementation on exercise-induced oxidative damage. It was reported that in rats vitamin E supplementation (10,000 IU/kg diet) did not prevent injury in soleus muscle even though susceptibility of the muscle to oxidative stress was reduced.[61] Trained marathon runners were given α-tocopherol (400 IU/day) and ascorbic acid (200 mg/day) for 4.5 weeks prior to a marathon race.[62] There were no differences in plasma lipid peroxides or lactate dehydrogenase 24 h after the race compared to the subjects who had received a placebo. However, a significantly smaller increase of serum CK was observed in the supplemented groups compared to the placebo group.

In conclusion, exercise increases oxygen consumption and oxidative stress, which can be detected in bodily fluids and tissues. In both animals and humans, dietary vitamin E supplementation may prevent the oxidative stress associated with exercise. However, it appears that short-term vitamin E supplementation cannot totally overcome the overwhelming oxidative stress produced from exhaustive exercise such as marathon running.

V. TRAINING EFFECTS ON ANTIOXIDANT ENZYMES

In addition to the antioxidant vitamins, cells possess intrinsic antioxidant-scavenging enzymes. These enzymes are important aids in the neutralization of the potential damage caused by ROS. During aerobic exercise, whole-body oxygen consumption can increase with the well-described increase in reactive oxygen molecules. In addition to dietary sources of antioxidant vitamins, a well-developed system of antioxidant enzymes exists within skeletal muscle which attenuates oxidative reactions in this metabolically active tissue. Individuals who exercise on a regular basis may repeatedly undergo bouts of oxidative stress; however, there is overwhelming evidence that regular exercise can improve cardiorespiratory fitness and muscle function,[63] even in older individuals,[64] and reduce all-cause mortality and death rates from cardiovascular disease and cancer.[65,66] In view of the overwhelmingly beneficial effects of regular physical activity, mechanisms must be in place that can limit the potentially toxic effects of oxygen radicals generated during exercise.

Superoxide dismutase (SOD), CAT, GSH peroxidase (GPX), and GSH reductase (GRS) all participate in eliminating ROS and preventing cellular injury and are present in skeletal muscle. SOD acts to catalyze the formation of H_2O_2 from $O_2 \cdot^-$. CAT acts to reduce H_2O_2 to water (H_2O) and molecular oxygen (O_2). GPX catalyzes H_2O_2 to H_2O and reduces lipid peroxides to their corresponding alcohol. GRS reduces oxidized glutathione disulfide in the presence of the reducing agent NADPH with the formation of GSH.

The antioxidant enzymes are specifically localized in cellular organelles and the cytosol within skeletal muscle and their activities also appear to be fiber type dependent. Cross-sectional data from young male volunteers has demonstrated a relationship between oxidative capacity and the activities of the free radical-scavenging enzymes. Jenkins et al.[67] observed a significant correlation between skeletal muscle CAT and whole-body maximal oxygen uptake ($r = 0.7$, $p < .01$ for CAT). Activities of SOD and CAT are tissue specific and are related to the oxidative capacities of various tissues.[67] In skeletal muscle, SOD is present in both mitochondria and cytosol; however, slow oxidative fibers and cardiac muscle appear to have higher total SOD activity than fast muscle, probably due to the marked differences in oxidative capacity of these fibers as previously cited.[68,69] CAT is primarily found in peroxisomes, but its activity varies over tenfold in different muscle fiber types, being lowest in fast muscle and highest in cardiac muscle.[68,69] GSX is localized within mitochondria and cytosol.[70] GSX activity also appears to be fiber-type dependent with the highest activities reported in cardiac and slow oxidative muscle fibers.[69,71] GSR also appears to be higher in slow oxidative muscle fibers.[69]

Exercise training studies have revealed changes in some but not all of these antioxidant enzyme systems. Caladera and co-workers[72] first reported increases in muscle, liver, and heart CAT activity after an acute exercise bout in the rat. Higuchi et al.[68] reported no increase in CAT activity and no significant increase in cytosolic SOD activity following a 3-month run-training program (2 h/day, 5 days/week) in female rats. However, mitochondrial levels of SOD increased 37% in slow oxidative muscle and 14% in fast muscle along with the twofold increases in markers of mitochondrial oxidative capacity. These results suggested that, coupled with the increased oxidative capacity and flux, skeletal muscle mitochondria increase their expression of SOD to minimize the generation of ROS in response to the increased metabolic activity of repeated contractile activity. Despite the increases in mitochondrial SOD activity, these increases were outpaced by the near doubling of the mitochondrial oxidative capacity in response to training, indicating that radical species may still exert damaging effects in exercise-trained animals and that the antioxidant scavenging capacity in exercise-trained mitochondria may still not be adequate.

Alessio and Goldfarb[73] reported significant exercise-induced increases in CAT activity in both red and white muscle from rats after 10 weeks of exercise training. In addition to the changes they observed in antioxidant enzymes, they also reported that exercise training reduced lipid peroxidation (MDA production) induced by exercise in white (fast) quadriceps muscle as well as in liver. However, in contrast to the results of Higuchi et al.,[68] they reported no effects of exercise on total SOD activity. These apparent discrepancies are difficult to resolve but may be related to measurement of total SOD activity and mitochondrial SOD activity as reported by Higuchi et al.[68] Studies by Laughlin et al.[69] and Ji et al.[74] have also demonstrated no significant change in SOD activity using a similar exercise training protocol or an acute bout of exercise.

GPX and GRS activities also appear to be fiber-type dependent with higher activities in more oxidative muscle fibers.[69,71] GPX activity has been shown to increase in response to acute exercise and exercise training.[71,75,76]

The functional consequences of increased antioxidant scavenger enzymes by exercise training has also been examined in relation to toxicity of the chemotherapeutic agent doxo-rubicin (Adriamycin) in cardiac muscle. Although the effects of doxorubicin on superoxide generation in myocardial tissue have recently been questioned,[77] Kanter et al.[78] observed that mice who had been subjected to swim training for 21 weeks had less cardiotoxicity to this agent, which is known to generate ROS, despite no significant increase in myocardial anti-oxidant enzymes in the drug-treated groups. The reduced cardiotoxicity did appear to be associated with increased antioxidant scavenger enzymes, particularly in the blood and liver. A higher training intensity protocol may be necessary to induce changes in cardiac muscle antioxidant enzymes. Powers and co-workers[79] have reported an approximately 25% increase in ventricular SOD activity in response to high and moderate, but not low, intensity training (10 weeks at 30, 60, or 90 min/day at low, moderate, or high intensity) in the rat. Both an acute bout of exercise and exercise training have also been shown to increase SOD, CAT, and GPX in rat heart mitochondria.[80]

Fewer studies have examined the effects of exercise on hepatic antioxidant enzymes. An early study by Pyke et al.[81] reported an 80% depletion of liver GSH levels following exhaustive exercise in rats. An acute bout of exercise has been shown to increase liver CAT[73] and GPX.[82,83] Studies on the effects of exercise training on hepatic antioxidant enzymes are not in agreement. Higuchi et al.[68] reported no changes in liver CAT and SOD activity following 3 months of treadmill exercise training. Kanter et al.[78] have reported significant increases in liver CAT, SOD, and GPX following 21 weeks of swim training in mice. Sen et al.[75] observed an increase in hepatic glutathione-S-transferase activity with exercise training in dogs. In this same study, no training-induced increases in hepatic GPX or GRS were observed. It is possible that the relatively small increase in hepatic oxygen uptake during exercise and the relatively high baseline antioxidant enzyme levels in liver preclude a further increase in these enzymes with exercise training. However, the reduction in blood flow in the splanchnic area during exercise may have potential effects on ROS generation in the liver.

Biological aging is thought to be influenced by the generation of ROS.[84,85] Studies in rats have shown significant increases in the antioxidant enzymes with advancing age in skeletal muscle.[82,86] SOD, CAT, and GPX are all increased in rat muscle by 31 months. Acute exercise and exercise training in older animals has been shown to increase GPX activity in muscle in some but not all studies.[87,88]

The majority of exercise and training studies examining adaptations and activation of the antioxidant enzymes have focused on submaximal and aerobic activities. Only one study has compared high-intensity interval training to continuous submaximal exercise training in rodents. Criswell et al.[89] trained young rats for 12 weeks with a continuous (45 min at 70% $\dot{V}O_2$max) or an intermittent protocol (6 × 5 min at 80 to 95% $\dot{V}O_2$max). Both exercise training protocols increased SOD activity. However GPX activity was only increased in the interval-trained group in soleus muscle. No changes in antioxidant activity were observed in the gastrocnemius or rectus femoris muscles after training. From this one study, it appears that induction of the antioxidant enzymes is relatively similar regardless of whether a con-tinuous or interval protocol is employed. Further studies should examine the effects of higher exercise training intensities and resistance training programs on antioxidant enzymes in muscle. High-intensity exercise, particularly eccentric contraction, has been shown to induce oxidative bursts from increased circulating neutrophils[57] which may upregulate muscle SOD and other antioxidant enzymes.

In summary, it appears that both acute exercise and exercise training in animal models increase antioxidant enzyme levels in skeletal muscle and, if the training is of a high intensity, can also increase antioxidant enzyme activity in cardiac muscle. With the exception of one cross-sectional study,[67] no studies have been conducted in human subjects examining the effects of acute exercise and/or training on antioxidant enzymes. Aging is associated with increases in antioxidant enzymes; however, controversy still exists as to whether exercise training further upregulates the expression of these free radical-scavenging enzymes. Older individuals who participate in regular exercise may have higher requirements for antioxidant vitamins such as vitamin E to compensate for the deficit of endogenous antioxidants. In addition, further studies need to be conducted to understand the interaction between these various antioxidant scavengers in relation to free-radical production and antioxidant vitamin status.

VI. VITAMIN E AND PERFORMANCE

As with any nutritional supplement that has a potential interaction with metabolic functions during exercise, some studies have examined the role of vitamin E as a possible ergogenic or performance-enhancing agent. Although it is well established that during exercise measures of free-radical generation and lipid peroxidation increase, and that vitamin E supplementation reduces free radical production and indices of lipid peroxidation, there is little evidence to suggest that the reduction in free-radical formation and/or lipid peroxide formation will enhance exercise performance or hasten recovery from exercise.

In male prisoners performing hard physical labor, a vitamin E-deficient diet induced a rapid drop in plasma tocopherol, suggesting an increased dietary requirement for vitamin E in individuals engaged in physically demanding occupations.[90] However, studies on supplementing individuals who already consume an adequate intake of vitamin E have not shown ergogenic effects. Two studies by Sharman et al.[91,92] reported no significant effects of vitamin E supplementation (400 mg α-tocopherol acetate per day) on swimming (400 m) and running (1 mi run) performance in a group of boys who participated in 6 weeks of swim training compared to control subjects who participated in an identical training without supplementation. These results were also confirmed by Lawrence et al.[93] who fed a group of well-trained swimmers 600 IU of vitamin E (α-tocopheryl acetate) or placebo for 6 months and found no differences in 500-yd performance times. Similar effects of vitamin E have been reported by other investigators.[94,95] Sumida et al.[55] supplemented male college students with 300 mg of vitamin E (α-tocopheryl acetate) for 4 weeks and observed no effects of vitamin E supplementation on maximal aerobic capacity or exercise time to exhaustion during an incremental cycle ergometer exercise test. Despite the absence of effect on aerobic capacity or performance, the subjects had lower postexercise increases in lipid peroxidation and serum β-glucoronidase levels after vitamin E supplementation, suggesting an enhanced radical quenching effect and less subsequent oxidative damage.

Low atmospheric pressures, such as those encountered during high-altitude expeditions, may increase lipid peroxidation during exercise and increase antioxidant requirements. In one study, Simon-Schnass and Pabst[96] observed a significant reduction in expired pentane production in mountaineers supplemented with 200 mg of vitamin E per day during residence at high altitude (43 days at 5000 m). In addition, there was a small but statistically significant improvement in the percentage of $\dot{V}O_2max$ at which the anaerobic threshold occurred. The mechanisms by which vitamin E exerts a performance-enhancing effect at high altitude are not known. These results require further confirmation before widespread recommendations about vitamin supplementation for athletes competing or training at high altitude are made.

Studies have also been conducted examining the effects of vitamin E supplementation of exercise performance in elite athletes. Rokitzki et al.[62] studied the effects of vitamin E supplementation (330 mg/day) on exercise tolerance in elite male cyclists. They reported no effects of vitamin E supplementation on the blood lactate response or the heart rate response to an incremental exercise test on a cycle ergometer, despite lower measures of lipid peroxidation during exercise in the vitamin E-supplemented group.[62] More recently, Snider et al.[97] have reported that ingestion of a multivitamin supplement (100 mg coenzyme Q10, 500 mg cytochrome C, 100 mg inosine, and 200 IU vitamin E) for 4 weeks had no effect on exercise time to exhaustion at 70% $\dot{V}O_2$max (90 min treadmill running, stationary cycling to exhaustion) in competitive triathletes.

With the exception of one study conducted at high altitude,[96] no studies have shown a performance-enhancing effect with vitamin E supplementation, and its use by athletes to enhance performance cannot be objectively confirmed at present, and should not be recommended. However, in those studies which also measured indices of lipid peroxidation, vitamin E supplementation universally lowered peroxidation. The long-term beneficial consequences of this reduced lipid peroxidation are not known and certainly warrant future study. In addition, individuals and athletes who by their dietary habits consume low levels of antioxidants in their diets may be at increased risk for the effects of oxygen radicals and their subsequent harmful effects.

VII. SURVEY OF VITAMIN E INTAKE IN ATHLETES

Coupled with proper training and sound coaching, nutrition is the cornerstone to success in athletic performance. Researchers and athletes have strived for decades to perfect nutritional manipulations to achieve success in sport (for a complete review see Singh[98]). With the well-described increases in ROS production during exercise, coaches and athletes (as well as scientists) have speculated about the possibilities of vitamin E supplementation during heavy training. Also, given the fact that many high-caliber endurance athletes require and often consume a diet high in carbohydrate,[99] questions have arisen regarding the adequacy of their vitamin E intake.

Although nutritional survey methods for assessing micronutrient requirements are not always the most desirable method of assessing vitamin status, several studies have examined the nutrient intakes of athletes. A survey of 22 dietary intake studies of elite endurance and power athletes revealed generally adequate intakes of vitamin E.[100] However, 60 to 90% of the male athletes and 80 to 100% of the female athletes reported multivitamin and mineral supplementation.[100] Other studies have also reported a high prevalence of vitamin supplement use among athletes.[101-104] In a randomized, controlled, double-blind placebo trial of multivitamin supplementation on nutritional and running performance, Weight et al.[105,106] observed no improvements in nutritional status or running performance with nine months of supplementation. Despite the relatively high carbohydrate intake, particularly in endurance-trained athletes, vitamin E status appears to be adequate.

Although there are no proven effects of vitamin E supplementation, the prevalence of vitamin use among athletes is high. Future studies are needed to assess whether antioxidant vitamins (specifically vitamin E) may speed recovery from muscle fatigue and stress after heavy training or enhance performance in specific environmental extremes.

VIII. CONCLUSION

Vitamin E is an essential micronutrient for normal muscle function. The majority of the U.S. population consumes foods that provide adequate amounts of vitamin E to meet the daily requirement for vitamin E. However, athletes, who usually maintain a different level of total calorie intake and have adapted to different dietary habits, may be at greater risk for antioxidant imbalance without supplement use — in particular, those who maintain a high-carbohydrate, low-fat regimen and engage in strenuous exercise. Physical activity alters skeletal muscle blood flow and increases oxygen consumption, possibly contributing to an increase in whole-body production of ROS by several mechanisms. Even though training increases endogenous antioxidant capacity to neutralize ROS and maintain the balance between oxidants and antioxidants, it may not be adequate to meet the challenge of this increased oxidative stress. Evidence indicates that vitamin E and other dietary antioxidants may have a complementary role in this situation; therefore, untrained individuals and the elderly may even benefit more when engaged in physical activity such as weekend workouts to which they are unaccustomed.

There is accumulating evidence from animal studies showing a reduction in oxidative stress from physical activity with vitamin E supplementation. However, very few studies have shown this effect in controlled human studies, and at present, limited evidence does not support the notion that vitamin E supplementation increases training capacity or improves performance in trained individuals. However, the long-term beneficial effects of vitamin E supplementation on lowering oxidative stress, which is known to be involved in many pathological processes, warrants further investigation.

ACKNOWLEDGMENTS

The authors would like to thank Timothy S. McElreavy, M.A., for preparation of this manuscript. This project has been funded at least in part with Federal funds from the U.S. Department of Agriculture, Agricultural Research Service, under contract number 53-K06-01. The contents of this publication do not necessarily reflect the views or policies of the U.S. Department of Agriculture, nor does mention of trade names, commercial products, or organizations imply endorsement by the U.S. government.

REFERENCES

1. Meydani, M., Antioxidant vitamins, *Front. Clin. Nutr.,* 4, 7, 1995.
2. Niki, E., Interaction of ascorbate and α-tocopherol, *Ann. N.Y. Acad. Sci.,* 498, 186, 1987.
3. Meydani, M., Vitamin E, *Lancet,* 345, 170, 1995.
4. Acuff, R.V., Thedford, S.S., Hidiroglou, N.N., Papas, A.M., and Odom, T.A.J., Relative bioavailability of RRR- and all-rac-α-tocopheryl acetate in humans: studies using deuteriated compounds, *Am. J. Clin. Nutr.,* 60, 397, 1994.
5. Traber, M.G., Cohn, W., and Muller, D.P.R., Absorption, transport and delivery to tissues, in: *Vitamin E in Health and Disease,* Fuchs, L.P.J., Ed., Marcel Dekker, New York, 1993, pp. 35-51.
6. Murphy, S.P., Subar, A.F., and Block, G., Vitamin E intake and sources in the United States, *Am. J. Clin. Nutr.,* 52, 361, 1990.
7. Lee-Kim, Y.C., Meydani, M., Kassarjian, Z., Blumberg, J.B., and Russell, R.M., Entrohepatic circulation of newly administered α-tocopherol in the rat, *Int. J. Vitam. Nutr. Res.,* 58, 284, 1988.
8. Meydani, M., Cohn, J.S., Macauley, J.B., McNamara, J.R., Blumberg, J.B., and Schaefer, E.J., Postprandial changes in the plasma concentration of α- and γ-tocopherol in human subjects fed fat-rich meals supplemented with fat-soluble vitamins, *J. Nutr.,* 119, 1252, 1989.

9. National Research Council, *Recommended Dietary Allowances,* 10th ed., National Academy Press, Washington D.C., 1989.

10. Lehmann, J., Martin, H.L., Lashley, E.L., Marshall, M.W., and Judd, J.T., Vitamin E in foods from high and low linoleic acid diets, *J. Am. Diet. Assoc.,* 86, 1208, 1986.

11. Bendich, A. and Machlin, L.J., The safety of oral intake of vitamin E: data from clinical studies from 1986-1991, in: *Vitamin E in Health and Disease,* Packer, L. and Fuchs, J., Eds., Marcel Dekker, New York, 1992, pp. 411-416.

12. Halliwell, B., A radical approach to human disease, in: *Oxygen Radicals and Tissue Injury,* Halliwell, B., Ed., FASEB, Bethesda, 1987, pp. 139-143.

13. Boveris, A., Cadenas, E., and Stoppani, A.O.K., Role of ubiquinone in mitochondrial generation of hydrogen peroxide, *Biochem. J.,* 156, 435, 1976.

14. Davies, K.J.A., Quintanilha, A.T., Brooks, G.A., and Packer, L., Free radicals and tissue damage produced by exercise, *Biochim. Biophys. Res. Commun.,* 107, 1198, 1982.

15. Petrone, W.F., English, D.K., Wong, K., and McCord, J.M., Free radicals and inflammation: superoxide dependent chemotactic factor in plasma, *Proc. Natl. Acad. Sci. U.S.A.,* 77, 1159, 1980.

16. Evans, W. and Cannon, J.G. The metabolic effect of exercise-induced muscle damage, in: *Exercise and Sports Sciences Reviews,* Holloszy, J.O., Ed., Williams & Wilkins, Baltimore, 1991, pp. 99-126.

17. Cannon, J.G. and Kluger, M.J., Endogenous pyrogen activity in human plasma after exercise, *Science,* 220, 617, 1983.

18. Kokot, K., Schaefer, R.M., Teschiner, M., Plass, G.U.R., and Heidland, A., Activation of leukocytes during prolonged physical exercise, *Adv. Exp. Med. Biol.,* 240, 57, 1988.

19. Morozov, V.I., Priiatikin, S., and Nazarov, I.B., Secretion of lysosome by blood neutrophils during physical exertion, *Fiziol. Zh. SSSR. im. I. M. Sechenova,* 75, 334, 1989.

20. Bast, A., Haenen, G.R., and Doelman, C.J.A., Oxidants and antioxidants: state of the art, *Am. J. Med.,* 91, 2S, 1991.

21. Azzi, A., Boscobonik, D., and Hensey, C., The protein kinase C family, *Eur. J. Biochem.,* 208, 547, 1992.

22. Meydani, M., Evans, W.J., Handelman, G., Biddle, L., Fielding, R.A., Meydani, S.N., Burrill, J., Fiatarone J., Fiatarone, M.A., Blumberg, J.B., and Cannon, J.G., Protective effect of vitamin E on exercise-induced oxidative damage in young and older adults, *Am. J. Physiol.,* 33, R992, 1993.

23. Pette, D. and Spamer, C., Metabolic properties of muscle fibers, *Fed. Proc.,* 45, 2910, 1986.

24. Riley, D.A., Ellis, S., and Bain, J.L., Catalase-positive microperoxisomes in rat soleus and extensor digitorum longus muscle fiber types, *J. Histochem. Cytochem.,* 36, 633, 1988.

25. Lammi-Keefe, C.J., Hegarty, P.V.J., and Swan, PB, Effect of starvation and refeeding on catalase and superoxide dismutase activities in skeletal and cardiac muscles from 12-month-old rats, *Experientia,* 37, 25, 1980.

26. Jenkins, R.R., Newsham, D., Rushmore, P., and Tengie, J., Effect of disuse on the skeletal muscle catalase of rats, *Biochem. Med.,* 27, 195, 1982.

27. Fry, J.M., Smith, G.M., and Speijers, E.J., Plasma and tissue concentrations of alpha- tocopherol during vitamin E depletion in sheep, *Br. J. Nutr.,* 69, 225, 1993.

28. Salviati, G., Betto, R., Margreth, A., Novello, F., and Bonetti, E., Differential binding of vitamin E to sarcoplasmic reticulum from fast and slow muscles of the rabbit, *Experientia,* 36, 1140, 1980.

29. Niyo, Y., Glock, R.D., Ramsey, F.K., and Ewan, R.C., Effects of intramuscular injections of selenium and vitamin E on selenium-vitamin E deficiency in young pigs, *Am. J. Vet. Res.,* 38, 1479, 1977.

30. Van Fleet, J.F. and Ferrans, V.J., Ultrastructural changes in skeletal muscle of selenium-vitamin E-deficient chicks, *Am. J. Vet. Res,* 37, 1081, 1977.

31. Van Fleet, J.F. and Ferrans, V.J., Ultrastructural alterations in skeletal muscle of ducklings fed selenium-vitamin E-deficient diet, *Am. J. Vet. Res.,* 38, 1399, 1977.

32. Chan, A.C. and Hegarty, P.V.J., Morphological changes in skeletal muscles in vitamin E-deficient and refed rabbits, *Br. J. Nutr.,* 38, 361, 1977.

33. Lazaro, R.P., Dentinger, M.P., Rodichok, L.D., Barron, K.D., and Satya-Murti, S., Muscle pathology in Bassen-Kornzweig Syndrome and vitamin E deficiency, *Am. J. Clin. Pathol.,* 86, 378, 1986.

34. Neville, H.E., Ringel, S.P., Guggenheim, M.A., Wehling, C.A., and Starcevich, J.M., Ultrastructural and histochemical abnormalities of skeletal muscle in patients with chronic vitamin E deficiency, *Neurology,* 33, 483, 1983.

35. Walsh, D.M., Kennedy, S., Blanchflower, W.J., Goodall, E.A., and Kennedy, D.G., Vitamin E and selenium deficiencies increase indices of lipid peroxidation in muscle tissue of ruminant calves, *Int. J. Vitam. Nutr. Res.,* 63, 188, 1993.

36. Brady, P.S., Brady, L.J., and Ullrey, D.E., Selenium, vitamin E, and the response to swimming stress in the rat, *J. Nutr.,* 109, 1103, 1979.

37. Dillard, C.J., Dumelin, E.E., and Tappel, A.L., Effect of dietary vitamin E on expiration of pentane and ethane by the rat, *Lipids,* 12, 109, 1977.

38. Salminen, A., Kainulainen, H., Arstila, A.U., and Vihko, V., Vitamin E deficiency and the susceptibility to lipid peroxidation of mouse cardiac and skeletal muscles, *Acta Physiol. Scand.,* 122, 56, 1984.

39. Federico, A., Battisti, C., Eusebi, M.P., de Stefano, N., Malandrini, A., Mondelli, M., and Volpi, N., Vitamin E deficiency secondary to chronic intestinal malabsorption and effect of vitamin supplement. A case report, *Eur. Neurol.,* 31, 366, 1991.

40. Pillai, S.R., Traber, M.G., Kayden, H.J., Cox, N.R., Toivio-Kinnucan, M., Wright, J.C., Braund, K.G., Whitley, R.D., Gilger, B.C., and Steiss, J.E., Concomitant brainstem anoxal dystrophy and necrotizing myopathy in vitamin E-deficient rats, *J. Neurol. Sci.,* 123, 64, 1994.

41. Smith, G.M., Fry, J.M., Allen, J.G., and Costa, N.D., Plasma indicators of muscle damage in a model of nutritional myopathy in weaned sheep, *Aust. Vet. J.,* 71, 12, 1994.

42. Shih, J.C.H., Jonas, R.H., and Scott, M.L., Oxidative deterioration of the muscle proteins during nutritional muscular dystrophy in chicks, *J. Nutr.,* 107, 1786, 1977.

43. De Villers, A., Simard, P., and Srivastava, U., Biochemical changes in progressive muscular dystrophy. X. Studies on the biosynthesis of protein and RNA in cellular fractions of the skeletal muscle of normal and vitamin E-deficient rabbits, *Can. J. Biochem.,* 51, 450, 1973.

44. Dayton, W.R., Schollmeyer, J.V., Chan, A.C., and Allen, C.E., Elevated levels of a calcium-activated muscle protease in rapidly atrophying muscles from vitamin E-deficient rabbits, *Biochim. Biophys. Acta,* 584, 216, 1979.

45. Jackson, M.J., Edwards, R.H.T., and Symons, M.C.R., Electron spin resonance studies of intact mammalian skeletal muscle, *Biochim. Biophys. Acta,* 847, 185, 1985.

46. Dillard, C.J., Litov, R.E., Savin, W.M., Dumelin, E.E., and Tappel, A.L., Effects of exercise, vitamin E, and ozone on pulmonary function and lipid peroxidation, *J. Appl. Physiol.,* 45, 927, 1978.

47. Quintanilha, A.T., Effects of physical exercise and/or vitamin E on tissue oxidative metabolism, *Biochem. Soc. Commun.,* 12, 403, 1984.

48. Starnes, J.W., Cantu, G., Farrar, R.P., and Kehrer, J.P., Skeletal muscle lipid peroxidation in exercised and food-restricted rats during aging, *J. Appl. Physiol.,* 67, 69, 1989.

49. Packer, L., Almada, A.L., Rothfuss, L.M., and Wilson, D.S., Modulation of tissue vitamin E levels by physical exercise, *Ann. N.Y. Acad. Sci.,* 399, 311, 1988.

50. Reznick, A.Z., Witt, E., Matsumoto, M., and Packer, L., Vitamin E inhibits protein oxidation in skeletal muscle of resting and exercised rats, *Biochem. Biophys. Res. Commun.,* 189, 801, 1992.

51. Tiidus, P.M. and Houston, M.E., Vitamin E status does not affect the responses to exercise training and acute exercise in female rats, *J. Nutr.,* 123, 834, 1993.

52. Salminen, A. and Vihko, V., Endurance training reduces the susceptibility of mouse skeletal muscle to lipid peroxidation in vitro, *Acta Physiol. Scand.,* 117, 109, 1983.

53. Viguie, C.A., Frei, B., Shigenaga, M.K., Ames, B.N., Packer, L., and Brooks, G.A., Antioxidant status and indexes of oxidative stress during consecutive days of exercise, *J. Appl. Physiol.,* 75, 566, 1993.

54. Kumar C.T., Reddy V.K., Prasad M., Thyagaraju K., and Reddanna P., Dietary supplementation of Vitamin E protects heart tissue from exercise-induced oxidant stress, *Mol. Cell. Biochem.,* 111, 109, 1992.

55. Sumida, S., Tanaka, K., Kitao, H., and Nakadomo, F., Exercise-induced lipid peroxidation and leakage of enzymes before and after vitamin E supplementation, *Int. J. Biochem.,* 21, 835, 1989.

56. Goldfarb, A.H., McIntosh, M.K., Boyer, B.T., and Fatours, J., Vitamin E effects on indices of lipid peroxidation in muscle from DHEA-treated and exercised rats, *J. Appl. Physiol.,* 76, 1630, 1994.

57. Cannon, J.G., Orencole, S.F., Fielding, R.A., Meydani, M., Meydani, S.N., Fiatarone, M.A., Blumberg, J.B., and Evans, W.J., The acute phase response in exercise: interaction of age and vitamin E on neutrophils and muscle enzyme release, *Am. J. Physiol.,* 259, R1214, 1990.

58. Cannon, J.G., Meydani, S.N., Fielding, R.A., Fiatarone, M.A., Meydani, M., Farhangmehr, M., Orencole, S.F., Blumberg, J.B., and Evans, W.J., Acute phase response in exercise. II. Associations between vitamin E, cytokines, and muscle proteolysis, *Am. J. Physiol.,* 260, R1235, 1991.

59. Babior, B.M., Kiphes, R.S., and Curnutte, J.T., Biological defense mechanisms. The production by leukocytes of superoxide, a potential bacterial agent, *J. Clin. Invest.,* 52, 741, 1973.

60. Hartmann, A., Niess, A.M., Grunert-Fuchs, M., Poch, B., and Speit, G., Vitamin E prevents exercise-induced DNA damage, *Mut. Res.,* 346, 195, 1995.

61. Warren, J.A., Jenkins, R.R., Packer, L., Witt, E.H., and Armstrong, R.B., Elevated muscle vitamin E does not attenuate eccentric exercise-induced muscle injury, *J. Appl. Physiol.,* 72, 2168, 1992.

62. Rokitzki, L., Logemann, E., Sagredos, A.N., Murphy, M., Wetzel-Roth, W., and Keul, J., Lipid peroxidation and antioxidative vitamins under extreme endurance stress, *Acta Physiol. Scan.,* 151, 149, 1994.

63. Saltin, B. and Rowell, L.B., Functional adaptations to physical activity and inactivity, *Fed. Proc.,* 39, 1506, 1980.

64. Fielding, R.A., The role of progressive resistance training and nutrition in the preservation of lean body mass in the elderly, *J. Am. Coll. Nutr.,* 14, 587, 1995.

65. Paffenbarger, R.S., Hyde, R.T., Wing, A.L., and Hsieh, C.-C., Physical activity, all-cause mortality, and longevity of college alumni, *N. Engl. J. Med.,* 314, 605, 1986.

66. Blair, S.N., Kohl, H.W., Paffenbarger, R.S., Clark, D.G., Cooper, K.H., and Gibbons, L.W., Physical fitness and all-cause mortality: a prospective study of healthy men and women, *J. Am. Med. Assoc.,* 262, 2395, 1989.

67. Jenkins, R.R., Friedland, R., and Howald, H., The relationship of oxygen uptake to superoxide dismutase and catalase activity in human skeletal muscle, *Int. J. Sportmed.,* 5, 11, 1984.

68. Higuchi, M., Cartier, L.J., Chen, M., and Holloszy, J.O., Superoxide dismutase and catalase in skeletal muscle: adaptive response in exercise, *J. Gerontol.,* 40, 281, 1985.

69. Laughlin, M.H., Simpson, T., Sexton, W.L., Brown, O.R., Smith, J.K., and Korthuis, R.J., Skeletal muscle oxidative capacity, antioxidant enzymes, and exercise training, *J. Appl. Physiol.,* 68, 2337, 1990.

70. Mbemba, F., Houbion, A., Raes, M., and Remacle, J., Subcellular localization and modification with ageing of glutathione, glutathione peroxidase and glutathione reductase activities in human fibroblasts, *Biochem. Biophys. Acta,* 838, 211, 1985.

71. Ji, L.L., Stratman, F.W., and Lardy, H.A., Antioxidant enzyme systems in rat liver and skeletal muscle, *Arch. Biochem. Biophys.,* 263, 150, 1988.

72. Caladera, C.M., Guarnieri, C., and Lazzari, F., Catalase and peroxidase activity of cardiac muscle, *Boll. Soc. Ital. Biol. Sper.,* 49, 72, 1973.

73. Alessio, H.M. and Goldfarb, A.H., Lipid peroxidation and scavenger enzymes during exercise: adaptive response to training, *J. Appl. Physiol.,* 64, 1333, 1988.

74. Ji, L.L., Stratman, F.W., and Lardy, H.A., Enzymatic downregulation with exercise in rat skeletal muscle, *Arch. Biochem. Biophys.,* 263, 137, 1988.

75. Sen, C.K., Marin, E., Kretzchmar, M., and Hanninen, O., Skeletal muscle and liver glutathione homeostasis in response to training, exercise, and immobilization, *J. Appl. Physiol.,* 73, 1265, 1992.

76. Powers, S.K., Criswell, D., Lawler, J., Ji, L.L., Martin, D., Herb, R.A., and Dudley, G., Influence of exercise and fiber type on antioxidant enzyme activity in rat skeletal muscle, *Am. J. Physiol.,* 266, R375, 1994.

77. Ji, L.L. and Mitchell, E.W., Effects of adriamycin on heart mitochondrial function in rested and exercised rats, *Biochem. Pharmacol.,* 47, 877, 1994.

78. Kanter, M.M., Hamlin, R.L., Unverferth, D.V., Davis, H.W., and Merola, A.J., Effect of exercise training on antioxidant enzymes and cardiotoxicity of doxorubicin, *J. Appl. Physiol.,* 59, 1298, 1985.

79. Powers, S.K., Criswell, D., Lawler, J., Martin, D., Lieu, F.K., Ji, L.L., and Herb, R.A., Rigorous exercise training increases superoxide dismutase activity in ventricular myocardium, *Am. J. Physiol.,* 265, H2094, 1993.

80. Somani, S.M., Frank, S., and Rybak, L.P., Responses of antioxidant system to acute and trained exercise in rat heart subcellular fractions, *Pharmacol. Biochem. Behav.,* 51, 627, 1995.

81. Pyke, S., Low, H., and Quintanilla, A., Severe depletion of liver glutathione during physical exercise, *Biochem. Biophys. Res. Commun.,* 139, 926, 1986.

82. Ji, L.L., Dillon, D., and Wu, E., Alteration of antioxidant enzymes with aging in rat skeletal muscle and liver, *Am. J. Physiol.,* 258, R918, 1990.

83. Lang, J.K., Gohill, K., Packer, L., and Burk, R.F., Selenium deficiency, endurance exercise capacity, and antioxidant status in rats, *J. Appl. Physiol.,* 63, 2532, 1987.

84. Harman, D., Aging: a theory based on free radical and radiation chemistry, *J. Gerontol.,* 11, 298, 1956.

85. Harman, D., Free radical theory of aging: the "free radical" diseases, *Age,* 7, 111, 1984.

86. Lammi-Keefe, C.J., Swan, P.B., and Hegarty, P.V.J., Copper-zinc and manganese superoxide dismutase activities in cardiac and skeletal muscles during aging in male rats, *Gerontology,* 30, 153, 1984.

87. Ji, L.L., Wu, E., and Thomas, D.P., Effect of exercise training on antioxidant and metabolic functions in senescent rat skeletal muscle, *Gerontology,* 37, 317, 1991.

88. Hammeren, J., Powers, S., Lawler, J., Criswell, D., Lowenthal, D., and Pollock, M., Exercise training-induced alterations in skeletal muscle oxidative and antioxidant enzyme activity in senescent rats, *Int. J. Sportsmed.,* 13, 412, 1993.

89. Criswell, D., Powers, S., Dodd, S., Lawler, J., Edwards, W., Renshler, K., and Grinton, S., High intensity training-induced changes in skeletal muscle antioxidant enzyme activity, *Med. Sci. Sports Exercise,* 25, 1135, 1993.

90. Bunnell, R.H., DeRitter, E., and Rubin, S.H., Effects of feeding polyunsaturated fatty acids with a low vitamin E diet on blood levels of tocopherol in men performing hard physical labor, *Am. J. Clin. Nutr.,* 28, 706, 1975.

91. Sharman, I.M., Down, M.G., and Sen, R.N., The effects of vitamin E and training on physiological function and athletic performance in adolescent swimmers, *Br. J. Nutr.,* 26, 265, 1971.

92. Sharman, I.M., Down, M.G., and Norgan, N.G., The effects of vitamin E on physiological function and athletic performance of trained swimmers, *J. Sports Med.,* 16, 215, 1976.

93. Lawrence, J.D., Bower, R.C., Riehl, W.P., and Smith, J.L., Effects of α-tocopherol acetate on the swimming endurance of trained swimmers, *Am. J. Clin. Nutr.,* 28, 205, 1975.

94. Shephard, R.J., Campbell, R., Pimm, P., Stuart, D., and Wright, G.R., Vitamin E, exercise, and the recovery from physical activity, *Eur. J. Appl. Physiol.,* 33, 119, 1974.

95. Watt, T., Romet, T.T., McFarlane, I., McGuey, D., Allen, C., and Goode, R.C., Vitamin E and oxygen consumption, *Lancet,* 2, 354, 1974.
96. Simon-Schnass, I. and Pabst, H., Influence of vitamin E on physical performance, *Int. J. Vitam. Nutr. Res.,* 58, 49, 1988.
97. Snider, I.P., Bazzarre, T.L., Murdoch, S.D., and Goldfarb, A., Effects of coenzyme athletic performance system as an ergogenic aid on endurance performance to exhaustion, *Int. J. Sports Nutr.,* 2, 272, 1992.
98. Singh, V.N., A current perspective on nutrition and exercise, *J. Nutr.,* 122, 760, 1992.
99. Costill, D.L., Carbohydrates for exercise: Dietary demands for optimal performance, *Int. J. Sportsmed.,* 9, 1, 1988.
100. Economos, C.D., Bortz, S.S., and Nelson, M.E., Nutritional practices of elite athletes: practical recommendations, *Sports Med.,* 16, 381, 1993.
101. Nowak, R.K., Knudsen, K.S., and Schulz, L.O., Body composition and nutrient intakes of college men and women basketball players, *J. Am. Diet. Assoc.,* 88, 575, 1988.
102. Van Erp-Baart, A.M., Saris, W.M., Binkhorst, R.A., Vos, J.A., and Elvers, J.W., Nationwide survey on nutritional habits in elite athletes. Mineral and vitamin intake, *Int. J. Sports Med.,* 10, S11, 1989.
103. Williams, M.H., Vitamin supplementation and athletic performance, *Int. J. Vitam. Nutr. Res.,* 30, 163, 1989.
104. Bazzarre, T.L., Scarpino, A., Sigmon, R., Marquart, L.F., Wu, S.M., and Izurieta, M., Vitamin-mineral supplement use and nutritional status of athletes, *J. Am. Coll. Nutr.,* 12, 162, 1993.
105. Weight, L.M., Noakes, T.D., Labadarios, D., Graves, J., Jacobs, P., and Berman, P.A., Vitamin and mineral status of trained athletes including the effects of supplementation, *Am. J. Clin. Nutr.,* 47, 186, 1988.
106. Weight, L.M., Myburgh, K.H., and Noakes, T.D., Vitamin and mineral supplementation: effect on the running performance of trained athletes, *Am. J. Clin. Nutr.,* 47, 192, 1988.

Chapter **11**

IRON

Brian W. Tobin
John L. Beard

CONTENTS

0-8493-8192-4/97/$0.00+$.50
© 1997 by CRC Press, Inc.

I. INTRODUCTION

Among all of the micronutrients, iron possesses the longest and best described history. Iron is the fourth most abundant terrestrial element, comprising approximately 4.7% of the Earth's crust in the form of the minerals hematite, magnetite, and siderite. Primordial iron compounds probably contributed to the catalytic generation of some of the atmospheric oxygen upon which most modern life forms depend.[1] Iron is an essential nutrient for all living organisms with the exception of certain members of the bacterial genera *Lactobacillus* and *Bacillus*. In all other life forms, iron is an essential component of, or cofactor for, hundreds of proteins and enzymes.

Based on extrapolations made from modern aboriginal societies, prehistoric humans probably had an adequate intake of iron.[2] The ancient Chinese, Egyptians, Greeks, and Romans, although ignorant of its nutritional importance, attributed therapeutic properties to iron.[3] These early observations document some of the first links between iron and physical activity. For example, the ancient Greeks administered iron to their injured soldiers to improve muscle weakness, which probably derived from hemorrhagic anemia.[4] Alchemists and physicians of the 16th century prescribed iron for medicinal use.[5,6] Iron salts were given to young women to treat what was then described as chlorosis, an anemia often due to iron or protein deficiency.[4] Curiously, those physicians who prescribed iron pills for anemia were unceremoniously ridiculed by their successors in the medical profession.[7,8]

II. IRON DEFICIENCY

A. DEFINITION AND CLASSIFICATION

Iron deficiency is the most common single nutrient deficiency disease in the world and is a major concern for approximately 15% of the world's population.[9] Approximately 6 to 11% of reproductive age females, 14% of 15 to 19-year-old females, and approximately 25% of pregnant women are iron-deficient in the U.S. and Canada depending on the assessment criteria.[10,11] These criteria attempt to distinguish between tissue iron stores depletion, iron-deficient erythropoiesis, and iron deficiency anemia. The commonly used definition for anemia, for whatever cause, is a low hemoglobin concentration (Hb). If iron deficiency is an underlying etiology, then by definition the individual must have depleted iron stores, a low plasma ferritin, or decreased stainable iron in bone marrow, and an inadequate delivery of iron to tissues as characterized by a low transferrin saturation, a high erythrocyte protoporphyrin concentration, and a elevated transferrin receptor concentration.[12,13]

Iron deficiency can be defined as that moment in time when body iron stores become depleted and a restricted supply of iron to various tissues becomes apparent.[14] The process of depletion of iron stores can occur rapidly or very slowly and is dependent on the balance between iron intake and iron requirements. Clearly, iron intake is dependent on food composition and the quantity of iron therein, with a number of inhibitors and a smaller number of enhancers of iron absorption now known to exist. Iron absorption increases in individuals who have depleted iron stores; it is this internal regulator of absorption that may be more important that any particular constituents of the food supply.[15]

The iron nutritional status of an individual and of populations is largely a function of the amount of dietary iron, the bioavailability of that iron, and the extent of iron losses. Many foods that are potentially good sources of iron are limited by the bioavailability of iron in those foods.[16] The bioavailability of iron is a function of its chemical form and the presence of food items that promote or inhibit absorption. Basal obligatory iron losses in humans are approximately 1 mg/day and must be replaced by an equivalent amount of iron derived from the diet. The typical Western diet provides an average of 6 mg of heme and nonheme iron per 1000 kcals of energy intake.[17,18] Heme iron is an important dietary source of iron because it is more effectively absorbed than nonheme iron; thus, vegetarians can be at risk for iron deficiency. From 5 to 35% of heme iron is absorbed from a single meal, whereas nonheme iron absorption from a single meal can range from 2 to 20% depending on the iron status of the individual and the ratio of enhancers to promoters in the diet. Thus, although it constitutes about 10% of the iron found in the diet, heme iron may provide up to 1/3 of total absorbed dietary iron.[19]

Nonheme iron, which constitutes 90% of the remaining dietary iron, accounts for 60% of the iron from animal sources and about 100% of the iron found in vegetable material. Iron fortification or iron contamination of food during preparation may account for as much as 10 to 15% of dietary nonheme iron.[20] The overall effect of foodstuffs on nonheme iron absorption is inhibitory. The rat, which has been the standard model of iron absorption for humans, appears to be less sensitive to these factors than humans, thus their influence may be underestimated.[21] Conversely, the long-term contributions of these enhancers and promoters to body iron stores may be more limited than first thought.

B. IRON ABSORPTION

The process of iron absorption can be divided into three stages: (1) uptake of luminal iron, (2) intraenterocyte transport, and (3) storage and extraenterocyte transfer. During the intestinal phase of digestion, iron binds to specific mucosal membrane sites, is internalized, and then is either retained by the mucosal cell or is transported to the basolateral membrane where it is bound to transferrin in the plasma pool. The process of iron absorption is controlled by intraluminal, mucosal, and somatic factors. A multitude of intraluminal factors affect the amount of iron available for absorption as either inhibitors or promoters. Mucosal factors include the amount of mucosal surface and intestinal motility. Somatic factors which influence iron absorption include erythropoiesis and hypoxia.

1. Luminal Phase

No absorption of iron occurs in the mouth, esophagus, or stomach. However, the stomach does contribute hydrochloric acid which removes protein-bound iron by denaturation, and solubilizes iron by reducing it from the ferric to the ferrous state. The majority of iron absorption takes place in the duodenum and upper jejunum. Factors which increase transit time through these areas decrease iron absorption.[22] A multitude of dietary factors affect iron absorption during this phase. Heme iron appears to be affected only by animal proteins which facilitate its absorption and calcium which inhibits its absorption.[23] In contrast to heme iron, a large number of factors affect nonheme iron absorption[24] and include bran, hemicellulose, cellulose, pectin, phytic acid found in wheat and soy products, and polyphenolic compounds.[25] The absorption of supplemental iron may be dependent upon the type of prepartation used. The amount of iron bioavailable from multimineral preparations, especially when calcium salts are used, is less than that absorbed during the administration of iron alone.[26,27] These preparations may provide less iron than suspected.

2. Mechanisms of Intestinal Cell Uptake

The complete pathway of iron absorption is largely unknown and is currently a matter of controversy. Basically, heme iron is taken up directly by the enterocyte and, after enzymatic action, is processed in a manner analogous to nonheme iron. Nonheme iron is transferred to binding proteins within the lumen. Specific transporters exist for nonheme iron-binding proteins on the luminal surface of enterocytes. Nonheme iron is transported to the enterocyte interior where it is bound to an iron-binding protein(s). This iron is either transferred to ferritin or to the basolateral side of the enterocyte. Since iron absorption increases with low iron stores and decreases with high iron stores, there may be genetic regulation of both receptors and binding proteins. This regulation appears to be exerted across the basolateral membrane in a manner which is correlated to whole-body iron stores. Iron is then either lost when the cell is sloughed or bound to transferrin in the circulation. Transport of absorbed iron through the enterocyte may involve a transferrin-like protein such as mobilferrin.[28] Since iron status increases the amount of iron retained by the enterocyte, ferritin may act as an "iron sink" for intestinal mucosal cells. Iron that is not transferred to the plasma is stored in mucosal cell ferritin and is lost when the enterocyte is subsequently shed.

C. CONSEQUENCES OF POOR IRON STATUS

Many organs show morphological, physiological, and biochemical changes with iron deficiency in a manner related to the turnover of essential iron-containing proteins. Sometimes this occurs even before there is any significant drop in Hb concentration.[29] Iron deficiency is associated with altered metabolic processes; among them are mitochondrial electron transport, neurotransmitter synthesis, protein synthesis, organogenesis, and others. The manifestations of these specific alterations have been noted in immune function, cognitive performance and behavior, thermoregulatory performance, energy metabolism, and exercise or work performance.[29,30]

1. Assessment of Iron Status
a. *Single Indicators*
The most applicable indicator currently available to monitor iron stores is serum ferritin (Table 1), where the concentration in plasma or serum is proportional to the amount of iron stored in tissue.[31] This measure, however, is highly variable and is affected by both acute and chronic inflammation. The result is a poor sensitivity to true depletion of iron reserves. Under normal circumstances, a serum ferritin level below 12 µg/l is diagnostic of depleted iron stores and in combination with a low Hb is indicative of iron deficiency anemia. However, given the fact that ferritin behaves as an acute phase reactant, this level is disproportionately elevated for each grade of marrow iron in patients with acute and chronic inflammation. It is now known that there is a considerable within-subject day-to-day variation in plasma ferritin concentrations and in other indicators of iron status such as plasma iron and transferrin saturation.[32] The coefficient of variation approaches 25 to 40% in young women and men and is independent of the size of the pool. Thus ferritin measures when used alone, must be evaluated with caution.

b. *Multiple Indicators*
The use of multiple indicators for the assessment of iron status has distinct advantages. Traditional models utilize Hb, transferrin saturation, protoporphyrin, and ferritin as a mechanism to improve the sensitivity of the diagnosis of iron deficiency anemia.[12] The NHANES II and III surveys used this approach with the generation of two basic models for the assignment of iron status. The mean corpuscular volume (MCV) model uses Hb, MCV, and erythrocyte protoporphyrin while the ferritin model replaces MCV with ferritin.[33] Assessment of plasma transferrin receptor concentrations may also be of diagnostic value for the assessment of iron deficiency anemia.[34] The amount of transferrin receptor detected by immunologic techniques is detectable in circulation and has been shown to vary in a reciprocal fashion with the iron status of the subject. This "receptor" fragment is lost into plasma and can be detected by a highly specific enzyme-linked immunosorbant assay. Serum transferrin receptor levels are increased in mild iron deficiency of recent onset.

2. Functional Iron
Four major classes of iron-containing substances carry out reactions in the mammalian system: iron-containing proteins (Hb and myoglobin), iron-sulfur enzymes, heme proteins, and iron-containing enzymes (non-iron sulfur, nonheme enzymes). In iron-sulfur enzymes,

TABLE 1   Indicators Used to Assess Iron Status

Indicator	Indicates	Disadvantages
Single Indicator		
Serum ferritin	Iron stores	Affected by inflammation
		Day to day variation
Hemoglobin	Anemia	Insensitive to iron depletion
Multiple Indicators		
Traditional model:	Iron stores	Complex vs. single indicator
Hb, TFS, FEP, ferritin	Iron-deficient erythropoiesis	
	Anemia	
MCV Model:	Iron-deficient erythropoiesis	Plasma iron not evaluated
Hb, MCV, FEP	Anemia	
	Type of anemia	
Ferritin model:	Iron stores	Type of anemia not known
Hb, ferritin, FEP	Iron-deficient erythropoiesis	
	Anemia	

Note: Hb: Hemoglobin, TFS: transferrin saturation, MCV: mean corpuscular volume, FEP: free erythrocyte protoporphyrin.

iron can be bound to sulfur in four possible arrangements (FeS, 2Fe-2S, 4Fe-4S, 3Fe-4S). However, in humans only three of these occur. In heme proteins, iron is bound to various forms of heme which differ not only in the composition of their side chains but also the methods whereby they are attached to proteins. In humans the predominant form of heme is protoporphyrin-IX.

a.   Oxygen Transport and Storage

The movement of oxygen from the environment to terminal oxidases is one of the key functions of iron in which dioxygen is bound to porphyrin ring iron-containing molecules, either as part of the prosthetic group of Hb within red blood cells or as the facilitator of oxygen diffusion in tissue, myoglobin. Hb is a tetrameric protein with two pairs of identical subunits whose ferrous iron reversibly binds dioxygen. The subunits react cooperatively with dioxygen with specific modulation by pH, pCO_2, organic phosphates, and temperature. These modulators determine the efficiency of transport of oxygen from the alveoli capillary interface in the lung to the red cell-capillary tissue interface in peripheral tissues. 2,3-Diphosphoglycerate is a product of accelerated metabolism in erythrocytes and decreases Hb-O_2 binding affinity. This causes a right shift of the dissociation curve, favoring unloading of oxygen into tissues in anemia. Myoglobin is the single chain hemoprotein in cytoplasm of cells and increases the rate of diffusion of dioxygen from capillary red blood cells to cytoplasm and mitochondria. The concentration of myoglobin in muscle is drastically reduced in tissue iron deficiency, thus limiting the rate of diffusion of dioxygen from erythrocytes to mitochondria.[29]

b.   Electron Transport

The cytochromes contain heme as the active site with the Fe-porphyrin ring functioning to reduce ferrous iron to ferric iron with the acceptance of electrons. The iron-sulfur proteins also act as electron carriers via the action of iron bound to either two or four sulfur atoms and cysteine side chains. The 40 different proteins that constitute the respiratory chain contain 6 different heme proteins, 6 iron-sulfur centers, 2 copper centers, as well as ubiquinone to connect NADH to oxygen. Several hundred enzyme activities have also been ascribed to the cytochrome P450 family of enzymes. As noted in the review of Dallman,[29] a good number of these enzymes will decrease in activity with iron deficiency.

3. Manifestations of Iron Deficiency

The overt physical manifestations of chronic iron deficiency are glossitis, angular stomatitis, koilonychia (spoon nails), blue sclera, esophageal webbing (Plummer-Vinson Syndrome), and anemia. Behavioral disturbances such as pica (abnormal consumption of dirt [geophagia] and ice [pagophagia]) are often present in iron deficiency. Physiological manifestations of iron deficiency include altered immune function, cognitive performance and behavior, thermoregulatory performance, energy metabolism, and exercise or work performance.[29,30] Many of these manifestations are not mutually exclusive, and may also occur only during certain stages of iron deficiency.

The progression of iron deficiency occurs in two steps related to depletion of iron stores prior to depletion of functional iron (Table 2): (1) bone marrow, spleen, and liver stores depletion and, (2) diminished erythropoiesis due to a negative iron balance leading to anemia and decreased activity of iron-dependent enzymes. Clinically, iron deficiency is frequently diagnosed by anemia secondary to long-term diminished erythropoiesis. Depletion of the storage iron pool is generally without influence on physiologic function with a few exceptions. Nearly all functional consequences are more strongly related to human "anemia" rather than tissue iron deficits. The challenge of separating O_2 transport/events from tissue iron deficits still looms large and its importance in exercise and sport will be discussed later in this chapter.

TABLE 2   Biochemical Values in Normal, Iron Depletion, and Iron Deficiency Anemia

	Normal	Iron Depletion	Iron Deficiency Anemia
Transferrin iron-binding capacity (µg/100 ml)	330	360	410
Plasma iron (µg/100 ml)	115	<115	<40
Plasma ferritin (ng/ml)	60	<12	<12
Transferrin saturation (%)	35	35	<16
Red blood cell protoporphyrin (µg/100 ml)	30	30	>100
Mean corpuscular volume (µ^3)			<80
Hematocrit (%)	>30	<30	<30

From Beard, J. L, Iron Fortification — Rationale and Effects, *Nutrition Today,* July/August, 1986. With permission.

Several of the well-known consequences of iron deficiency that occur after the depletion of iron stores are the decline in Hb concentration, the decrease in mean corpuscular Hb concentration, a decrease in the size and volume of the new red cells, reduced myoglobin, and reduced amounts of both Fe-S and heme iron-containing cytochromes within cells. Diffusion of dioxygen from Hb into tissue becomes limited due to fewer erythrocytes, increased membrane diffusivity, and a decreased tissue myoglobin concentration. In severe anemia, oxygen transport is clearly limiting to tissue oxidative function at anything but the resting condition[29] despite a right-shifted Hb-O_2 dissociation curve and increased cardiac output. Tissue extraction of oxygen is increased by this compensation and mixed venous PO_2 is significantly lower in anemic individuals. While Hb-O_2 affinity compensation is reasonable at sea level, just the opposite direction of compensation occurs in anemic individuals at high altitudes (4000 m). The Hb-O_2 dissociation curve is "left-shifted" in these hypobaric hypoxic conditions to increase O_2 loading in the lung at the expense of tissue delivery.[35] The very significant decrease in myoglobin and other iron-containing proteins in skeletal muscle in iron deficiency anemia contributes significantly to the decline in muscle aerobic capacity.[29]

A typical repair curve for muscle iron-containing and oxidative enzymes during iron repletion experiments has been described.[36] Pyruvate and malate oxidase were decreased to 35% of normal in iron-deficient muscle and improved to 85% of normal in 10 days of treatment. 2-Oxoglutarate oxidase was decreased to 47% of normal and improved to 90%; in contrast, succinate oxidase was only 10% of normal in iron deficiency and improved to only 42% of normal after 10 days. Cytoplasmic enzymes hexokinase and lactate dehydrogenase were unaffected by iron status. The 50 to 90% decrease in both the Fe-S enzymes and in the heme-containing mitochondrial cytochromes are consistent with many other observations over the last two decades.[29] What seems to determine the amount of decline in activity with cellular iron deprivation is the turnover rate of iron-containing proteins.

III. IRON AND EXERCISE

Given our knowledge of the physiology and biochemistry of iron deficiency and anemia, and its relation to oxygen transport and metabolic function, it is relevant to ask whether altered iron status could affect exercise performance. It is also important to delineate whether exercise itself may promulgate altered iron status, and whether such alterations are detrimental to athletic performance or to the health of an athlete. While a multitude of laboratories worldwide have contributed to a very broad-based accumulation of knowledge in these areas, an analysis of over two decades of research illustrates four central points. First, it is clear that reductions in heme and nonheme iron can detrimentally alter exercise performance. Second, it is documented that measures of heme and nonheme iron are altered in certain populations of chronically exercising individuals. Third, it has been illustrated that women may have an increased prevalence for exercise-related alterations in body iron. Fourth, although such alterations can be demonstrated, it is prudent to question whether these manifestations are specifically detrimental to the health or the athletic performance of the athlete.

In the following sections we review the literature supporting these contentions, and reiterate an often overlooked hypothesis regarding the influence of exercise on the distribution of body iron. We propose that alterations in heme and nonheme body iron do occur in certain populations of athletes, and that these manifestations occur in part due to a combination of transiently increased plasma volume, alterations in dietary intake, increased iron losses, and may also be influenced by an exercise-related redistribution of body iron.

A. IRON AND EXERCISE PERFORMANCE

The role of heme and nonheme iron in biologic function and work performance has been elucidated through human and animal experiments, and several classic reviews have been published.[8,37-39] For the purpose of the present discussion, however, a review of submaximal vs. maximal exercise performance is useful to delineate nonheme vs. heme iron contributions to athletic performance. Considering the effects of anemia vs. tissue iron deficiency is important in critically evaluating the functional role of iron in athletic performance, and proposing dietary recommendations specific to the athletic population.

1. Animal Studies

Iron plays a unique role in the transport of oxygen to tissues via heme compounds, and the generation of ATP from reducing equivalents via iron-dependent cytochrome enzymes. The availability of iron in Hb is thus critical to the functioning of the red blood cells and their ability to carry oxygen to tissues undergoing increased levels of oxidative metabolism. At the tissue level, many iron-dependent enzymes such as pyruvate oxidase, mitochondrial cytochromes, cytochrome p-450, ribonucleotide reductase, tyrosine and proline hydrolase, monoamine oxidase, catalase, glucose 6-phosphatase, and 6-phosphogluconate dehydrogenase[40,41] are responsible for metabolism of energetic substrates, energy transformation, and energy liberation. Therefore, it is not surprising that heme iron, when lacking, can profoundly alter physical work performance. What is intriguing, however, is that although nonheme iron associated with enzyme systems comprises only 1% of total body iron, profound deficits of these components per se may have detrimental effects upon athletic performance. Understanding the functional consequences of a deficit between heme and nonheme iron requires differentiating between anemia and iron deficiency when studying maximal exercise vs. endurance exercise performance at reduced exercise intensities.

A series of seminal investigations performed by Finch and co-workers[42] differentiated the effects of anemia from tissue iron deficiency in the rat. In a unique animal model, rats made iron-deficient were studied vs. control counterparts. Iron-deficient animals were then transfused with red blood cells from control donor rats to attain a normal hematocrit (HCT), while control animals had blood sequentially removed and plasma reinfused to reduce their packed-cell volume. This paradigm produced animals that were (1) iron-deficient and anemic, (2) iron-deficient without anemia, (3) anemic without iron deficiency, and (4) normal controls. Work performance of control and iron-deficient animals before and after exchange transfusion to Hb of approximately 12 to 14 g/dl was compared. These studies illustrated that with anemia, in both control and iron-deficient animals, there is a marked decrease in running ability. When iron-deficient and control animals were retransfused to a control Hb concentration there was an impressive recovery in running ability in the control animals at about 10 g/dl Hb concentration. However, the iron-deficient animals were still markedly impaired in running ability. These studies illustrated that muscle dysfunction does exist in iron deficiency anemia of sufficient severity, but that this dysfunction is ordinarily hidden by anemia.[42]

Davies et al.[43,44] extended the observations of Finch et al.[42] by further delineating the relative contributions of anemia and tissue iron deficiency to maximal work efforts vs. endurance performance. Using a similar experimental paradigm, these studies illustrated that maximal oxygen consumption is determined primarily by the oxygen-carrying capacity of the blood and is thus correlated to the degree of anemia. Endurance performance at reduced exercise intensities, however, is more closely related to tissue iron levels since a strong association is seen between the ability to maintain prolonged submaximal exercise and the activity of the oxidative enzyme pyruvate oxidase. Taken together, the studies of Finch et al.[42] and Davies et al.[43,44] illustrated that tissue iron is associated with endurance performance at submaximal workloads, whilst Hb-associated iron plays an important role in oxidative capacity and maximal aerobic work performance.

In order to more clearly delineate the influence of a specific concentration of Hb upon aerobic work capacity, Perkkio et al.[45] studied the effects of various levels of iron deficiency upon changes in work performance of rats. Maximal oxygen consumption was measured relative to Hb concentration to determine the functional consequences of anemia upon % $\dot{V}O_2$max. Maximal oxygen consumption declined 16% with a decrease in Hb from 14 to 8 g/dl, but fell more rapidly below a Hb of 7 g/dl.[45] Bouts of treadmill exercise to exhaustion illustrated that endurance capacity declines abruptly (73%) between a Hb of 10 and 8 g/dl. These data illustrated the concept of a Hb threshold in rats, below which exercise performance rapidly deteriorates.

2. Human Studies

Research with human subjects verifies the importance of iron to work performance yet does not necessarily directly support the concept of a Hb threshold phenomenon. In two separate studies, Gardner and co-workers[46,47] evaluated the physical work capacity and metabolic stress in iron-deficient workers of a tea farm in Sri Lanka. In one study, 13 men and 16 women with Hb levels of 4 to 12 g/dl were divided into either an iron treatment or placebo group.[46] Hematologic, cardiorespiratory, and exercise performance data were collected before, during, and after iron supplementation and compared to control subjects. The data showed that blood lactate during exercise is higher in placebo than controls. In addition, 15% more

O_2 was delivered per pulse in the iron-treated group, and peak exercise heart rates were reduced after iron treatment. It was apparent that work performance which requires a high rate of oxygen delivery is significantly affected by Hb levels.[46] In a second study, Gardner et al.[47] evaluated exercise performance in 75 female subjects with Hb levels from 6.1 to 15.9 g/dl. When performance time to exhaustion was measured, the lower Hb groups had the lowest exercise tolerance.

Research by Edgerton et al.[48] suggested that the decrement in work performance in iron-deficient anemic subjects was a reflection of the level of anemia rather than other non-Hb-related biochemical changes. When iron-deficient subjects were retransfused, work tolerance was the same as in those subjects who had the same posttransfusion Hb levels. Unlike the data of Perkkio et al.[45] these studies suggested a more linear relationship between Hb and work performance and thus do not necessarily support the presence of a Hb threshold phenomenon. Nonetheless, these studies taken together illustrate the importance of Hb-associated iron to aerobic work performance where delivery of oxygen to metabolic tissues is limiting at high-intensity work loads.

B. EXERCISE ALTERS IRON STATUS
1. Animal Studies

Animal studies illustrate both beneficial and detrimental effects of exercise on iron status and its functional consequences. In additional experiments to those previously reviewed, Perkkio and co-workers[49] further differentiated the effects of iron deficiency and exercise training on work performance in Sprague-Dawley rats. Treadmill exercise training intensity for control animals was matched over an eight-week period to that of iron-deficient animals. Iron-deficient exercised animals improved in endurance capacity relative to sedentary counterparts. These studies illustrated a beneficial effect of exercise upon the work performance of iron-deficient animals. The data suggest interactive adaptations in iron-deficient trained animals which enhance endurance performance and favor oxidative metabolism at rest. Willis et al.[50,51] extended these observations and subsequently determined iron-deficient trained animals will increase TCA cycle and electron transport chain capacity compared to sedentary counterparts. These studies illustrated a 15% increase in cytochrome C, a 15% increase in TCA cycle enzymes, and a 33% increase in the manganese superoxide dismutase. Thus, compensatory mechanisms favoring oxidative metabolism are apparently partially up-regulated in iron-deficient exercised animals, in an attempt to offset the effects of a compromised metabolic status.

In a series of experiments conducted in our own laboratories the interactive effects of iron and exercise were considered. These studies[52] illustrated that 12 weeks of submaximal exercise training per se (treadmill running) at 65 to 70% $\dot{V}O_2$max did not alter HCT, Hb, mean corpuscular Hb, red blood cell mass, or serum iron of iron-deficient exercised animals; however, an interactive effect of diet and exercise exerted a significant effect upon HCT. In addition to hematologic alterations, there were significant differences in the kinetic behavior of vascular iron. That is, the rate of clearance of iron from the plasma pool (fractional iron clearance) was increased 16% in iron-deficient exercised animals when compared to their sedentary iron-deficient controls. A portion of this increase could be attributed to an enhanced red blood cell uptake of radiolabeled iron (red cell-associated iron). We were unable to duplicate studies in humans, however, which suggested a more fragile red blood cell;[53] in our studies erythrocyte osmotic fragility was not altered by exercise. Taken together, the ferrokinetic data illustrated that iron-deficient exercised animals behaved in a manner characteristic of a heightened state of iron deficiency. The kinetic behavior of iron suggested that exercise exerts an independent effect upon vascular iron, and may alter certain aspects of the distribution of iron.

2. Human Studies

Early studies documented changes in the serum ferritin, Hb HCT, and serum iron-binding capacity of athletes involved in intense physical activity.[54-56] Several researchers coined the phrase "sports anemia" to characterize the hematologic changes occurring during periods of intense physical activity.[57,58] The exact nature of a true sports-related anemia and the relative contributions of altered blood volume vs. red blood cell mass, however, is still the subject of debate in the literature.[59] The reader is directed to more comprehensive reviews on iron and exercise.[60,61]

Several studies conducted as early as two decades ago documented altered iron status in athletes, yet questioned whether such alterations were physiologically detrimental. Wijn et al.[54] measured Hb, packed cell volume, serum iron, and iron-binding capacity of selected athletes and compared these to the hematologic profile of officials during the 1968 Olympic games. These data illustrated an iron-deficient anemia in 2% of male and 2.5% of female athletes and a mild anemia without signs of iron depletion in 3% of the athletic population. Defaux et al.[62] studied the serum ferritin, transferrin, haptoglobin, and iron levels in middle- and long-distance runners, elite rowers, and professional racing cyclists. Interestingly, runners had significantly lower ferritin, iron, and haptoglobin values than did the controls. The authors speculated that a recurring hemoglobinuria might produce diminished iron reserves in middle- and long-distance runners. Radomski et al.[63] evaluated hematologic changes in physically fit young soldiers who marched 35 km/day for 6 days at 35% of their $\dot{V}O_2$max. These studies showed that 4 days of marching produced a decrease in the number of erythrocytes, and in the HCT. This "sports anemia" persisted beyond day 6 into the postmarch period and was accompanied by decreases in Hb, mean corpuscular volume, mean corpuscular Hb concentration, and mean corpuscular Hb.[63] Dressendorfer and co-workers[64] presented data on RBC number, Hb, and related hematological factors in 12 marathon runners during a 20-day, 312-mi road race. These experiments demonstrated a significant decrease in RBC number and a decrease in Hb. However, the authors were among the first to suggest that the observed hematological manifestations may represent a pseudoanemia with no adverse functional consequences. Although the runners became marginally anemic during the race, their running speeds were not affected.[64]

Subsequent investigations have supported these early studies and have demonstrated a reduction in Hb and HCT in certain athletic populations.[65-67] It has been further documented that the incidence of altered iron status may be increased in distance runners;[65,68,69] however, others contend that such a relationship may not exist[70-72] or that alterations in iron status may be obscured by gender-specific manifestations. Those who engage in strength training seem to be marginally affected, with only slight, nonclinically significant alterations in iron status despite rigorous training regimens.[73,74] What seems to be a repeatable phenomenon, however, is a decreased serum ferritin concentration in athletes engaging in chronic aerobic activities such as distance running.[75-77] As a measure of iron stores in the absence of inflammation, a decrease in serum ferritin concentration would be indicative of prelatent iron deficiency prior to the development of overt anemia.[38,39] The functional consequences of such alterations will be discussed further in a later section of this chapter.

Several investigators have proposed mechanisms by which iron balance could be affected by intense physical exercise.[53,78-80] Explanations include increased gastrointestinal blood losses following running,[79] and hematuria as a result of erythrocyte rupture within the foot during running.[53,78] Brune et al.[80] has suggested that the iron losses in sweat would have little bearing upon the variation in total body iron stores seen with severe exercise.

C. GENDER DIFFERENCES IN IRON STATUS OF ATHLETES

There is a growing body of evidence which suggests that the prevalence of iron deficiency without anemia is increased in female athletes. Contributing to this observation is an increased iron loss through regular menstrual function as well as putative dietary factors. Given these observations, if exercise does further compromise iron status then it would logically follow that the population of chronically exercising female athletes may be at greater risk for developing iron deficiency.

Newhouse and colleagues[81-83] elucidated the implications of iron deficiency in female athletes. The most compelling evidence for iron depletion is the observation of altered serum ferritin concentrations, which are generally lower in female athletes. Studies by several groups[60,76,84-86] documented a greater incidence of decreased serum ferritin in female runners. Estimates of deficiency prevalence from these separate studies illustrate a range of decreased serum ferritin vs. controls. Three cited studies[83] demonstrate that 35% of female athletes have a serum ferritin concentration <12 µg/l,[76] 82% are <25 µg/l,[86] or 60% are <30 µg/l,[81] values higher than sedentary counterparts from the nonathletic female population. Although estimations of the precise prevalence rates differ, an increased incidence of reduced serum ferritin seems to be a repeatable observation between laboratories in this population.

Fogelhom[87] recently reviewed studies[69,70,88-90] comparing female controls vs. athletic populations, and also suggested that suboptimal serum ferritin concentrations are more likely to be found in female than male athletes. These results may be influenced by menstrual flow, and may additionally be affected by dietary iron intake. This contention is supported by studies[77] which indicate that female runners consuming a lactovegetarian diet exhibit a higher incidence of serum ferritin depletion than nonvegetarian counterparts. Taken together these investigations illustrate a statistically significant difference between female athletes and control populations. What these investigations do not demonstrate, however, is a clinically subnormal or reduced serum ferritin concentration concurrent with a demonstrated functional consequence in the absence of overt anemia.

D. FUNCTIONAL CONSEQUENCES OF EXERCISE-RELATED IRON ALTERATIONS

A number of investigators have illustrated a higher prevalence of iron deficiency without anemia in certain populations of chronically exercising individuals. It is suggested that gender differences may in part explain a portion of these observed data. However, the overt hyperchromic microcytic anemia of classic iron deficiency, which clinically presents with a reduction in oxygen-carrying capacity, decreased oxidative metabolism, and reduced exercise performance, is likely not of ubiquitous concern for athletic populations. One reason for this position is that the marginal decrements in Hb and HCT documented by laboratories worldwide do not appear to be a phenomenon which can be disassociated from the transient blood volume alterations which confound determinations of iron status.[91] Thus, the following section will focus on delineating a series of experiments which illustrate the functional consequences of decreased tissue iron upon exercising individuals. Given that alterations in tissue-associated iron seem to be more prevalent an observation,[83,87] the potential influence of these alterations upon the nonheme pool of body iron will be examined relative to exercise performance. Relevant to these discussions are a series of investigations which illustrate effects of iron deficiency upon metabolic systems other than those directly related to oxygen transport and illustrate alterations in substrate utilization and delivery.

1. Iron Deficiency and Fuel Homeostasis

Aside from the role that heme iron plays in transporting oxygen to tissues, tissue iron deficiency may influence basic processes of energy metabolism (Table 3). One of the first studies to demonstrate this was performed by Henderson et al.,[92] who illustrated that irondeficient animals are characterized by an increased basal metabolic rate and increased glucose oxidation. The laboratories of Brooks et al.[93] later confirmed that iron-deficient rats have an enhanced reliance upon glucose as a metabolic substrate and that this phenomenon is characterized by enhanced glucose turnover and oxidation. With an increased reliance upon glucose, however, it would stand to reason that mechanisms would be required to insure adequate delivery of substrate for metabolism. Support of this concept was demonstrated by Farrell et al.,[94] who illustrated that a part of the increased utilization of glucose in iron-deficient animals may be explained by enhanced insulin sensitivity. Borel and colleagues[95] later expanded on this observation and demonstrated a left-shifted glucose-insulin sensitivity curve in iron-deficient rats through the use of hyperinsulinemic-euglycemic glucose clamp experiments. Assuming that the glucose transporter function of iron-deficient animals is analogous to the general population, such adaptations would physiologically favor the uptake of blood glucose into the cytosol via insulin-dependent glucose transporters.[96-98] Taken together, these experiments illustrate an increased reliance upon glucose as a metabolic substrate, and a putative up-regulation of mechanisms responsible for the transport of glucose from the plasma into the cytosol of insulin-dependent tissues in iron-deficient animals. A titration of body iron stores against the observed level of these dependent variables has not yet been accomplished in humans. However, the studies described suggest a pivotal role of iron in the maintenance of fuel homeostasis and aerobic metabolism beyond that ascribed to the delivery of oxygen to metabolically active tissue beds. More importantly, they suggest that decrements in body iron may favor the reprioritization of fuel homeostasis in favor of pathways which provide increased production and delivery of glucose carbon for entry into the TCA cycle.[99,100]

TABLE 3   Physiological Effects of Exercise with Anemia and/or Iron Deficiency

Anemia	Iron Deficiency
Decreased oxygen delivery	Increased glucose oxidation
Decreased $\dot{V}O_2$max	Increased lactic acid production
Decreased endurance performance	Increased RQ
Decreased oxidative metabolism	Decreased endurance performance?
Increased glucose oxidation	
Increased lactic acid production	
Increased RQ	

Note: $\dot{V}O_2$max: maximal oxygen consumption; RQ: Respiratory quotient (moles CO_2 produced/moles O_2 consumed).

2.   Tissue Iron and Exercise Performance

In view of studies which suggest significant detrimental effects of exercise on iron status, it is salient to reiterate that exercise, per se, may beneficially influence nonheme iron-associated metabolic machinery. That iron-deficient exercise-trained animals demonstrate beneficial adaptations to exercise was illustrated by Willis et al.[50,51,101] Iron-deficient trained animals had increased TCA cycle activity, pyruvate carboxylation, and electron transport chain capacity compared to sedentary counterparts. Increased cytochrome C, TCA cycle enzymes, and manganese superoxide dismutase were also observed in trained iron-deficient animals. These investigations support the concept that increases in iron-associated systems which require an enhanced delivery of glucose as a metabolic substrate are more prevalent in animals whose iron status is compromised by physical activity. They also support the speculation that the iron-related adaptations observed in chronically exercising individuals may not be entirely detrimental, but may compensatorily favor up-regulation of metabolic pathways which enhance delivery of substrates prerequisite for enhanced work performance.[102]

One cannot discount, however, that a severe decrement in tissue-associated iron in the presence of overt iron deficiency anemia can be detrimental to work performance. The seminal studies which illustrated a profound, rapid effect of iron supplementation upon exercise capacity were performed by Willis and colleagues.[103] These studies built upon the work of

Finch et al.[42] and Davies et al.[43,44] by creating an experimental paradigm where anemia effects could also be considered separate from the role of nonheme iron. In these studies ionic iron was supplied to iron-deficient rats to evaluate influences of non-Hb-associated iron upon exercise capacity.[103] Work time to fatigue at submaximal exercise intensities was evaluated, thus delineating the effects of iron supplementation upon oxidative metabolism. Rats made iron-deficient were given an intraperitoneal injection of iron dextran (50 mg/kg) and endurance time was measured 15 and 18 h after treatment. These experiments illustrated a substantial increase in exercise time to exhaustion, suggesting that iron as a cofactor in the enzyme systems of oxidative metabolic pathways plays a central role in endurance, submaximal exercise performance.

What one must critically consider, however, is whether a decrement in serum ferritin to levels indicative of a clinically defined deficiency (<12 µg/l) or higher, would have a deleterious effect upon athletic performance in the absence of overt anemia. Several studies probe this issue. Studies of $\dot{V}O_2$max of iron-deficient women[104,105] who demonstrate anemia, illustrate that although circulating lactic acid is reduced following iron supplementation, no change in $\dot{V}O_2$max is observed. Newhouse and Clement[83] later illustrated that raising the serum ferritin from 12.3 to 37.7 µg/l did not enhance maximal work capacity. A more recent study by Lukaski et al.[106] investigated the effects of a depletion and repletion of iron stores upon maximal work capacity, without the induction of overt anemia. Serum ferritin was reduced from 26 to 6 µg/l by repeated venisection. These studies illustrated no change in $\dot{V}O_2$max at the reduced serum ferritin concentration (Hb 12 ± 2 g/dl), yet an increased CO_2 production and elevated post-exercise lactate were observed. These studies in human female subjects extended earlier studies[92,94,95] by indirectly indicating an increased reliance upon glucose as a metabolic substrate in iron depleted, nonanemic subjects. Consistent with the earlier studies of Finch et al.[42] and Davies et al.,[43,44] these data support the concept that heme iron is a primary determinant of maximal exercise performance, and nonheme tissue associated iron is more closely correlated to performance at less than maximal workloads.

While a number of laboratories have demonstrated equivocal results in maximal work performance with iron supplementation,[81,107-110] a singular study by Rowland et al.[105] illustrated that increasing serum ferritin can enhance endurance performance. This one study seems to stand alone. Thus, what remains to be consistently verified is whether endurance performance at workloads of say 35 to 65% of $\dot{V}O_2$max would be detrimentally affected by iron deficiency without anemia. A titration of serum ferritin values in the 5 to 50 µg/l range vs. work time to exhaustion at submaximal exercise intensities has yet to be performed by any laboratory, and could importantly shed light on this unresolved issue.

E. BODY IRON REDISTRIBUTION IN ATHLETES MAY CONTRIBUTE TO ALTERED IRON STATUS

By far, the majority of studies which address effects of exercise upon iron status assume that either a decreased uptake or an increased loss may be responsible for altered iron status of athletes. An additional possibility is that the distribution of body iron might also be affected by exercise (Table 4). The first studies which suggested a redistribution of body iron to exercise-related organs were performed by Ohira and colleagues.[111] These experiments confirmed the effects of tissue iron deficiency in rats and demonstrated that the distribution of iron may be influenced by iron deficiency in organs which play a central role in exercise performance. For the vast majority of muscles and organs, both non-Hb tissue iron and mitochondrial iron concentrations show similar decrements as a result of iron deficiency.[111] Tracer studies performed with ^{59}Fe illustrated that the heart and soleus muscle showed an increased incorporation of radio-iron tracer into the mitochondrion of the iron-deficient animals. These data suggested that the kinetics of distribution of iron uptake seem to reflect the ability of the organism to preferentially utilize iron in those organs and tissues directly related to work performance.[111]

TABLE 4   Putative Effects of Exercise on Body Iron Status

Iron Balance	Iron Distribution
Decreased iron intake	Increased mobilzation of storage iron
Decreased iron absorption	Increased iron incorporation into muscle
Increased iron losses	Redistribution of iron
Intravascular hemolysis	Loss from hepatocytes
Gastrointestinal blood losses	Uptake into RE system
Increased iron loss in sweat	Altered kinetic behavior of vascular iron

Note: Re: reticuloendothelial.

An alternative hypothesis which may in part explain exercise related iron alterations was first presented by Magnussen et al.[65] who postulated that a diminished body iron may not be the sole mechanism contributing to altered iron status of athletes. Magnussen suggested that a redistribution of iron from the reticuloendothelial cells to the hepatocytes might explain a reduced serum ferritin. This possibility is indirectly supported by the studies of Ohira et al.[111] and our own investigations,[52] which demonstrated alterations in the kinetic behavior and distribution of vascular iron in exercised iron-deficient rats. In the latter studies, the rate of disappearance of iron from the plasma pool was increased, and the uptake of iron by red blood cells was increased. Such observations are consistent with a hyperplastic bone marrow and increased circulating reticulocytes, and also may indicate an enhanced delivery of iron to extravascular sites possessing a transferrin receptor.

Other studies additionally support the notion that iron redistributions may occur with exercise. If acute or chronic physical activity does trigger an acute phase response through muscle damage or altered hormonal status, then a redistribution of iron may be favored.[112,113] In support of this hypothesis are data which illustrate increases in acute phase proteins including ferritin, secondary to modulations by the cytokines IL-1, or TNF-α.[114,115] In an inflammatory response, the release of iron to serum transferrin is inhibited secondary to an increased serum ferritin synthesis. Such conditions are characteristic of the anemia of chronic disease.[116] Whether such mechanisms are operative in chronically or acutely exercising individuals, and whether such alterations might contribute to the altered iron status of athletes remains to be determined. Such a hypothesis is nonetheless intriguing, and is consistent with previously mentioned kinetic data in animals[52,111] and supports the initial postulate by Magnussen.[65] A more concrete verification of this hypothesis would certainly warrant a reexamination of the accepted contention that body iron balance is primarily determined by the rate of iron absorption from the gastrointestinal tract.[117] It is interesting to consider that iron balance, as defined by input minus output, may need to be evaluated separate from the compartmental distribution of body iron in chronically exercising individuals, given that comparisons of iron losses to iron intake may not clearly differentiate the adequacy of the iron status of athletes.[118]

IV. RECOMMENDATIONS

The Recommended Dietary Allowances (RDA) established by the Food and Nutrition Board of the National Academy of Sciences-National Research Council were revised most recently in 1989.[119] These recommendations are designed for the maintenance of good nutrition of practically all healthy people, and they define intakes of iron for infants, children, men, and women, and also consider additional needs during pregnancy and lactation. For men ages 11 to 18, the RDA is 12 mg/day; for those older than 19 years, 10 mg/day. Women who are not pregnant or lactating should consume 15 mg/day at ages 11 to 50, and those who are older than 51 should consume 10 mg/day. There are no specific recommendations regarding intake of iron for those engaging in vigorous physical activity or sport. Thus, in lieu of such a recommendation a list of nutritional priorities may be useful to preclude altered iron status in athletes. From the data presented in this review, the following recommendations broadly apply to the three groups which appear to be at greatest risk of developing altered body iron given the data available. These recommendations do not assume that a deficiency will exist in these populations when consuming the RDA. However, a deficiency may be more likely, thus warranting closer dietary monitoring and regularly scheduled hematologic evaluations in these at-risk groups.

1. *Female athletes* are advised to pay particular attention to maintaining an adequate consumption of iron in their diet.
2. *Distance runners* should also pay attention to maintaining an adequate consumption of iron-rich foods.
3. *Vegetarian athletes* should be particularly vigilant to include iron-rich foods in their diet.

For all three groups, monitoring of dietary intake, and good nutritional counseling by a Registered Dietitian (RD) may preclude a negative iron balance and should be the first line of action in the prevention of iron deficiency. Indiscriminant pharmacologic intervention should be viewed as an undesirable means of achieving adequate iron intake since, in the least, it marginalizes the importance of promoting good nutritional habits in the athletic population. From the above priorities it is apparent that the female runner who consumes a vegetarian diet would likely be at greatest risk for a negative iron balance. Therefore, it is advisable that these women consider regular evaluation of nutritional intake to preclude iron deficiency. The RDA of 15 mg/day is suggested (ages 11 to 50). However, if iron intake cannot be adjusted by dietary means and if hematologic evaluation warrants, then iron supplements may be desirable.

The use of supplements, however, must be a judicious choice based not upon the likelihood of anemia, but ideally upon hematologic evaluation. At present, approximately 40% of adults utilize over-the-counter mineral or vitamin-mineral products.[120] However, it should be noted that the optimal dose of iron is still unresolved, as is the most effective means of administration of that dose of iron. The amount of iron bioavailable from multimineral preparations, especially when calcium salts are used, is less than that absorbed during the administration of iron alone.[26,27] Using these complex preparations may provide less iron than suspected, and warrant a careful reexamination with regard to efficacy. Clinically utilized oral iron preparations contain ferrous sulfate, hydrated or gluconated, or ferrous gluconate, or ferrous fumarate.[121] These preparations contain from 37 to 106 mg elemental iron. Supplementation is not without consequence, however; the use of high doses of supplemental iron is often associated with gastrointestinal distress and constipation, with a subsequent decline in compliance. In those genetically predisposed, hemochromatosis may develop following iron supplementation. Iron toxicity may even develop in those not genetically predisposed when ingesting dosages of 75 mg or more.[122] In addition, accidental poisoning via iron supplements is one of the most common causes of pediatric poisoning in the U.S., with toxic doses estimated as low as 60 mg/kg body weight for infants and children.[121]

V. CONCLUSION

In summary, it is clear that a decreased HCT and Hb will impair delivery of oxygen to tissues and lead to a reduced maximal oxygen uptake. Supplementation of individuals to normal HCT verifies the effects of heme iron on $\dot{V}O_2$max. However, the effects of iron supplementation upon the athletic performance of those with clinically low serum ferritin is less clear, although limited evidence seems to suggest improved endurance performance and a decreased reliance upon glucose as an oxidative substrate. Whether such adaptations are beneficial at a subclinically reduced serum ferritin has not been established. Thus, it seems prudent to use in athletes the current guidelines for establishing a diagnosis of iron depletion (serum ferritin <12 µg/l). The use of multiple indicators (Hb, transferrin saturation, free erythrocyte protoporphyrin, serum ferritin) improve the sensitivity of detecting iron deficiency anemia and can be utilized to minimize misdiagnosis in the face of acute inflammation. In view of previously demonstrated alterations in neurologic and cognitive function with iron deficiency, studies of subclinical iron deficiency should be pursued to delineate the effects of deficiency upon these less-studied consequences of altered iron status in athletes. It may also be desirable to pursue investigations into iron distribution in athletes, so as to delineate altered iron balance from iron redistribution as an operative factor which may influence the hematologic profile of those individuals who engage in regular strenuous physical activity.

REFERENCES

1. de Duve, C., Prelude to a cell, *The Sciences*, 30, 22, 1990.
2. Eaton, S. B. and Konner, M., Paleolithic nutrition. A consideration of its nature and current implications, *N. Engl. J. Med.*, 312, 283, 1985.
3. Vannotti, A. and Delachaux, A., Iron Metabolism and Its Clinical Significance, Grune & Stratton, New York, 1949.
4. Hughes, E. R., Human iron metabolism, in: *Metal Ions in Biological Systems. Iron in Model and Natural Compounds*, Sigel, H., Ed., Marcel Dekker, New York, 1977.
5. MacKay, C., *Memoirs of Extraordinary Popular Delusions*, Richard Bently, London, 1841.
6. Marks, G. and Beatty, W. K., *The Precious Metals of Medicine*, Charles Scribner & Sons, New York, 1975.
7. Cule, J., The iron mixture of Dr. Griffith, *Pharm J.*, CXCVIII, 399, 1967.
8. Scrimshaw, N. S., Functional consequences of iron deficiency in human populations, *J. Nutr. Sci. Vitaminol.*, 30, 47, 1984.
9. DeMaeyer, E. and Adiels-Tegman, M., The prevalence of anemia in the world, *World Health Stat. Q.*, 38, 302, 1985.
10. Expert Scientific Working Group, Summary of a report on assessment of the iron nutritional status of the United States population, *Am. J. Clin. Nutr.*, 42, 1318, 1985.
11. Seoane, N. A., Roberge, A. G., Page, M., Allard, C., and Bouchard, C., Selected indices of iron status in adolescents, *J. Can. Diet. Assoc.*, 46, 298, 1985.
12. International Nutritional Anemia Consultative Group, Measurements of iron status, Report of the Nutrition Foundation, Washington, D.C., 1985.
13. Skikne, B. S., Flowers, C. H., and Cook, J. D., Serum transferrin receptor: a quantitative measure of tissue iron deficiency, *Blood*, 75, 1870, 1990.
14. Bothwell, T. H., Charlton, R. W., Cook, J. B., and Finch, C. A., *Iron Metabolism in Man*, Blackwell Scientific, Oxford, 1979, Chaps. 1–3.
15. Cook, J. D., Dassenko, S. A., and Lynch, S. R., Assessment of the role of nonheme-iron availability in iron balance, *Am. J. Clin. Nutr.*, 54, 717, 1991.
16. Beard, J. L. and Dawson, H., Chapter on iron, in: *Handbook of Nutritionally Essential Elements*, Sunde, R. and O'Dell, B., Eds., Marcel Dekker, New York, 1966.
17. Wretland, A., in: *Iron Deficiency*, Hallberg, L., Ed., Academic Press, London, 1970.
18. Takkunen, H., and Seppänen, R., Iron deficiency and dietary factors in Finland, *Am. J. Clin. Nutr.*, 28, 1141, 1975.
19. Bjorn-Rasmussen, E., Hallberg, L., Isaksson, B., and Arvidsson, B., Food iron absorption in man. Application of the two-pool extrinsic tag method to measure heme and nonheme iron absorption, *J. Clin. Invest.*, 53, 247, 1974.
20. Cook, J. D. and Reusser, M. E., Iron fortification: an update, *J. Food Sci.*, 48, 1340, 1983.

21. Reddy, M. B. and Cook, J. D., Assessment of dietary determinants of nonheme-iron absorption in humans and rats, *Am. J. Clin. Nutr.*, 54, 723, 1991.

22. Conrad, M. E., Regulation of iron absorption, in: *Essential and Toxic Trace Elements in Human Disease: An Update*, 2nd ed., Prasad, A. S., Ed., Wiley-Liss, New York, 1993.

23. Hallberg, L., Rossander-Hulten, L., Brune, M., and Gleerup, A., Inhibition of haem-iron absorption in man by calcium, *Br. J. Nutr.*, 69, 533, 1993.

24. Carpenter, C. E. and Mahoney, A. W., Contributions of heme and nonheme iron to human nutrition, *Crit. Rev. Food Sci. Nutr.*, 31, 333, 1992.

25. Davis, C. D., Malecki, E. A., and Greger, J. L., Interactions among dietary manganese, heme iron, and nonheme iron in women, *Am. J. Clin. Nutr.*, 56, 926, 1992.

26. Seligman, P. A., Caskey, J. H., Frazier, J. L., Zucker, R. M., Podell, E. R., and Allen, R. H., Measurements of iron absorption from prenatal multivitamin-mineral supplements, *Obstet. Gynecol.*, 61, 356, 1983.

27. Hallberg, L., Brune, M., Erlandsson, M., Sandberg, A.-S., and Rossander-Hulten, L., Calcium: effect of different amounts on nonheme and heme-iron absorption in humans, *Am. J. Clin. Nutr.*, 53, 112, 1991.

28. Nichols, G. M., Pearce, A. R., Alverez, X., Bibb, N. K., Nichols, K. Y., Alfred, C. B., and Glass, J., The mechanisms of nonheme iron uptake determined in IEC-6 rat intestinal cells, *J. Nutr.*, 122, 945, 1992.

29. Dallman, P. R., Biochemical basis for the manifestations of iron deficiency, *Annu. Rev. Nutr.*, 6, 13, 1986.

30. Beard, J., Neuroendocrine alterations in iron deficiency, in: *Progress in Food and Nutritional Science,* Chandra, R. K., Ed., Pergamon Press, Elmsford, NY, 1990, 45-82.

31. Lipschitz, D. A., Cook, J. D., and Finch, C. A., A clinical evaluation of serum ferritin as an index of iron stores, *N. Engl. J. Med.*, 290, 1213, 1974.

32. Borel, M. J., Smith, S. M., Beard, J. L., and Derr, J., Day-to-day variation in iron status parameters in healthy men and women, *Am. J. Clin. Nutr.*, 54, 729, 1991.

33. Beaton, G. H., Corey, P. N., and Steele, C., Conceptual and methodological issues regarding the epidemiology of iron deficiency and their implications for studies of the functional consequences of iron deficiency, *Am. J. Clin. Nutr.*, 50, 575, 1989.

34. Carriaga, M. T., Skikne, B. S., Finley, B., Cutler, B., and Cook, J. D., Serum transferrin receptor for the detection of iron deficiency in pregnancy, *Am. J. Clin. Nutr.*, 54, 1077, 1991.

35. Beard, J. L., Haas, J. D., Tufts, H., Spielvogel, E., Vargas, E., and Rodriguez, C., Iron deficiency anemia and steady-state work performance at high altitude, *J. Appl. Physiol.*, 64, 1878, 1988.

36. Azevedo, J. L., Willis, W. T., Turcotte, L. P., Rovner, A. S., Dalman, P. R., and Brooks, G. A., Reciprocal changes of muscle oxidases and liver enzymes with recovery from iron deficiency, *Am. J. Physiol.*, 256, E401, 1989.

37. Bowering, J. and Sanchez, A. M., A conspectus of research on iron requirements of man, *J. Nutr.*, 7, 987, 1976.

38. Finch, C. A., and Huebers, M. D., Perspectives in iron metabolism, *N. Engl. J. Med.*, 25, 1520, 1982.

39. Cook, J. D. and Lynch, S. R., The liabilities of iron deficiency, *Blood*, 68, 803, 1986.

40. Dallman, P. R., Manifestations of iron deficiency, *Semin. Hematol.*, 19, 19, 1982.

41. Arthur, C. K. and Isbuster, J. P., Iron deficiency: misunderstood, misdiagnosed, and mistreated, *Curr. Ther.*, 23, 1986.

42. Finch, C. A., Miller, L., Inamdar, A. R., Person, R., Seiler, K., and Mackler, B., Iron deficiency in the rat: physiological and biochemical studies of muscle dysfunction, *J. Clin. Invest.*, 58, 447, 1976.

43. Davies, K. J. A., Maquire, J. J., Brooks, G. A., and Dallman, P. R., Muscle mitochondrial bioenergetics, oxygen supply, and work capacity during dietary iron deficiency and repletion, *Am. J. Physiol.*, 242, E418, 1982.

44. Davies, K. J. A, Donovan, C. M., Refino, C. J., Brooks, G. A., Packer, L., and Dallman, P. R., Distinguishing effects of anemia and muscle iron deficiency on muscle bioenergetics in the rat, *Am. J. Physiol.*, 246, E535, 1984.

45. Perkkio, M. V., Jansson, L. T., Brooks, G. A., Refino, C. J., and Dallman, P. R., Work performance in iron deficiency of increasing severity, *J. Appl. Physiol.*, 58, 1477, 1985.

46. Gardner, G. W., Edgerton, V. R., Barnard, R. J., and Bernauer, E. H., Cardiorespiratory, hematological and physical performance responses of anemic subjects to iron treatment, *Am. J. Clin Nutr.*, 28, 982, 1975.

47. Gardner, G. W., Edgerton, V., Senewiratne, B., Barnard, R., and Ohira, Y., Physical work capacity and metabolic stress in subjects with iron deficiency anemia, *Am. J. Clin. Nutr.*, 30, 910, 1977.

48. Edgerton, V. R., Ohira, Y., Hettiarachi, J., Senewiratne, B., Gardner, G. W., and Barnard, R. J., Elevation of hemoglobin and work tolerance in iron-deficient subjects, *J. Nutr. Sci. Vitaminol.*, 27, 77, 1981.

49. Perkkio, M. V., Jansson, L. T., Henderson, S., Refino, C., Brooks, G. A., and Dallman, P. R., Work performance in the iron-deficient rat: improved endurance with exercise training, *Am. J. Physiol.*, 249, E306, 1985.

50. Willis, W. T., Brooks, G. A., Henderson, S. A., and Dallman, P. R., Effects of iron deficiency and training on mitochondrial enzymes in skeletal muscle, *J. Appl. Physiol.*, 62, 2442, 1987.

51. Willis, W. T., Dallman, P. R., and Brooks, G. A., Physiological and biochemical correlates of increased work performance in trained iron-deficient rats, *J. Appl. Physiol.*, 65, 256, 1988.

52. Tobin, B. W. and Beard, J. L., Interactions of iron deficiency and exercise training in male Sprague-Dawley rats. Ferrokinetics and hematology, *J. Nutr.*, 119, 1340, 1989.

53. Siegel, A. J., Hennekens, C. H., Solomon, H. S., and Van Boeckel, B., Exercise-related hematuria, findings in a group of marathon runners, *J. Am. Med. Assoc.*, 241, 391, 1979.

54. Wijn, J. F., De Jongste, J. L., Mosterd, W., and Willebrand, D., Hemoglobin, packed cell volume, and iron binding capacity of selected athletes during training, *Nutr. Metab.*, 13, 129, 1971.

55. Ehn, L., Carlmark, B., and Hoglund, S., Iron status in athletes involved in intense physical activity, *Med. Sci. Sport. Exercise*, 12, 61, 1980.

56. Wells, C. L., Stern, J. R., and Hecht, L. H., Hematological changes following a marathon race in male and female runners, *Eur. J. Appl. Physiol.*, 48, 41, 1982.

57. Pate, R. R., Sports anemia and its impact on athletic performance, in *Nutrition and Athletic Performance*, Bull Publishing, Palo Alto, CA, 1982, 202.

58. Clement, D. B. and Sawchuck, L. L., Iron status and sports performance, *Sports Med.*, 1, 65, 1984.

59. Sweringen, J. V., Iron deficiency in athletes: consequence or adaptation in strenuous activity, *J. Orthoped. Sport Phys. Ther.*, 7, 192, 1986.

60. Newhouse, I. J. and Clement, D. B., Iron status in athletes. An Update, *Sports Med.*, 5, 337, 1988.

61. Weaver, C. M. and Rajaram, S., Exercise and iron status, *J. Nutr.*, 122, 782, 1992.

62. Dufaux, B., Hoederath, A., Streitberger, I., Hollman, W., and Assman, G., Serum ferritin, transferrin, haptoglobin and iron in middle and long distance runners, elite rowers, and professional racing cyclists, *Int. J. Sports Med.*, 2, 43, 1981.

63. Radomski, M. W., Sabiston, B. H., and Isoard, P., Development of sports anemia in physically fit men after daily sustained submaximal exercise, *Aviat. Space Environ. Med.*, 51, 41, 1980.

64. Dressendorfer, R. H., Wade, C. E., and Amsterdam, E. A., Development of a pseudoanemia in marathon runners during a 20-day road race, *J. Am. Med. Assoc.*, 246, 1215, 1981.

65. Magnussen, B., Hallberg, L., Rossander, L., and Swolin, B., Iron metabolism and "sports anemia". II. A hematological comparison of elite runners and control subjects, *Acta. Med. Scand.*, 216, 157, 1984.

66. Balaban, E. P., Cox, J. V., Snell, P., Vaughan, R. H., and Frenkel, E. P., The frequency of anemia and iron deficiency in the runner, *Med. Sci. Sports Exercise*, 21, 643, 1989.

67. Fogelholm, G. M., Himberg, J. J., Alopaeus, K., Gref, C. G., Laasko, J. T., Lehto, J. J., and Mussalo-Rauhamaa, H., Dietary and biochemical indices of nutritional status in male athletes and controls, *J. Am. Coll. Nutr.*, 11, 181, 1992.

68. Casoni, I., Borsetto, C., Cavicchi, A., Martinelli, S., and Conconi, F., Reduced hemoglobin concentration and red cell hemoglobinization in Italian marathon and ultramarathon runners, *Int. J. Sports Med.*, 6, 176, 1985.

69. Pate, R. R., Miller, B. J., Davis, J. M., Slentz, C. A., and Klingshirn, L. A., Iron status of female runners, *Int. J. Sport Nutr.*, 3, 222, 1993.

70. Haymes, E. M. and Spillman, D. M., Iron status of women distance runners, sprinters, and control women, *Int. J. Sports Med.*, 10, 430, 1989.

71. Lampe, J. W., Slavin, J. L., and Apple, F. S., Iron status of active women and the effect of running a marathon on bowel function and gastrointestinal blood loss, *Int. J. Sports Med.*, 12, 173, 1991.

72. Rowland, T. W., Stagg, L., and Kelleher, J. F., Iron deficiency in adolescent girls. Are athletes at increased risk?, *J. Adol. Health*, 12, 22, 1991.

73. Fogelholm, M. and Lahtinen, P., Nutritional evaluation of a sailing crew during a transatlantic race, *Scand. J. Med. Sci. Sports*, 1, 99, 1991.

74. Spodaryk, K., Haematological and iron-related parameters of male endurance and strength trained athletes, *Eur. J. Appl. Physiol.*, 67, 66, 1993.

75. Dickson, D. N., Wilkinson, R. L., and Noakes, T. D., Effects of ultra-marathon training and racing on hematologic parameters and serum ferritin levels in well-trained athletes, *Int. J. Sports Med.*, 3, 111, 1982.

76. Deuster, P. A., Kyle, S. B., Moser, P. B., Vigersky, R. A., Singh, A., and Schoomaker, E. B., Nutritional survey of highly trained women runners, *Am. J. Clin. Nutr.*, 45, 954, 1986.

77. Snyder, A. C., Dvorak, L. L., and Roepke, J. B., Influence of dietary iron source on measures of iron status among female runners, *Med. Sci. Sports Exercise*, 21, 7, 1989.

78. Weight, L. M., Byrne, M. J., and Jacobs, P., Haemolytic effects of exercise, *Clin. Sci.*, 81, 147, 1991.

79. Stewart, J. G., Ahlquist, D. A., McGill, D. B., Ilstrup, D. M., Schwartz, S., and Owen, R. A., Gastrointestinal blood loss and anemia in runners, *Ann. Intern. Med.*, 100, 843, 1984.

80. Brune, M., Magnussen, B., Persson, H., and Hallberg, L., Iron losses in sweat, *Am. J. Clin. Nutr.*, 4, 438, 1986.

81. Newhouse, I. J., Clement, D. B., Taunton, J. E., and McKenzie, D. C., The effects of prelatent and latent iron deficiency on physical work capacity, *Med. Sci. Sports Exercise*, 21, 3, 263, 1989.

82. Newhouse, I. J., Clement, D. B., and Lai, C., The effects of iron supplementation and discontinuation on serum copper, zinc, calcium, and magnesium levels in women, *Med. Sci. Sports Exercise*, 25, 562, 1993.

83. Newhouse, I. J., and Clement, D. B., The efficacy of iron supplementation in iron depleted women, in *Sports Nutrition: Minerals and Electrolytes*, Kies, C. V. and Driskell, J. A., Eds., CRC Press, Boca Raton, FL, 1995, 47.

84. Magazanik, A., Weinstein, Y., Dlin, R. A., Derin, H., Schwartzman, S., and Allalouf, D., Iron deficiency caused by 7 weeks of intensive physical exercise, *Eur. J. Appl. Physiol.*, 57, 198, 1988.

85. Colt, E. and Heyman, B., Low ferritin levels in runners, *J. Sports Med.*, 24, 13, 1984.

86. Clement, D. B. and Asmundson, R. C., Nutritional intake and hematological parameters in endurance runners, *Phys. Sports Med.*, 10, 37, 1982.

87. Fogelholm, M., Inadequate iron status in athletes: an exaggerated problem?, in *Sports Nutrition: Minerals and Electrolytes*, Kies, C. V. and Driskell, J. A., Eds., CRC Press, Boca Raton, FL, 1995, 81.

88. Risser, W. L., Lee, E. V., Poindexter, H. B., Steward, W., West, M., Pivarnik, J. M., Risser, J. M. H., and Hickson, J. F., Iron deficiency in female athletes: its prevalence and impact on performance, *Med. Sci. Sports Exercise*, 20, 116, 1988.

89. Durstine, J. L., Pate, R. R., Sparling, P. B., Wilson, G. E., Senn, M. D., and Bartoli, W. P., Lipid, lipoprotein, and iron status of elite woman distance runners, *Int. J. Sports Med.*, 8, S119, 1987.

90. Hemmingson, P., Bauer, M., and Birgegard, G., Iron status in elite skiers, *Scand. J. Med. Sci. Sports*, 1, 174, 1991.

91. Weight, L. M., "Sports Anemia." Does it exist?, *Sports Med.*, 16, 1, 1993.

92. Henderson, S. A., Dallman, P. R., and Brooks, G. A., Glucose turnover and oxidation are increased in the iron-deficient rat, *Am. J. Physiol.*, 250, E414, 1986.

93. Brooks, G. A., Henderson, S. A., and Dallman, P. R., Increased glucose dependence in resting, iron-deficient rats, *Am. J. Physiol.*, 253, E461, 1987.

94. Farrell, P. A., Beard, J. L., and Druckenmiller, M., Increased insulin sensitivity in iron-deficient rats, *J. Nutr.*, 118, 1104, 1988.

95. Borel, M. J. Beard, J. L., and Farrell, P. A., Hepatic glucose production and insulin sensitivity and responsiveness in iron-deficient anemic rats, *Am. J. Physiol.*, 264, E380, 1993.

96. Joost, H. G. and Weber, T. M., The regulation of glucose transport in insulin-sensitive cells, *Diabetologia*, 32, 831, 1989.

97. Bell, G. I., Kayano, T., Buse, J. B., Burant, C. F., Takeda, J., Lin, D., Fukumoto, H., and Seina, S., Molecular biology of mammalian glucose transporters, *Diabetes Care*, 13, 198, 1990.

98. Napoli, R., Hirshman, M. F., and Horton, E. S., Mechanisms of increased skeletal muscle glucose transport activity after an oral glucose load in rats, *Diabetes*, 44, 1362, 1995.

99. Zinker, B. A., Dallman, P. R., and Brooks, G. A., Augmented glucoregulatory hormone concentrations during exhausting exercise in mildly iron-deficient rats, *Am. J. Physiol.*, 265, R863, 1993.

100. Linderman, J. K., Brooks, G. A., Rodriguez, R. E., and Dallman, P. R., Maintenance of euglycemia is impaired in gluconeogenesis-inhibited iron-deficient rats at rest and during exercise, *J. Nutr.*, 124, 2131, 1994.

101. Willis, W. T., Chengson, J. R., and Dallman, P. R., Hepatic adaptations to iron deficiency and exercise training, *Am. J. Physiol.*, 73, 510, 1992.

102. Lauffer, R. B., Exercise as prevention: Do the health benefits derive in part from lower iron levels?, *Med. Hypoth.*, 35, 103, 1991.

103. Willis, W. T., Gohil, K., Brooks, G. A., and Dallman, P. R., Iron deficiency: improved exercise performance within 15 hours of iron treatment in rats, *J. Nutr.*, 120, 909, 1990.

104. Shoene, R. B., Escaourrou, P., Robertson, H. T., Nilson, K. L., Parsons, J. R., and Smith, N. J., Iron repletion decreases maximal exercise lactate concentrations in female athletes with minimal iron-deficiency anemia, *J. Lab. Clin. Med.*, 102, 306, 1983.

105. Rowland, T. W., Deisworth, M. B., Green, G. M., and Kelleher, J. F., The effect of iron therapy on the exercise capacity of non anemic iron-deficient adolescent runners, *Am. J. Dis. Child.*, 142, 165, 1988.

106. Lukaski, H. C., Hall, C. B., and Siders, W. A., Altered metabolic response of iron-deficient women during graded, maximal exercise, *Eur. J. Appl. Physiol.*, 63, 140, 1991.

107. Fogelholm, M., Jaakola, L., and Lampisjarvi, T., Effects of iron supplementation in female athletes with low serum ferritin concentration, *Int. J. Sports Med.*, 13, 158, 1992.

108. Powell, P. D. and Tucker, A., Iron supplementation and running performance in female cross-country runners, *Int. J. Sports Med.*, 12, 462, 1991.

109. Klingshirn, L. A., Pate, R. R., Bourque, S. P., Davis, J. M., and Sargent, R. G., Effect of supplementation on endurance capacity in iron-depleted women, *Med. Sci. Sports Exercise*, 24, 819, 1992.

110. Matter, M., Stittfall, T., Graves, J., Myburgh, K., Adams, B., Jacobs, P., and Noakes, T. D., The effect of iron and folate therapy on maximal exercise performance in female marathon runners with iron and folate deficiency, *Clin. Sci.*, 72, 415, 1987.

111. Ohira, Y., Hegenauer, J., Slatman, P., and Edgerton, V. R., Distribution and metabolism of iron in muscles of iron-deficient rats, *Biol. Trace Elem. Res.*, 4, 45, 1982.

112. Cannon, J. G. and Kluger, M. J., Endogenous pyrogen activity in human plasma after exercise, *Science*, 220, 617, 1983.

113. Taylor, C., Rogers, G., Goodman, C., Baynes, R. D., Bothwell, T. H., Bezwoda, W. R., Kramer, F., and Hattingh, J., Hematologic, iron related, and acute-phase protein responses to sustained strenuous exercise, *J. Appl. Physiol.*, 62, 464, 1987.

114. Torti, S. V., Kwak, E. L., Miller, S. C., Miller, L. L., Ringold, G. M., Myambo, K. B., Young, A. P., and Torti, F. M., The molecular cloning and characterization of murine ferritin heavy chain, a tumor necrosis factor-inducible gene, *J. Biol. Chem.*, 263, 12638, 1988.

115. Kwak, E. L., Larochelle, D. A., Beaumont, C., Torti, S. V., and Torti, F. M., Role for NF-kappa B in the regulation of ferritin H by tumor necrosis factor-alpha, *J. Biol. Chem.*, 270, 15285, 1995.

116. Torti, S. V. and Torti, F. M., Iron and ferritin in inflammation and cancer, *Adv. Inorg. Biochem.*, 10, 119, 1994.

117. Conrad, M. E. and Umbreit, J. N., A concise review: Iron absorption — The mucin-mobilferrin integrin pathway. A competitive pathway for metal absorption, *Am. J., Hematol.*, 42, 67, 1993.

118. Aggett, P., Scientific considerations in the formulation of the RDI, *Eur. J. Clin. Nutr.*, 44, 37, 1990.

119. Food and Nutrition Board, National Research Council, *Recommended Dietary Allowances*, 10th ed., National Academy Press, Washington, D.C., 1989, 195.

120. Food and Nutrition Board, National Institute of Medicine, Iron Deficiency Anemia: Recommended Guidelines for the Prevention, Detection, and Management Among U.S. Children and Women of Childbearing Age, National Academy Press, Washington, D.C., 1993, 11.

121. Ries, C. A. and Santi, D. V., Agents used in anemias, in Basic and Clinical Pharmacology, Katzung, B. G., Ed., Appleton and Lange, Norwalk, CT, 1992, 453.

122. Haymes, E. M., Trace minerals and exercise, in Nutrition in Exercise and Sport, Wolinsky, I. and Hickson, J. F., Eds., CRC Press, Boca Raton, FL, 1994, 231.

Chapter 12

ZINC

Henry C. Lukaski

CONTENTS

I. INTRODUCTION

Individuals who seek the benefits of exercise generally pursue information about the role of diet in enhancing performance and optimizing health. Although the quantity of information in the public press promoting the value of certain foods and nutritional products for health and fitness enhancement is considerable, the amount of data from valid scientific studies to support these claims is quite limited. Information about the needs of mineral elements, particularly zinc (Zn), for physically active individuals is minimal.[1] Practical limitations contribute to the difficulty in conducting human studies to examine the interaction of dietary Zn and performance.

Zn is a mineral element that chemically combines in the +2 valence state. As a transition element, Zn has the ability to form stable complexes with side chains of proteins and nucleotides, with a specific affinity for thiol and hydroxy groups and for ligands containing nitrogen; Zn generally forms complexes with a tetrahedral arrangement of ligands around the metal. In this capacity, the Zn ion acts as a good electron acceptor, but does not participate in direct oxidation-reduction reactions. These characteristics serve to explain the principal biological function of Zn, that is, its varied roles in regulation of body metabolism.

Zn is essential for the function of more than 200 enzymes in various species.[2] At least one Zn-containing enzyme is found in each of the six major categories of enzymes designated by the International Union of Biochemistry Commission on Enzyme Nomenclature.

Zn has several recognized functions in Zn-metalloenzymes including catalytic, structural, and regulatory roles.[3] A catalytic function specifies that Zn participates directly in facilitating the action of the enzyme. If the Zn is removed by chelates or other agents, the enzyme becomes inactive. Carbonic anhydrase is an enzyme in which Zn plays a catalytic role.[4]

In a structural role, Zn atoms are required to stabilize the quaternary structure of the enzyme protein and to maintain the integrity of the complex enzyme molecules but not impact enzyme activity. Zn plays a structural role in the enzymes superoxide dismutase and protein kinase c.[2]

The importance of Zn in biological systems is reflected by the numerous functions and activities on which Zn exerts a regulatory role.[5] Zn is involved extensively in macronutrient metabolism. It is required for nucleic acid and protein metabolism and, hence, the fundamental processes of cell differentiation, particularly replication. Similarly, Zn is needed for glucose utilization and the secretion of insulin. Because of this role in glucose homeostasis, Zn also affects lipid metabolism; Zn-deficient animals display decreased *de novo* lipid synthesis.[6] Thus, Zn status impacts energy substrate utilization.

Zn exerts regulatory actions in various aspects of hormone metabolism.[5] Zn is required for the production, storage, and secretion of individual hormones including growth and thyroid hormones, gonadotrophins and sex hormones, prolactin, and corticosteroids. Zn status also regulates the effectiveness of the interaction of some hormones at receptor sites and end-organ responsiveness.

Integrated biological systems also require Zn for optimal function.[7] Adequate dietary Zn is necessary for proper taste perception, reproduction, immunocompetence, skin integrity, wound healing, skeletal development, brain development, behavior, vision, and gastrointestinal function in humans. It is apparent, therefore, that Zn is an essential nutrient which regulates many physiological and psychological functions and is required to promote human health and to optimize well-being.

II. ZINC METABOLISM

A. ZINC IN THE HUMAN BODY

Zn is present in all organs, tissues, fluids, and secretions of the body. More than 95% of Zn in the body is found within cells. Zn is associated with all organelles of the cell but only

60 to 80% of cellular Zn is localized in the cytosol; the remainder has been shown to be specifically bound to membranes which may be important in defining the effects of Zn deficiency on cellular function.[8] The concentration of Zn in extracellular fluids is very low; plasma Zn concentration is approximately 0.65 μmol/l. If the body plasma concentration is 45 ml/kg body weight,[9] then a 70-kg man has about 3 l of plasma which contains only 3 mg of Zn, or about 0.1% of the body Zn content.

The Zn concentration in various organs and tissues of the body is variable (Table 1). Although the concentration of Zn in skeletal muscle is not large, the substantial mass of skeletal muscle makes it the principal reservoir of Zn in the body. Bone and skeletal muscle account for almost 90% of the body Zn content.

TABLE 1   Approximate Zinc Concentration and Content of Some Organs and Tissues in a Healthy Adult Man (70/kg)

Tissue or Organ	Zinc Concentration (μmol/g)[a]	(μg/g)[a]	Total Zinc Content (mmol)	(g)	Percentage of Body Zinc
Skeletal muscle	0.78	51	24	1.53	57
Bone	1.54	100	12	0.77	29
Skin	0.49	32	2	0.16	6
Liver	0.89	58	2	0.13	5
Brain	0.17	11	0.6	0.04	1.5
Kidneys	0.85	55	0.3	0.02	0.7
Heart	0.35	23	0.15	0.01	0.4
Hair	2.30	150	<0.15	<0.01	0.1
Plasma	0.02	1	<0.15	<0.01	0.1

[a]   Wet weight.

Modified from International Commission on Radiological Protection, *Report on the Task Group of Reference Man.*, Pergamon Press, Oxford, 1975. With permission.

The Zn concentration of muscles varies with their metabolic functions. The highest Zn concentrations are found in skeletal muscles that are highly oxidative, with a large proportion of slow-twitch fibers.[10] The rat soleus muscle, which contains 63% slow-twitch fibers, contains about 300 μg Zn per gram dry weight. Conversely, the extensor digitorum longus, which is primarily a fast-twitch glycolytic muscle, has only 100 μg Zn per gram dry weight.[11] Interestingly, the Zn content of skeletal muscles generally is not reduced with restricted dietary Zn, except for small decreases in the soleus. The size and number of various types of muscle fibers, however, may be reduced and their relative distribution altered, with a characteristic decrease of the slow-twitch oxidative and an increase in the fast-twitch glycolytic fibers.[10,11] Thus, as a reservoir of body Zn, skeletal muscle is relatively unresponsive to changes in dietary Zn.

Because the concentration of Zn in bone is quite large relative to other body tissues and organs, and the amount of bone is very substantial, the skeleton is a major depot of Zn (Table 1). This store of Zn is impacted adversely by dietary Zn restriction. The decline in bone Zn is more responsive to dietary Zn intake than that of other tissues and may better reflect the gradual decline in overall Zn status of the body than does plasma Zn concentrations. Studies in growing rats fed Zn-deficient diets found a 50% reduction in bone Zn; short-term Zn supplementation of Zn-deficient rats significantly increased bone Zn.[12] In adult male rats, however, bone Zn only responded to a minor degree to dietary Zn.[5]

B. ZINC HOMEOSTASIS
1. Absorption
The amount of Zn in the body represents a dynamic balance between the Zn intake and losses (Figure 1). Zn is absorbed principally along the small intestine with only negligible

amounts absorbed in the stomach and the large intestine. The quantity of Zn in the intestines is a combination of dietary Zn and Zn-containing endogenous secretions that aid in digestion. Pancreatic secretions are a major source of endogenous Zn. Other sources include biliary and gastro-duodenal secretions, transepithelial flux of Zn from mucosal cells into the small intestine, and mucosal cells sloughed into the gut.[5] Thus, the amount of Zn in the lumen of the small intestine after a meal exceeds the quantity of Zn from the meal because of endogenous secretions.

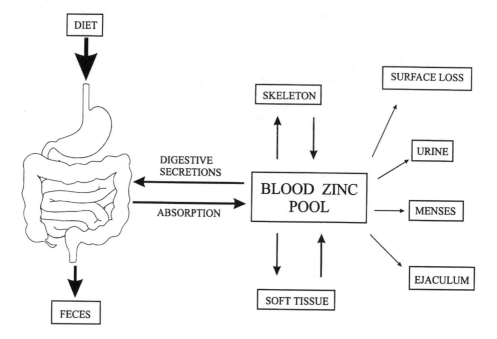

FIGURE 1 Components of human zinc metabolism.

During digestion, secreted enzymes release Zn from the food and endogenous Zn from various ligands. The free Zn can form coordination complexes with various exogenous and endogenous ligands such as amino acids, organic acids, and phosphates.[13] The amino acids, histidine and cysteine, are preferred amino acid ligands. It has been shown that Zn-histidine complexes are very efficiently absorbed, more so than Zn sulfate.[14] Other compounds such as iron and phytate, found in the intestinal milieu, can compete with Zn for mucosal binding sites or form insoluble complexes that inhibit Zn absorption.[15]

Zn enters mucosal cells by a mechanism that is not well understood.[16] It is thought that Zn enters the mucosal cell by a carrier-mediated process, saturable at higher luminal Zn concentrations, and by diffusion. Within the mucosal cell, Zn is released at the serosal surface, where it binds with albumin, then is transported by the portal blood to the liver.

The total body content of Zn is controlled partially by the regulation of the efficiency of intestinal absorption of Zn. Numerous studies in animals and humans have reported an inverse relationship between dietary Zn and Zn absorption.[17] Thus, the regulation of Zn absorption by the mucosal cell provides a general control of total body Zn.

2. Excretion

Control of Zn excretion in feces represents another regulatory mechanism for maintenance of body Zn. In normal dietary circumstances, the feces are the major route of Zn excretion. In healthy humans with an average intake of 10 to 14 mg of Zn per day, more than 90% of dietary Zn is excreted in the feces.[5] Some of the Zn in the feces is from endogenous secretions. Studies indicate that 2.5 to 5 mg of Zn are secreted into the duodenum after a meal.[15] Much of the Zn secreted into the lumen of the gut is absorbed and returned to the body. The amount of Zn secreted into the gut varies with the Zn content of the meal. Endogenous fecal Zn excretion is directly related to dietary Zn intake.[17] In humans, endogenous fecal Zn losses may range from 1 mg/d with very low Zn intakes to more than 5 mg/d with extremely large Zn intakes.[18,19] In contrast to absorption, endogenous fecal Zn excretion represents a sensitive control to balance Zn retention to metabolic needs.

Other routes of Zn excretion are present in humans (Figure 1). About 0.4 to 0.5 mg of Zn are excreted daily in the urine.[5] Urinary Zn originates from the ultrafilterable portion of plasma Zn and represents a fraction of previously absorbed dietary Zn. Dietary Zn affects urinary Zn losses only under conditions of extreme intakes and results in corresponding changes in Zn output in the urine.[5]

Zn also is lost from the skin and in various secretions. Surface losses, which include sloughing of the skin, sweat, and hair, contribute only 1 mg of Zn loss daily. A marked change in Zn intake results in parallel changes in surface Zn loss.[20] Other minor sources of Zn loss include seminal and menstrual secretions. An ejaculum of semen includes about 1 mg of Zn.[18] Total menstrual losses of Zn may reach 0.5 mg per menstrual period.[22]

The elimination of absorbed Zn from the body has been approximated with two-component model.[5] In humans, an initial or rapid phase has a half-life of 12.5 days and a slower turnover phase of about 300 days. The initial rapid phase represents liver uptake of circulating Zn and its quick release into the circulation. The slower turnover rate reflects the different rates of turnover in various organs, excluding the liver. The most rapid rates of Zn uptake and turnover are found in the pancreas, liver, kidney, and spleen, with slower rates in erythrocytes and muscle. Zn turnover is slowest in bone and the central nervous system.

Manipulation of dietary Zn impacts zinc turnover. In rats, dietary Zn restrictions promotes retention of Zn in soft tissues and organs but not in bone.[23] In humans, the turnover of the slow Zn pool is increased by ingestion of pharmacologic amounts (100 mg) of Zn.[24] These homeostatic actions serve to maintain soft tissue Zn concentrations despite variations in dietary Zn.

3. Transport

Distribution of absorbed Zn to the extrahepatic tissues occurs primarily in the plasma which contains approximately 3 mg of Zn or about 0.1% of total body Zn.[25] Zn is partitioned among α_2-macroglobulin (40%), albumin (57%), and amino acids (3%) in plasma. Zn is loosely bound to albumin and amino acids; these fractions are responsible for transport of Zn from the liver to tissues. The amino acid-bound Zn constitutes the ultrafilterable fraction that is filtered at the kidneys and excreted in the urine. Because the total amount of Zn present in tissue is far greater than the Zn in the plasma, relatively small changes in tissue Zn content, such as the liver, can have striking effects on the plasma Zn concentration. Importantly, because all absorbed Zn is transported from the plasma to tissues, the exchange of Zn from plasma into tissues is very rapid to maintain relatively constant plasma Zn concentrations (Figure 1).

III. ASSESSMENT OF HUMAN ZINC NUTRITIONAL STATUS

A deficiency of Zn progresses in a pattern which is different than that for most nutrients.[26] In general, an insufficient intake of an essential nutrient initially induces a mobilization of body stores or functional reserves. As depletion persists, tissue nutrient concentrations decrease which results in deterioration in one or more nutrient-dependent metabolic functions. Therefore, growth reduction is a late manifestation of the nutritional deficiency. In contrast, when dietary Zn is decreased, the initial response is a reduction in growth by children and a decrease in endogenous losses of Zn as a means to conserve tissue Zn. If the dietary deficiency is mild, homeostasis may be reestablished after adjusting growth and Zn excretion with no further impairment of function or biochemical changes. When dietary Zn is severely restricted, however, the body cannot restore homeostasis by adjusting endogenous losses and growth, consequently generalized impairment of organ and tissue function develops quickly.

Although severe dietary Zn deficiency can be induced in animals, it is rarely present in humans with the exception of infants and children with acrodermatitis enteropathica, patients fed total parenteral nutrition solutions lacking Zn, and experimental human Zn depletion. Evidence of moderate or mild Zn deficiency is difficult to demonstrate because of the lack of a sensitive and specific indicator of human Zn nutriture.[27]

Two general approaches have been used to assess human Zn status. One strategy has been to measure static indices, including concentrations of Zn in tissues or body fluids or measurements of biochemical surrogates for Zn nutriture in the form of Zn-containing enzymes and proteins. Another approach involves the measurement of dynamic indices that reflect the biological performance of Zn-dependent physiological or psychological functions.

Although frequently measured, plasma and serum Zn concentrations have been shown to be relatively insensitive to modest changes in dietary Zn and changes in body Zn.[28] Because whole-body Zn content is conserved in Zn deficiency, plasma and serum Zn are not reliable indicators of human Zn status. Further, plasma Zn is unresponsive to changes in dietary Zn unless the Zn intake is so low that homeostasis cannot be reestablished. It is more realistic to describe plasma Zn as a component of a labile, nutritionally available pool of total body Zn.[28] Any decrease in plasma Zn concentration, therefore, should be interpreted as a decrease in the size of the labile Zn pool. Use of this concept is limited, however, by the findings that metabolic factors also influence the labile Zn pool. Infection, food intake, stress, brief duration fasting, and hormonal status can alter the distribution of Zn among the tissues and thus influence the amount of Zn in the plasma.[25]

Other static indices of human Zn status have failed to be useful. Eryhthrocyte Zn concentration is relatively unresponsive to mild or moderate Zn deficiency.[27] The Zn concentration in various populations of leukocytes also is not sensitive to changes in Zn status.[29] Timed urinary Zn excretion rates are decreased in severe Zn deficiency but are not responsive to more moderate changes in dietary Zn.[28] Therefore, current biochemical methods of assessment of human Zn status remain a limitation for routine clinical evaluation of Zn nutritional status.

IV. ZINC NUTRITURE OF PHYSICALLY ACTIVE ADULTS

Attempts to evaluate the Zn status of physically active individuals have been complicated by the use of different experimental designs and reliance on indirect indices of Zn nutritional status. The lack of an integrated assessment of factors affecting Zn homeostasis in physically active individuals contributes to the deficit of knowledge about Zn requirements for physical activity.

A. PLASMA ZINC CONCENTRATION

Awareness of potentially adverse effects of physical activity on human Zn nutritional status began with the observation that some endurance runners had significantly decreased serum Zn concentrations as compared to nontraining men.[30] About 25% of 76 competitive male runners had serum Zn concentrations less than 11.5 µmol/l, the lower limit designated for the range of normal values. Importantly, serum Zn concentration was inversely related to weekly training distance. The investigators speculated that dietary habits, including avoidance of animal products and consumption of carbohydrate-rich foods which are low in Zn, and possible increased losses of Zn in sweat, may have predisposed the runners to hypozincemia.

Similar findings of reduced plasma Zn concentrations have been reported for some, but not all, groups of highly trained athletes. In a survey of elite German athletes,[31] there was no difference between serum Zn concentrations of athletes and sex-matched nonathletes. However, hypozincemia, defined as serum Zn concentration less than 12 μmol/l, was observed in about 25% of the athletes. Among female marathon runners, plasma Zn values were clustered at the low end of the range of normal values, with 22% of the values less than 12 μmol/l.[32,33] In contrast, no differences in plasma Zn concentrations were found in comparisons of male and female collegiate athletes with age-matched nontraining students.[34,35] One explanation for these divergent results is that Zn intake may have been inadequate in the athletes with decreased circulating Zn concentrations.

B. DIETARY ZINC

Based on self-reported food and beverage consumption (Table 2), athletes generally consume Zn in amounts exceeding 70% of the Recommended Dietary Allowance (RDA)[36] of 15 and 12 mg/d for men and women, respectively. However, a significant proportion of participants in some activities, including long-distance running and gymnastics, may consume less than 10 mg of Zn daily. Marginal intake is more widespread among female, as compared to male, athletes who restrict food intake. This behavior is characteristic among groups of athletes who participate in activities in which physical appearance is a component of performance evaluation.[39-41]

TABLE 2   Zinc Intake and Plasma Zinc Concentrations of Athletes and Control Subjects

Study	Activity	Sex	Dietary Zinc (mg/d)	Plasma Zinc (μmol/l)
Lukaski et al.[34]	Football, basketball, hockey, track and field	Male	16.3 ± 1.5[a]	13.3 ± 1.1
	Untrained	Male	13.7 ± 1.7	13.1 ± 1.2
Deuster et al.[39]	Running	Female	10.3 ± 0.7	10.1 ± 0.4
	Untrained	Female	10.0 ± 0.7	11.1 ± 0.4
Lukaski et al.[35]	Swimming	Female	12.4 ± 0.8	12.6 ± 0.5
	Untrained	Female	9.8 ± 0.9	12.8 ± 0.4
	Swimming	Male	17.9 ± 1.0	14.3 ± 0.5
	Untrained	Male	15.2 ± 1.0	12.8 ± 0.5
Fogelholm et al.[37]	Endurance	Male	17.7[b]	13.6[b]
	Untrained	Male	14.1[b]	13.8[b]
Fogelholm et al.[38]	Skiing	Female	15.8[b]	12.7[b]
	Untrained	Female	10.5[b]	12.6[b]
	Skiing	Male	21.9[b]	14.1[b]
	Untrained	Male	14.1[b]	14.3[b]

[a]   Mean ± SE.
[b]   Mean.

A general relationship between dietary Zn and plasma Zn in athletes is evident. On the average, athletes who consume at least 70% of the RDA for Zn apparently have plasma Zn concentrations within the range of normal values (Table 2). This observation is independent of sex and sporting activity. Thus, if an individual consumes adequate dietary Zn, regardless of activity status, plasma Zn is within normal values.[38] Conversely, if dietary Zn is marginal, then plasma Zn concentration will decline;[32,39] the apparent threshold for plasma Zn to decline is 4 mg of Zn per day.[42] Thus, low dietary Zn is associated with a reduced labile pool of Zn in the plasma, and may reflect impaired Zn status.

C. ZINC LOSSES
1. Surface Loss

Exercise is a stressor that might perturb body Zn homeostasis because it is associated with increased Zn excretion. Estimates of whole-body Zn loss in sweat in men consuming controlled dietary Zn at 12.7 mg/d and not involved in vigorous activity were variable at 0.8 ± 0.2 (mean ± SE) mg/d and represented about 5% of daily Zn intake.[43] When acute bouts of submaximal exercise (30 min/d) were coupled with daily heat exposure (7.5 h at 37.8°C) for 18 d, Zn loss estimated from measurements of arm sweat of 3 men decreased appreciably after the first 4 days of acclimatization from 13.7 to 2.2 mg/d, which represented about 18% of the daily Zn intake of 12.5 mg.[44]

The concentrations of Zn in sweat depends on the location from which sweat is collected during exercise and the ambient temperature. Zn concentration in sweat collected from 12 men during 30 to 40 min of strenuous ergocycle work ranged from 12.7 μmol/l at the abdomen as compared to about 7 μmol/l at the arm, chest, and back.[45] The variation in sweat Zn concentration by site was considerable, ranging from 50 to 100% among the participants. Arm sweat Zn concentration after 1 h of low-intensity ergocycle work was lower at 35°C than at 25°C (0.8 vs. 1.3 μmol/l) but sweat Zn losses were similar (1.15 vs. 1.06 μg/min) in male and female athletes during submaximal cycle ergometer exercise, indicating that differences in rate of sweating tend to normalize surface Zn losses.[46] Exercise intensity and duration, therefore, contribute to differences in estimates of Zn loss in sweat. Furthermore, the large variability in estimates of surface loss of Zn suggests contamination of samples may be a problem when evaluating the reported magnitude of Zn lost during exercise.

Increased excretion of Zn in sweat during exercise coincides with moderate reductions in circulating Zn. Men and women exposed to heat for one week have decreased serum Zn concentrations.[47] Similarly, men participating in a 20-d marathon road race demonstrated a tendency toward a decrease in serum Zn concentration.[48] It is unclear if the slight reductions in serum Zn reflect differences in dietary Zn or a modest expansion of plasma volume as an adaptation to chronic exposure to a stressor.

2. Urinary Excretion

Increased Zn excretion in the urine with exercise also has been reported. Studies of untrained men participating in short-duration activity (10 min of stair-climbing to exhaustion) or trained men participating in a 10-mi road race observed a 50 to 60% increase in urinary Zn loss during the first hour after exercise as compared to a similar period of time before the exercise.[49] Similarly, Anderson et al.[50] reported a 50% increase in urinary Zn excretion on the day of exercise as compared to the day before in men performing a 6-mi run. In contrast, another study[51] found no differences in urinary Zn output when trained and untrained men performed high-intensity (90% peak work capacity), brief duration bouts of treadmill running (30 s run followed by 30 s rest). Urinary Zn excretion, however, returns to preexercise values on the day following the exercise bouts.[50] Therefore, acute increases in urinary Zn excretion are homeostatically regulated with commensurate reductions in urinary Zn on the day following the exercise bout.

D. ZINC REDISTRIBUTION DURING EXERCISE

Exercise is a potent stressor that influences circulating Zn concentrations in the blood. In general, short-duration, high-intensity activities induce an immediate increase in plasma and serum Zn concentrations.[42,49,52] Longer duration activities, such as distance runs or skiing, tend to have no immediate effect on plasma or serum Zn, but decreases have been observed in the hours after the activity.[49,50] These changes in circulating Zn have been interpreted as evidence of redistribution of Zn in the body.

There are limited data to support the hypothesis that exercise induces Zn redistribution. Plasma Zn concentrations, determined before and immediately after graded ergocycle work capacity tests, changed in response to dietary Zn.[42] Although preexercise plasma Zn values were within the range of normal values, they decreased significantly when dietary Zn was reduced and increased significantly when dietary Zn was increased (Figure 2). Postexercise plasma Zn concentrations increased significantly after exercise; they responded similarly to the preexercise values to changes in dietary Zn. As compared to the control period when dietary Zn was adequate, the change in plasma Zn concentration in response to exercise was significantly smaller (8%) when dietary Zn was restricted and significantly larger (19%) when dietary Zn was increased. To correct for the effects of hemoconcentration, plasma Zn concentrations were adjusted for changes in hematocrit and hemoglobin to yield values of change in plasma Zn content. The adjusted values, which were positive when dietary Zn was adequate and negative when Zn intake was low (Figure 2), have been interpreted to indicate altered Zn mobilization, presumably a release of Zn from muscle Zn stores in association with exercise-induced catabolism when dietary Zn was inadequate.[42] This postulated explanation is consistent with data from animals studies in which slow-twitch muscle Zn was reduced in response to restricted Zn intake.[11]

Alternatively, exercise-induced changes in plasma Zn may be explained by release of Zn from erythrocytes. Ohno et al.[52] found that erythrocyte Zn concentration decreased immediately after short-duration, high-intensity ergocycle exercise and returned to preexercise values within 1 h. A significant correlation was reported between erythrocyte Zn and α_2-macroglobulin Zn in plasma after exercise. Thus, brief physical exercise apparently induces the movement of Zn into the plasma.

Although it is clear that a transient redistribution of Zn occurs during exercise, the mechanism is unclear. Immune factors, such as cytokines, have been shown to change circulating Zn concentrations of rats.[53] In addition, exercise has been shown to induce metallothionein in liver and to exert small but significant increases in hepatic Zn with concomitant decreases in plasma Zn.[54]

V. ZINC SUPPLEMENTATION

Zn supplements are used by some athletes to improve performance. Singh et al.[33] found that 21% of elite female runners consumed Zn supplements to enhance their performance. Although there is evidence that Zn is needed for optimal muscle function,[55] the effects of supplemental Zn on performance are equivocal.

A. PERFORMANCE-ENHANCING EFFECTS

Isaacson and Sandow[56] demonstrated that added Zn enhances *in situ* contraction of frog skeletal muscle. This ergogenic effect was associated with increased tension without tetanus and prolonged contraction and relaxation periods of the muscle twitch. Thus, ionic Zn in the physiologic range is a potentiator of muscle contraction and relaxation. The effects of supplemental Zn on muscle function were examined in adult male rats receiving Zn (2 or 4 mg/d) dissolved in water for 30 days.[57] Contraction was induced by electrical stimulation of the gastrocnemius muscle and fatigue was determined. Rats supplemented with 4, as compared to 2 mg Zn per day, had a greater time to fatigue (19.8 ± 1.0 vs. 16.2 ± 0.8 s). Although these findings suggest that oral Zn supplements, at least in rodents, may increase muscle stamina by prolonging muscle contraction, there is no indication that the observed change in performance resulted from an improvement in muscle Zn status or increased activity of Zn-dependent enzymes.

TABLE 3 Content and Estimated Percent of Recommended Dietary Allowance (RDA) of Zinc in Selected Foods

Foods	Serving Size[a]	Zinc[b,c] (mg)	% RDA[d] Men	% RDA[d] Women
Meats and fish				
Chuck blade roast, braised	3 oz (85 g)	8.7	58	73
Beef, ground lean, broiled	3 oz (85 g)	5.3	35	44
Steak, T-bone	3 oz (85 g)	4.6	31	38
Beef, eye of round, roasted	3 oz (85 g)	4.0	27	33
Pork shoulder blade, broiled	3 oz (85 g)	4.3	29	36
Pork loin chop, broiled	3 oz (85 g)	1.9	13	16
Chicken, drumstick, fried	3 oz (85 g)	2.7	18	23
Chicken, dark meat, fried	3 oz (85 g)	1.8	12	15
Chicken, breast meat, fried	3 oz (85 g)	0.9	6	8
Turkey, dark meat, roasted	3 oz (85 g)	3.8	25	32
Turkey, light meat, roasted	3 oz (85 g)	1.7	11	14
Tuna, canned in oil	3 oz (85 g)	0.8	5	7
Haddock, breaded, fried	3 oz (85 g)	0.5	3	4
Lobster, cooked moist heat	3 oz (85 g)	2.5	17	21
Shrimp, boiled	3 oz (85 g)	1.3	9	11
Dairy products				
Yogurt, nonfat/fruit flavored	6 oz (170 g)	1.3	9	11
Milk, lowfat, 2%	1 cup (244 g)	0.9	6	8
Cottage cheese, lowfat, 2%	1/2 cup (113 g)	0.5	3	4
Cereals				
Raisin bran	3/4 cup (38 g)	1.1	7	9
Corn flakes	1 cup (25 g)	0.1	1	1
Grains				
Bagel, whole wheat	3 in (55 g)	1.3	9	11
Whole wheat bread	1 slice (28 g)	0.5	3.	4
Macaroni, boiled	1/2 cup (70 g)	0.4	3	3
Fruits				
Banana	8 3/4 in (114 g)	0.2	1	2
Orange, raw	medium (131 g)	0.1	1	1
Vegetables				
Spinach, boiled, drained	1/2 cup (90 g)	0.7	5	6
Potato, white, baked w/skin	2–3 in (122 g)	0.4	3	3
Broccoli, chopped, raw	1/2 cup (44 g)	0.2	1	2
Carrots, raw	7.5 in (72 g)	0.2	1	2
Tomato	2 in (76 g)	0.1	1	1
Beans and Legumes				
Pork and beans	1/2 cup (126 g)	7.4	49	62
Kidney beans	1/2 cup (86 g)	1.0	7	8
Mixed dishes				
Beef cheeseburger, bun	4 oz (95 g)	6.8	45	57
Chile con carne	1 cup (253 g)	3.6	24	30
Lasagna	1 cup (250 g)	3.3	22	28
Spaghetti, meatball, and tomato sauce	1 cup (248 g)	2.6	17	22
Macaroni and cheese, prepared from box	3/4 cup (147 g)	1.3	9	11

[a] English units with metric units in parentheses.

[b,c] Values estimated by using data provided by U.S. Department of Agriculture.[72-73]

[d] Food and Nutrition Board, National Academy of Sciences.[36]

There is limited information about the effects of Zn supplementation on human muscle strength and endurance. A group of 16 middle-aged women received a Zn supplement (135 mg/d) and a placebo in a double-blind, cross-over design study.[58] Muscle strength and endurance were measured with an isokinetic, one-leg exercise test using a standardized dynamometer before and after 14 d of experimental treatment. As compared to placebo,

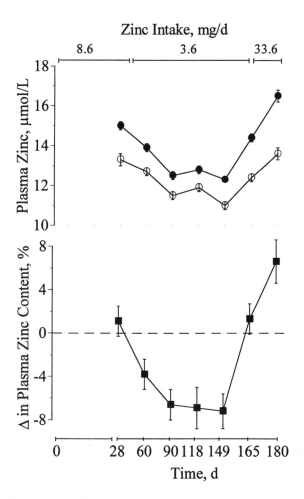

FIGURE 2 Effects of dietary zinc on plasma zinc concentrations before (open circles) and immediately after (closed circles) graded, maximal ergocycle exercise (upper panel), and changes in plasma zinc content after the same exercise in healthy men (lower panel). Data are mean ± SE. From Lukaski, H. C., Bolonchuk, W. W., Klevay, L. M., et al., *Am. J. Physiol.,* 247, E88, 1984. With permission.

Zn supplementation significantly increased dynamic isokinetic strength and isometric endurance. Because these types of muscular strength and endurance require recruitment of fast-twitch glycolytic muscle fibers, it may be hypothesized that Zn supplementation enhanced activity of the Zn-containing enzyme, lactate dehydrogenase. Unfortunately, because neither dietary Zn nor Zn status was determined, it is unclear whether Zn supplementation had a physiological or pharmacological effect on the measured indices of performance.

The effects of graded dietary Zn or peak work capacity also has been evaluated. In untrained men fed diets containing variable Zn contents (3.6, 8.6, and 33.6 mg Zn per day), peak oxygen uptake, determined during graded maximal ergocycle exercise, was not affected.[42] Similarly, rats fed diets containing 5 as compared to 50 mg Zn per kilogram of diet for 3 weeks had significantly decreased serum Zn concentrations (10 vs. 19 μmol/l) without a decrease in endurance assessed with treadmill running to exhaustion.[59] It remains to be determined if Zn supplementation has any impact on aerobic performance of trained athletes.

B. ANTIOXIDANT EFFECTS

Recent studies in animals and *in vitro* support the hypothesis that Zn possesses antioxidant properties.[60] Results from some human studies indicate that Zn supplementation may benefit only individuals with impaired Zn status. Insulin-dependent diabetic patients with low plasma Zn concentrations supplemented with 30 mg Zn (as Zn gluconate) daily for 3 months had significant increases in plasma Zn and selenium-dependent glutathione peroxidase, and reductions in plasma thiobarbituric acid reactants and plasma copper.[61] In contrast, Zn supplementation (50 mg/d as Zn sulfate for 28 days) of healthy men with normal serum Zn concentrations increased serum Zn with no measurable changes on *in vitro* low-density lipoprotein oxidation.[62] Beneficial effects of Zn supplementation on physiological function are manifest, therefore, only when Zn status is reduced.

C. ADVERSE EFFECTS OF ZINC SUPPLEMENTATION

Zn supplements should be used with caution and under the guidance of a physician or a registered dietitian. Copper absorption is impaired by Zn supplements providing 22.5 mg/d,[63] even when the supplement is taken independently of meals.[64] Erythrocyte superoxide dismutase activity, an index of copper status, is decreased within 12 days of ingesting 50 mg of supplemental Zn daily.[65] Larger doses of Zn supplements, 160 mg/d, taken for 16 weeks, reduce high-density lipoprotein (HDL) concentrations.[66] It has been suggested that use of Zn supplements ranging from 17 to 50 mg/d is sufficient to prevent an exercise-induced increase in HDL concentration.[67] It is recommended that if Zn supplements are used, the Zn consumed should not exceed 15 mg/d.[67]

D. SUPPLEMENTATION AND PERFORMANCE TRIALS

Generalized trials of the effects of vitamin and mineral supplementation on human physical performance have reported negligible results. A group of 30 male, trained long-distance runners participated in a 9-month cross-over design experiment in which supplements or placebos were consumed for 3 months, followed by a 3-month period in which no experimental treatment was given; then the treatments were reversed for the final 3 months.[68,69] On the basis of laboratory and field performance tests, there was no measurable ergogenic effect of multiple vitamin and mineral supplementation. Analyses of self-reported dietary records indicated that nutrient intakes, exclusive of supplements, were at least 70% of RDA or estimated safe and adequate daily dietary intake values. Blood biochemical measurements of nutritional status were within ranges of normal values.

Similar results were reported in other studies[70,71] of 86 competitive Australian athletes (50 men and 36 women) training in basketball, gymnastics, swimming, and rowing and receiving either a placebo or a commercially prepared vitamin and mineral supplement designed for athletes. During the 7- to 8-month experimental period there was no significant change in serum Zn concentration in either the supplemented or the placebo group (17.1 and 17.8 μmol/l, respectively). Dietary Zn, exclusive of supplementation, was consistent with recommended dietary intake for Australians. Performance, as assessed with a battery of general and sport-specific tests, was not impacted by the supplementation. Therefore, the results of these well-controlled and extensive trials[68-71] clearly indicate that general supplementation of individuals with adequate dietary intake of Zn provides no measurable improvement of Zn status or physical performance.

VI. DIETARY ZINC

A. ZINC IN FOODS

Zn content is a major determinant of the adequacy of various foods as sources of Zn.[72,73] Commonly consumed foods in the U.S. have a highly variable content of Zn (Table 3). Animal products (meat, fish, and poultry) have the greatest concentration of Zn and provide the principal source (about 49%) of Zn in the U.S. diet.[74] The richest source of Zn is oysters. Meat from fish has a smaller concentration of Zn than most muscle meats. Milk and milk products are important sources of Zn, particularly for infants and children, and contribute 19% of the daily Zn intake. Importantly, adipose tissue or fat in animal and diary products has negligible Zn content. The content of Zn consequently is high in cheese and low in butter and cream.

Cereals represent significant sources of energy and Zn in many areas throughout the world. Large differences in the Zn content, depending on the cereal type and including the variety, class, and location of production have been reported. For example, the Zn content of wheat has been found to range from 15 to 102 mg/kg depending on the strain, and from 219 to 61 mg/kg for the same variety of wheat grown in different locations and different years.[75] It is estimated that cereal and grain products provide about 13% of the dietary Zn in the U.S.[74] Data for the Zn content of legumes consumed by humans are limited. As with cereals, factors such as variety, strain, and growing location impact the Zn content of legumes.

Fruits and vegetables have modest contents of Zn (1 to 8 mg/kg) because of the high water content of the produce. Because these products provide limited energy intake, their contribution to total daily Zn intake is minimal.

B. PROCESSING AND PREPARATION OF FOODS

The amount of Zn present in foods is affected by how the fresh product is processed and prepared. Unfortunately, knowledge of nutrient losses during food processing and preparation is limited and generally restricted to vitamins.

The food process that has a major impact on Zn intake is refinement of cereals and grains. Because Zn is located in the outer layers, the germ and bran, of grain and cereal kernels, large losses of Zn occur during milling and extraction. For example, about 80% of Zn in wheat is lost during the milling process.[76] Similar losses occurs during the polishing of rice and in the refining of sugar.

Other pretreatments of foods before cooking or consumption, and cooking procedures themselves, can influence the Zn content of a meal. Use of galvanized cookware and storage of foods in Zn oxide-lined cans adds Zn to foods.[77] Zn losses may be significant (20%) from foods into water used for preparation, and from foods stored in cans into the storage media.[78]

C. Zinc Bioavailability

The quantity of dietary Zn that is absorbed by a human is a function of the Zn status of the individual, amount of Zn ingested, and the bioavailability of the Zn from the meal. Bioavailability refers to the combined effects of various promoters and inhibitors of Zn absorption in the foods present in a meal.[13] Various nutrients and food components impact human Zn bioavailability.

The amount and type of protein affects human Zn absorption. Zn absorption is positively related to the amount of protein in a meal and Zn bioavailability is generally better from foods of animal than plant origin.[17] Factors that impact Zn bioavailability from plant foods are fiber and phytic acid.

Fiber in the form of bran has been found to reduce Zn absorption[79,80] or to have no effect.[81] Differences in particle size of the bran has been suggested to be a factor in these conflicting results.[81] In humans, Zn absorption from wholemeal bread was less than half (17%) of that from white bread (38%), but the Zn content of the wholemeal bread was three times greater than that of the white bread, so the total Zn absorbed was greater from the wholemeal bread.[82]

Phytic acid also has been shown to interfere with human Zn absorption. Stable isotope studies in humans showed a 50% reduction in Zn absorption when 3 g/d of sodium phytate was added to the diet.[83]

Zn absorption is inhibited in humans by the presence of excesses of certain minerals. When inorganic salts of iron and Zn are given, Zn absorption is decreased.[84] Zn absorption from food was not affected by large amounts of heme iron.[85,86]

VII. CONCLUSIONS

Zn is an essential nutrient that has biological roles in protein, carbohydrate, and lipid metabolism and, hence, is needed for health and optimal performance. Experimental evidence describing the interaction of dietary Zn and physical activity in humans is limited. Athletes who consume adequate amounts of dietary Zn have plasma or serum Zn concentrations that are within the range of normal values. Conversely, athletes who restrict food intake, and concomitantly dietary Zn, have low concentrations of Zn in the circulation. As compared to nonexercise conditions, exercise induces increased losses of Zn in the sweat and urine that represent a small and perhaps significant percentage of daily Zn intake. Because the body tends to maintain the Zn content by selectively adjusting absorption and endogenous excretion of Zn, and an adaptation in urinary Zn output occurs on the day following a bout of exercise, the losses of Zn associated with heavy exercise probably are compensated. Proper selection of a variety of foods, including animal products and unprocessed grains and cereals with varied zinc content will ensure an adequate Zn intake. Unequivocal evidence of beneficial effects of Zn supplementation on physical performance of humans is lacking.

Consumption of Zn supplements by individuals with adequate Zn status may cause harm by inducing copper deficiency. Without biochemical or physical evidence of altered Zn status, individuals should avoid the use of Zn supplements in amounts exceeding 15 mg/d. Consumption of supplemental Zn in amounts greater than 15 mg/d can lead to impaired copper absorption and decreased HDL cholesterol. Because Zn impacts many diverse biological functions, physically active people should attempt to consume a balanced diet to ensure an adequate Zn intake and thus optimize health and physical performance.

ACKNOWLEDGMENT

Cyndy O'Brien-Nimens, L.R.D., is recognized for contributing the data on the zinc content of foods commonly consumed in the U.S.

REFERENCES

1. Lukaski, H. C., Micronutrients (magnesium, zinc and copper): are mineral supplements needed?, *Int. J. Sports Nutr.,* 5, S74, 1995.
2. Vallee, B. L. and Falchuk, K. H., The biochemical basis of zinc physiology, *Physiol. Rev.,* 73, 79, 1993.
3. Vallee, B. L. and Auld, D. S., Active zinc binding sites of zinc metalloenzymes, in *Matrix Metalloproteinases and Inhibitors, Matrix Supplement 1,* Birkedal-Hansen, H., Werb, Z., Welgus, H., and van Wart, H., Eds., Gustav Fischer, Stuttgart, 1992, 5.
4. Vallee, B. L. and Auld, D. S., Zinc coordination, function and structure of zinc enzymes and other proteins, *Biochemistry,* 29, 5647, 1990.
5. Hambidge, K. M., Casey, C. E., and Krebs, N. F., Zinc, in *Trace Elements in Human and Animal Nutrition,* 5th ed., Vol. 2, Mertz, W., Ed., Academic Press, Orlando, FL, 1986, 1.
6. Reeves, P. G. and O'Dell, B. L., Effect of zinc deficiency on glucose metabolism in meal-fed rats, *Br. J. Nutr.,* 49, 441, 1983.
7. Mills, C. F., Ed., *Zinc in Human Biology,* International Life Science Institute, London, 1989.

8. Bettger, W. J. and O'Dell, B. L., A critical physiological role of zinc in the structure and function of biomembranes, *Life Sci.,* 28, 1425, 1981.

9. International Commission on Radiological Protection, Report No. 23, *Report on the Task Group on Reference Man,* Pergamon Press, Oxford, 1975.

10. Maltin, C. A., Duncan, L., Wilson, A. B., and Hesketh, J. E., Effect of zinc on muscle fiber type frequencies in the post-weanling rat, *Br. J. Nutr.,* 50, 597, 1983.

11. O'Leary, M. J., McClain, C. J., and Hegarty, P. V. J., Effect of zinc on the weight, cellularity and zinc concentration of different skeletal muscles in the post-weaning rat, *Br. J. Nutr.,* 42, 487, 1979.

12. Jackson, M. J., Jones, D. A., and Edwards, R. H. T., Tissue zinc as an index of body zinc status, *Clin. Physiol.,* 2, 333, 1982.

13. Sandström, B. and Lönnerdal, B., Promoters and antagonists of zinc absorption, in *Zinc in Human Biology,* Mills, C. F., Ed., International Life Science Institute, London, 1989, 57.

14. Schölmerich, J., Freudemann, A., Köttgen, E., Wietholtz, H., Steiert, B., Löhle, E., Häussinger, D., and Gerok, W., Bioavailability of zinc from zinc-histidine complexes. I. Comparison with zinc sulfate in healthy men, *Am. J. Clin. Nutr.,* 45, 1480, 1987.

15. King, J. C. and Keen, C. L., Zinc, in *Modern Nutrition in Health and Disease,* 9th ed., Shils, M. E., Olson, J. A., and Shike, M., Eds., Lea & Febiger, Philadelphia, PA, 214.

16. Cousins, R. J., Absorption, transport and hepatic metabolism of copper and zinc: special reference to metallothionein and ceruloplasmin, *Physiol. Rev.,* 65, 238, 1985.

17. Johnson, P. E., Zinc absorption and excretion in humans and animals, in *Inflammation and Drug Therapy Series,* Vol. 4, Copper and Zinc in Inflammation, Milanino, R., Rainsford, K. D., and Velo, G. P., Eds., Kluwer Academic, Amsterdam, 1989, 103.

18. Baer, M. T. and King, J. C., Tissue zinc levels and zinc excretion during experimental zinc depletion in young men, *Am. J. Clin. Nutr.,* 39, 556, 1984.

19. Jackson, M. J., Jones, D. A., Edwards, R. H. T., Swainbank, I. G., and Coleman, M. L., Zinc homeostasis in man: studies using a new stable isotope-dilution technique, *Br. J. Nutr.,* 51, 199, 1984.

20. Prasad, A. S., Schulbert, A. R., Sandstead, H. H., Miale, A., and Farid, Z., Zinc, iron and nitrogen content of sweat in normal and zinc-deficient men, *J. Lab. Clin. Med.,* 62, 84, 1963.

21. Milne, D. B., Canfield, W. K., Mahalko, J. R., and Sandstead, H. H., Effect of dietary zinc on whole body surface loss of zinc: impact on estimation of zinc retention by balance method, *Am. J. Clin. Nutr.,* 38, 181, 1983.

22. Hess, F. M., King, J. C., and Margen, S., Zinc excretion in young women on low zinc diet and oral contraceptive agents, *J. Nutr.,* 107, 1610, 1977.

23. Coppen, D. E. and Davies, N. T., Studies on the effect of dietary zinc dose on ^{65}Zn absorption in vivo and on effects of zinc status on ^{65}Zn absorption and body loss in young rats, *Br. J. Nutr.,* 57, 35, 1987.

24. Aamodt, R. L., Rumble, W. F., Babcock, A. K., Foster, D. M., and Henkin, R. I., Effects of oral zinc loading on zinc metabolism in humans. I. Experimental studies, *Metabolism,* 31, 326, 1982.

25. Cousins, R. J., Systemic transpsort of zinc, in *Zinc in Human Biology,* Mills, C. F., Ed., International Life Science Institute, London, 1989, 79.

26. Golden, M. H. N., The diagnosis of zinc deficiency, in *Zinc in Human Biology,* Mills, C. F., Ed., International Life Science Institute, London, 1989, 323.

27. Solomons, N. W., On the assessment of zinc and copper nutriture in man, *Am. J. Clin. Nutr.,* 32, 856, 1979.

28. King, J. C., Assessment of zinc status, *J. Nutr.,* 120, 1474, 1990.

29. Milne, D. B., Ralston, N. V. C., and Wallwork, J. C., Zinc content of cellular components of blood: methods for cell separation and analysis evaluated, *Clin. Chem.,* 31, 65, 1985.

30. Dressendorfer, R. H. and Sockolov, R., Hypozincemia in runners, *Phys. Sportsmed.,* 8, 97, 1980.

31. Haralambie, G., Serum zinc in athletes during training, *Int. J. Sports Med.,* 2, 135, 1981.

32. Deuster, P. A., Dyle, S. B., Moser, P. B., Vigersky, R. A., and Schoonmaker, E. B., Nutritional survey of highly trained women runners, *Am. J. Clin. Nutr.,* 45, 954, 1986.

33. Singh, A., Deuster, P. A., and Moser, P. B., Zinc and copper status of women by physical activity and menstrual status, *J. Sports Med. Phys. Fitness,* 30, 247, 1990.

34. Lukaski, H. C., Bolonchuk, W. W., Klevay, L. M., Milne, D. B., and Sandstead, H. H., Maximal oxygen consumption as related to magnesium, copper and zinc nutriture, *Am. J. Clin. Nutr.,* 37, 407, 1983.

35. Lukaski, H. C., Hoverson, B. S., Gallagher, S. K., and Bolonchuk, W. W., Physical training and copper, iron and zinc status of swimmers, *Am. J. Clin. Nutr.,* 51, 1093, 1990.

36. Food and Nutrition Board, National Research Council, *Recommended Dietary Allowances,* 10th ed., National Academy Press, Washington, D.C., 1989, 30.

37. Fogelholm, M., Laasko, J., Lehto, J., and Ruokonen, I., Dietary intake and indicators of magnesium and zinc status in male athletes, *Nutr. Res.,* 11, 1111, 11991.

38. Fogelholm, M., Rehunen, S., Gref, C.-G., Laasko, J. T., Lehto, J. J., Ruokonen, I., and Himberg, J.-J., Dietary intake and thiamin, iron and zinc status in elite skiers during different training periods, *Int. J. Sports Nutr.,* 2, 351, 1992.

39. Deuster, P. A., Day, B. A., Singh, A., Douglass, L., and Moser-Veillon, P. B., Zinc status of highly trained women runners and untrained women, *Am. J. Clin. Nutr.,* 49, 1295, 1989.

40. Benson, J., Gillien, D. M., Bourdet, K., and Loosli, A. R., Inadequate nutrition and chronic calorie restriction in adolescent ballerinas, *Phys. Sportsmed.,* 13, 79, 1985.

41. Loosli, A. R., Benson, J., Gillien, D. M., and Bourdet, K., Nutrition habits and knowledge in competitive adolescent female gymnasts, *Phys. Sportsmed.,* 14, 118, 1986.

42. Lukaski, H. C., Bolonchuk, W. W., Klevay, L. M., Milne, D. B., and Sandstead, H. H., Changes in plasma zinc content after exercise in men fed a low-zinc diet, *Am. J. Physiol.,* 247, E88, 1984.

43. Jacob, R. A., Sandstead, H. H., Munoz, J. M., Klevay, L. M., and Milne, D. B., Whole-body surface loss of trace elements in normal males, *Am. J. Clin. Nutr.,* 34, 1379, 1981.

44. Consolazio, C. F., Nutrition and performance, in *Progress in Food and Nutrition Science,* Vol. 7, Johnson, R. E., Ed., Pergamon Press, Oxford, 1983.

45. Aruoma, O. I., Reilly, T., MacLaren, D., and Halliwell, B., Iron, copper and zinc in human sweat and plasma: effect of exercise, *Clin. Chim. Acta,* 177, 81, 1988.

46. Tipton, K., Green, N. R., Waller, M., and Haymes, E. M., Mineral losses from sweat in athletes exercising at two different temperatures, *FASEB J.,* 6, A768, 1991.

47. Uhari, M., Pakarinen, A., Hietala, J., Nurmi, T., and Kouvalainen, K., Serum iron, copper, zinc, ferritin, and ceruloplasmin after intense heat exposure, *Eur. J. Appl. Physiol.,* 51, 331, 1983.

48. Dressendorfer, R. H., Wade, C. E., Keen, C. L., and Scaff, J. H., Plasma mineral levels in marathon runners during a 20-day road race, *Phys. Sportsmed.,* 10, 113, 1982.

49. van Rij, A. M., Hall, M. T., Dohm, G. L., Bray, J., and Pories, W. J., Changes in zinc metabolism following exercise in human subjects, *Biol. Trace Elem. Res.,* 10, 99, 1986.

50. Anderson, R. A., Polansky, M. M., and Bryden, N. A., Strenuous running: acute effects on chromium, copper, zinc, and selected clinical variables in urine and serum of male runners, *Biol. Trace Elem. Res.,* 6, 327, 1984.

51. Anderson, R. A., Bryden, N. A., and Polansky, M. M., Acute exercise effects on urinary losses and serum concentration of copper and zinc of moderately trained and untrained men consuming a controlled diet, *Analyst,* 120, 867, 1995.

52. Ohno, H., Yamashita, K., Doi, R., Yamamura, K., Kondo, T., and Taniguchi, N., Exercise-induced changes in blood zinc and related proteins, *J. Appl. Physiol.,* 58, 1453, 1985.

53. Cannon, J. G. and Kluger, M. J., Engogenous pyrogen activity in human plasma after exercise, *Science,* 220, 617, 1983.

54. Oh, S. H., Deagen, J. T., Whanger, P. D., and Weswig, P. H., Biological function of metallothionein. V. Its induction in rats by various stresses, *Am. J. Physiol.,* 234, E282, 1978.

55. Wang, J. and Pierson, R. N., Distribution of zinc in skeletal muscle and liver tissue in normal and dietary controlled alcoholic rats, *J. Lab. Clin. Med.,* 85, 50, 1975.

56. Isaacson, A. and Sandow, A., Effects of zinc on responses of skeletal muscle, *J. Gen. Physiol.,* 46, 655, 1963.

57. Richardson, J. H. and Drake, P. D., The effects of zinc on fatigue of striated muscle, *J. Sports Med.,* 19, 133, 1979.

58. Krotkiewski, M., Gudmundsson, P., Backström, and Mandroukas, K., Zinc and muscle strength and endurance, *Acta Physiol. Scand.,* 116, 309, 1982.

59. McDonald, R. and Keen, C. L., Iron, zinc and magnesium nutrition and physical performance, *Sports Med.,* 5, 171, 1988.

60. Bray, T. M. and Bettger, W. J., The physiological role of zinc as an antioxidant, *Free Rad. Biol. Med.,* 8, 281, 1990.

61. Faure, P., Benhamou, P. Y., Halimi, S., and Roussel, A. M., Lipid peroxidation in insulin-dependent diabetic patients with early retina degenerative lesions: effects of an oral zinc supplementation, *Eur. J. Clin. Nutr.,* 149, 282, 1995.

62. Gatto, L. M. and Samman, S., The effect of zinc supplementation on plasma lipids and low-density lipoprotein oxidation in males, *Free Rad. Biol. Med.,* 19, 517, 1995.

63. Hackman, R. M. and Keen, C. L., Changes in serum zinc and copper levels after zinc supplementation in running and non-running men, in *Sport Health and Nutrition,* Katch, F. I., Ed., Human Kinetics, Champaiagn, IL, 1986, 89.

64. Van den Hamer, C. J. A., Hoogeraad, T. U., and Klompjan, E. R. K., Persistence of the antagonistic effect of zinc on copper absorption after cessation of zinc supplementation for more than five days, *Biol. Trace Elem. Res.,* 1, 99, 1984.

65. Abdallah, S. M. and Samman, S., The effect of increasing dietary zinc on the activity of superoxide dismutase and zinc concentration in erythrocytes of healthy female subjects, *Eur. J. Clin. Nutr.,* 47, 327, 1993.

66. Hooper, P. L., Visconti, L., Garry, P. J., and Johnson, G. E., Zinc lowers high-density lipoprotein cholesterol levels, *J. Am. Med. Assoc.,* 244, 1960, 1980.

67. Goodwin, J. S., Hunt, W. C., Hooper, P., and Garry, P. J., Relationship between zinc intake, physical activity and blood levels of high-density lipoprotein cholesterol in a healthy elderly population, *Metabolism,* 34, 519, 1985.

68. Weight, L. M., Noakes, T. D., Labadarios, D., Graves, J., Jacobs, P., and Berman, P. A., Vitamin and mineral status of trained athletes including the effects of supplementation, *Am. J. Clin. Nutr.,* 47, 186, 1988.

69. Weight, L. M., Myburgh, K. H., and Noakes, T. D., Vitamin and mineral supplementation: effect on the running performance of trained athletes, *Am. J. Clin. Nutr.,* 47, 192, 1988.

70. Tellford, R. D., Catchpole, E. A., Deakin, V., McLeay, A. C., and Plank, A. W., The effect of 7 to 8 minths of vitamin/mineral supplementation on the vitamin and mineral status of athletes, *Int. J. Sports Nutr.,* 2, 123, 1992.

71. Tellford, R. D., Catchpole, E. A., Deakin, V., Hahn, A. G., and Plank, A. W., The effect of 7 to 8 months of vitamin/mineral supplementation on athletic performance, *Int. J. Sports Nutr.,* 2, 135, 1992.

72. USDA, Consumer Nutrition Data Set 456-3, U.S. Department of Agriculture, Hyattsville, MD, 1977.

73. USDA, Composition of Foods, Agriculture Handbook 8.1-12, U.S. Department of Agriculture, Hyattsville, MD, 1976-1984.

74. Life Sciences Research Office, Federation of American Societies for Experimental Biology, Nutrition Monitoring in the United States — An Update Report on Nutrition Monitoring, U.S. Department of Agriculture, U.S. Department of Health and Human Services, DHHS Publ. No. (PHS) 89-1255, U.S. Government Printing Office, Washington, D.C., 1989, 71.

75. Davis, K. R., Peters, L. J., Cain, R. F., LeTourneau, D., and McGinnis, J., Evaluation of the nutrient composition of wheat. III. Minerals, *Am. Assoc. Cereal Chem.,* 29, 246, 1984.

76. Schroeder, H. A., Loss of vitamins and trace minerals resulting from processing and preservation of foods, *Am. J. Clin. Nutr.,* 24, 562, 1971.

77. Henriksen, L. K., Mahalko, J. R., and Johnson, L. K., Canned foods: appropriate in trace element studies?, *J. Am. Diet. Assoc.,* 85, 563, 1985.

78. Schmitt, H. A. and Weaver, C. M., Effects of laboratory scale processing on chromium and zinc in vegetables, *J. Food Sci.,* 47, 1693, 1982.

79. Sandberg, A.-S., Hasselbland, C., Hasselbland, K., and Hulten, L., The effect of wheat bran on the absorption of minerals in the small intestine, *Br. J. Nutr.,* 48, 185, 1982.

80. Schwartz, R., Apgar, B. J., and Wien, E. M., Apparent absorption and retention of Ca, Cu, Mg, Mn, and Zn from a diet containing bran, *Am. J. Clin. Nutr.,* 43, 444, 1986.

81. Van Dokkum, W., Wesstra, A., and Schippers, F. A., Physiological effects of fibre-rich types of bread. I. The effect of dietary fibre from bread on the mineral balance of young men, *Br. J. Nutr.,* 47, 451, 1982.

82. Sandström, B., Arvidsson, B., Cederblad, Å., and Björn-Rasmussen, E., Zinc absorption from composite meals. I. The significance of wheat extraction rate, zinc, calcium, and protein content in meals based on bread, *Am. J. Clin. Nutr.,* 33, 739, 1980.

83. Turnland, J. R., King, J. C., and Keyes, W. R., A stable isotope study of zinc absorption in young men: effects of phytate and cellulose, *Am. J. Clin. Nutr.,* 40, 1071, 1984.

84. Solomons, N. W. and Jacob, R. A., Studies on the bioavailability of zinc in humans: effects of heme and nonheme iron on the absorption of zinc, *Am. J. Clin. Nutr.,* 34, 475, 1981.

85. Solomons, N. W., Pineda, O., Viteri, F., and Sandstead, H. H., Studies on the bioavailability of zinc in humans: mechanisms of the intestinal interaction of nonheme iron and zinc, *J. Nutr.,* 113, 337, 1983.

86. Valberg, L. S., Flanagan, P. R., and Chamberlain, M. J., Effects of iron, tin and copper on zinc absorption in humans, *Am. J. Clin. Nutr.,* 40, 536, 1984.

Chapter 13

COPPER

Philip G. Reeves

CONTENTS

I. INTRODUCTION

During the past few years a sustained interest in trace element nutrition and metabolism as it relates to athletic performance has developed. The current belief is that athletes require more minerals than a more sedentary individual, that athletes do not eat a balanced diet, and that low consumption of some trace elements will lower performance. Whether these beliefs have substance in fact is still under consideration. However, for all the minerals covered in this volume, copper (Cu) may be one of the most important ones concerning athletic conditioning and performance. It is a "Jekyll and Hyde" of the mineral nutrients, because it serves as an essential component of the antioxidant system, but at the same time it also can be toxic by causing the generation of free radicals.

Cu is one of the transition metals. It has valence states of +1 or +2 and is highly reactive in oxidation-reduction reactions. Because of this property, nature has devised means to assure that very little free Cu is present in the tissues of animals or humans. Most of the Cu is bound to small ligands such as amino acids and peptides, and to proteins. Cu can interact with other metals near it in the periodic table. Some of these include iron, zinc, and cadmium. This interaction often involves the substitution of the other metals in enzyme active sites or metal transport sites normally reserved for Cu, and inhibits Cu's function there. Sometimes Cu can interfere with the metabolism of the other metals.

Cu is involved in many chemical reactions in the body that may be more prominently involved with oxygen consumption and stress, conditions that become exaggerated during participation in vigorous exercise. For example, Cu is necessary for full activity of cytochrome c oxidase, the enzyme in a chain of reactions that transfers electrons from cytochrome c to oxygen, which leads to the production of water during metabolism. Cu is also an active component of superoxide dismutase, an enzyme involved in free-radical quenching and elimination, thus lessening free-radical damage in the tissues. Cu is required for hemoglobin formation and in the prevention of anemia. Cu plays a major role in the acute phase response to stress situations.

Cu is also involved in cardiovascular and neuronal development and function. Cu is an active component of enzymes that cross-link collagen and elastin in the vascular system, lung, and other organs. Cu deficiency in young rats causes lung damage similar to emphysema. The trace element is intimately involved in enzyme systems that generate brain and somatic neurotransmitters. Cu deficiency in animals produces a Parkinson-like disease syndrome.

On the other hand, Cu can be toxic. Free Cu can participate in the superoxide-driven Fenton reaction to produce the free radical, HO·, from hydrogen peroxide. This radical is strongly reactive at the site of formation. Cu is more reactive than iron in causing DNA damage, which suggests that the free Cu concentrations in the body should be carefully controlled.

The preceding is presented to show the broad involvement of Cu in metabolism. The following will go into more detail on where we might obtain Cu in the diet, how it is absorbed into the body, how much is in the body, how it functions biochemically and physiologically, and what its dietary requirements are. This chapter attempts to relate each point to athletic training and performance, where applicable. For an in-depth review of Cu and its metabolism, please refer to Mason,[1] O'Dell,[2] and Linder.[3]

II. COPPER CONCENTRATIONS IN FOODS AND COPPER INTAKES BY ATHLETES

A. FOOD COPPER

Of all the minerals known to have a physiological function in the body, Cu perhaps is one of the most limiting in the human diet. The Food and Nutrition Board (FNB) of the National Research Council (NRC) of the U.S. National Academy of Sciences, in their 1980 deliberation,[4] could not agree on a recommended dietary allowance (RDA) for Cu. Instead, they established a value called "the safe and adequate daily dietary intake" (ESADDI) for Cu that has a range of 2.0 to 3.0 mg/day for individuals over the age of 11. The Canadian estimate for an adequate intake of Cu is 1.0 to 2.0 mg/day.[5] Although much more data had accumulated over the ensuing 9 years, the FNB again in 1989 could not choose an RDA for Cu but instead lowered the ESADDI to 1.5 to 3.0 mg/day.[6]

The normal intake of Cu by humans is relatively low compared to the ESADDI. Klevay et al.[7] chemically analyzed the amount of Cu in 849 individual Western-type diets consisting of foods from Belgium, Canada, the U.K., and the U.S. They found that the mean intake of Cu per day was 1.48 mg with 95% of the values falling between 0.46 and 3.64, and 32% of the diets provided less than 1.01 mg of Cu per day. They concluded that selecting a diet with less than the ESADDI is easy for an individual in the Western world if the diet is not balanced with a variety of foods. Johnson et al.[8] reported an intake of 1.3 mg of Cu per day for men and 0.95 mg/day for women between the ages of 19 and 40 consuming self-selected diets. However, when intake was expressed on the basis of caloric density, women were taking in about 15% more Cu than men. But again, these values fall short of the lowest ESADDI value for Cu.

Not many staple foods including breads, vegetable, fruits, or even meats, contain much Cu. Lawler and Klevay[9] suggested that foods containing more than 2 mg of Cu per kilogram of edible portion are good sources of dietary Cu. Table 1 lists some common foods and their Cu contents.[10,11] Milk, considered by some to be the perfect food, has one of the lowest concentrations of Cu. Some fruits and vegetables have moderate quantities of Cu, with potatoes and beans the highest. Nuts and seeds have high amounts of Cu compared with other foods, and seeds such as sunflower kernels are an excellent source of Cu. However, these foods also contain a very high amount of fat, up to 40%.

The foods containing the highest amount of Cu are liver and Pacific oysters. A person can obtain more than 100% of the ESADDI with a 3-oz serving of these foods. On the other hand, other meats and fish have low concentrations of Cu. It seems an unfortunate quirk of nature to have the highest amount of Cu in foods that are expensive (oysters), contain high fat (nuts and seeds), and/or disliked by most of the U.S. and Canadian public (liver). However, clever disguises of the latter and/or substitutions of these foods for others in combination dishes would not only improve one's nutritional Cu status but provide a host of other required nutrients as well. Wheat flour is not very high in Cu; however, wild rice, if eaten regularly, can provide a moderate amount of Cu in the diet.

B. COPPER INTAKE IN ATHLETES

We are often concerned that persons undergoing strenuous exercise, or prolonged training and sports competition are not taking in enough of the required nutrients to sustain nutritional status, thus affecting performance. Recently, the Australian Institute of Sport undertook a study[12] to decide if vitamin/mineral supplementation of a normal diet would affect the vitamin and mineral status of athletes. There were 86 athletes, male and female, who participated in various sports activities for 8 months. One half of the group took a supplement that contained 13 known essential vitamins and 8 essential minerals (Cu was not included). After eight months of training and participating, none of the mineral supplements changed the overall mineral status of the athletes when measured as a change in blood concentration of the mineral and compared with those not receiving the supplements. Of the vitamins supplemented, only thiamine, B_6, and B_{12} in blood were elevated because of the supplementation. Before the sports activities began, only 7% of the participants were considered below the laboratory acceptable range for blood Cu concentration. However, at the end of the sports activities, no participant was below normal whether he or she took the supplements or not. Throughout the study, personal and group dietary counseling sessions were carried out to ensure that each athlete maintained a well-balanced diet. Therefore, one could interpret the results of this study to mean that if athletes maintain a well-balanced diet of a variety of foods, they do not require extra supplementation with vitamins and minerals. In addition, a corresponding study using the same subjects showed that the vitamin and mineral supplementation had no significant effects on performance.[13]

Another recent study looked at the dietary patterns and nutritional knowledge of recreational triathletes.[14] They found that over an 11-week training period, women consumed an average ± SD of 1.5 ± 0.5 mg of Cu per day, and men 1.8 ± 0.7. This represented 75 and 90% of the lowest range of the ESADDI for Cu for the 1980 version of the RDAs, respectively. However, when compared with the 1989 version, the average values were not lower than the

TABLE 1   Content and Estimated Percent of the Safe and Adequate Daily Dietary Intake (ESADDI) of Cu in Selected Foods by Serving Size

Foods	Serving Size	Cu (mg)[a]	% ESADDI[b]
Meats and fish			
Liver, cooked	3 oz	3.842	256
Oysters, Pacific, cooked	3 oz	2.279	152
Oysters, Atlantic, cooked	3 oz	1.220	81
Trout, broiled	3 oz	0.204	14
Duck, roasted w/skin	3 oz	0.193	13
Beef, sirloin roast	3 oz	0.105	7
Chicken, roasted	3 oz	0.068	5
Pork loin, roasted	3 oz	0.069	5
Salmon, coho, broiled	3 oz	0.076	5
Whitefish, broiled	3 oz	0.078	5
Fruits and vegetables			
Potato, white, baked w/skins	1 med	0.616	41
White beans, boiled	1 cup	0.514	34
Lentils, boiled	1 cup	0.497	33
Avocado, raw	1 med	0.460	31
Kidney beans, boiled	1 cup	0.428	28
Asparagus tips, steamed	1 cup	0.308	21
Potato, sweet, baked	1 sm	0.237	16
Mushrooms, raw	$^1/_2$ cup	0.172	11
Nuts, grains, and seeds			
Sunflower kernels, oil roasted	2 oz	1.037	69
Walnuts, fresh	2 oz	0.787	52
Almonds, dry roasted	2 oz	0.694	46
Wheat germ	$^1/_2$ cup	0.458	31
Peanuts, oil roasted	2 oz	0.381	25
Wild rice, cooked	1 cup	0.200	13
Barley, cooked	1 cup	0.165	11
Whole wheat bread	2 slices	0.172	11
White rice, cooked	1 cup	0.108	7
Oatmeal, cooked	1 cup	0.129	9
Milk, 1% fat	1 cup	0.025	2
Brewer's yeast	$^1/_2$ oz	0.700	47
Molasses, brown	1 fl oz	0.225	15

[a]   Values were generated from nutrition data sets provided by the U.S. Department of Agriculture.[10,11]

[b]   The Food and Nutrition Board of the National Research Council of the U.S. National Academy of Sciences recommends an ESADDI in the range of 1.5 to 3.0 mg of Cu per day.[6] These values are calculated based on the low end of this range.

ESADDI. When they looked at the frequency at which the athletes consumed diets with Cu below the 1980 ESADDI, they found that when consuming a normal diet without vitamin/mineral supplements, 90% of the women and 65% of the men were below the ESADDI for Cu. With vitamin/mineral supplementation, these values decreased to about 50% for both groups. These values would have been much lower, however, if they had compared the data with the 1989 ESADDI. Because they measured no Cu status indicators during the study, it is impossible to decide if these seemingly low Cu intakes affected the Cu status of the athletes. Based on the Australian studies[12,13] and the fact that the Australian diet is not very different from the U.S. diet, it seems unlikely that any low status would have been observed, except perhaps in individuals who were consistently taking in extremely low amounts of dietary Cu. Based on the standard deviation of the data, Cu intakes for some of the women in the U.S. study[14] were below the low range of the ESADDI. Bazzarre et al.[15] also showed that both men and women athletes consuming diets that provided an estimated average of 2.5 ± 3.6 mg/day of Cu (mid-range of the 1989 ESADDI), had serum Cu concentrations of about 22.6 ± 5.3 μmol/l (normal range, 14.2 to 23.6 μmol/l). With the large SD, it can be safely assumed that some of the subjects were ingesting diets with low concentrations of Cu. Therefore, it would have been of interest to determine the correlation between Cu intake and Cu concentrations in serum.

In a well-controlled study, Lukaski et al.[16] found no correlation between Cu intake of male and female swimmers and control nonswimmers and Cu status indicators measured before and after extensive training. The daily intake of Cu averaged 1.15 ± 0.36 mg/day for female nonswimmers and 1.35 ± 0.40 for female swimmers. Males averaged about 1.7 ± 0.54 for both swimmers and non-swimmers; this was significantly higher than for women. When intake was calculated on the basis of caloric intake, there were no significant differences in intake between men and women. Plasma concentrations of Cu ranged from 13.8 ± 3.2 to 15.9 ± 5.2 μmol/l for females whether they were swimmers or not, and the concentrations for males ranged from 13.2 ± 1.6 to 14.3 ± 2.0. In another study by Lukaski et al.,[17] collegiate male and female free-style swimmers reported intakes of Cu of 1.8 ± 0.2 and 1.3 ± 0.2 mg/day, respectively. Their serum Cu concentrations were 13.9 ± 1.3 for the males and 15.9 ± 2.5 for the females. Based on these studies, reported 6 years apart, it seems that Cu intake and serum Cu concentrations are very consistent among young athletes.

Rigorously controlled studies in our laboratory were performed on nonathletic women age 18 to 36.[18] They consumed natural ingredient diets with as little as 0.65 ± 0.05 mg/day of Cu for 7 weeks and developed signs of low Cu status. When compared with values from controls consuming 1.45 mg/day of Cu, low dietary Cu resulted in a 9% reduction in plasma Cu concentration and a 19% reduction in plasma ceruloplasmin activity. The subjects fed the low Cu diets were in negative balance with respect to Cu. When supplemented with 2.65 mg/day of Cu for 5.5 weeks, they came back into Cu balance. These data suggest that the basal Cu requirement for nonathletic women is higher than 0.65 mg/day, but lower than 1.5 mg/day. Other studies from our laboratory suggest that the requirement for adult human males is about 1.6 mg/day when body surface losses of Cu are considered.[19] However, the concentration of dietary Cu at which signs of low status could develop would depend on the length of time subjects were consuming a particular amount of Cu. Therefore, in studies such as these, the experimental periods may be too short to find an indication of low status at higher concentrations of dietary Cu.

III. COPPER BIOAVAILABILITY

Bioavailability is defined as how much of a nutrient is absorbed from the gut and how it is utilized in metabolic processes. However, in many studies this term may only refer to absorption. In humans as well as other mammals, the amount of Cu absorbed from the gut varies with the amount of Cu in the diet. On a percentage basis, there is an inverse relationship between dietary Cu and absorption. However, the net amount of Cu absorbed actually increases as dietary Cu increases, up to a point. With data referred to by Turnlund et al.,[20] it can be predicted by using a hyperbolic curve fit analysis of Cu absorbed vs. Cu intakes over a range of 0.8 to 7.5 mg/day that the maximal amount of Cu absorbed will be approximately 1.1 mg/day, with the one-half maximal rate at 1.2 mg of Cu intake per day. This suggests that a person taking in the lowest ESADDI amount (1.5 mg/day) will absorb only 0.6 mg of Cu and those taking in the highest amount (3.0 mg/day) will absorb about 0.8 mg.

Although some foods may contain moderate amounts of Cu, the availability of the Cu for absorption and utilization may not be realized because of other factors in the food. Some of the inhibiting factors include fructose, ascorbic acid, iron, and zinc. Phytate, common in most plant foods, is an enhancing factor. For the most part, the ESADDI accounts for the effect of other dietary components on Cu absorption.

A. CARBOHYDRATES AND COPPER ABSORPTION

It has been known for years that sucrose or fructose in the diet of laboratory animals such as the rat can intensify the effects of low dietary Cu.[21-23] Some evidence suggests that dietary fructose reduces the absorption of Cu from the gut of rats.[24-26] Van den Berg et al.[25] showed that fructose, compared to glucose, lowers the solubility of Cu in the gut and may contribute to low absorption of Cu. However, the detrimental effects of fructose on Cu metabolism has not been successfully demonstrated for other species including the pig[27,28] or the human.[29,30] Nonetheless, with the ever-increasing use of high-fructose syrups in foods, including sports beverages, there may be some future concern about the effects of long-term use of this carbohydrate on Cu metabolism in humans.

B. ASCORBIC ACID AND COPPER ABSORPTION

Van Campen and Gross[31] were the first to show that dietary ascorbic acid (vitamin C) attenuates the absorption of Cu from the gut of mammals. The mechanism is probably related to the chemical reduction of Cu from +2 to +1 oxidation state by ascorbic acid, a strong reducing agent. Van den Berg's group[32,33] did extensive work on the effects of ascorbic acid on Cu absorption, and showed that ascorbic acid lowered the amount of soluble Cu in the small intestine of rats and impaired Cu absorption. Finley and Cerklewski[34] found that young men fed 500 mg of ascorbic acid 3 times a day showed a gradual decrease in plasma Cu and ceruloplasmin activity over 64 days of treatment. When the ascorbic acid supplement was removed, both parameters rebounded within 20 days. Milne et al.[35] were able to demonstrate a negative effect of dietary ascorbic acid on Cu status in nonhuman primates but did not see further effects on Cu status when adult women were given 1500 mg of ascorbic acid and only 0.6 mg of Cu per day for 42 days.[18] Based on these studies, it is highly likely that long-term supplementation with high doses of ascorbic acid could lead to reduced absorption of Cu and the eventual lowering of Cu status, especially in those individuals that habitually consume a diet relatively low in Cu. Therefore, such supplementation practices are not recommended unless the intake of Cu is also relatively high.*

C. OTHER MINERALS AND COPPER ABSORPTION

The mineral components of the diet affect Cu availability. Mineral elements with similar electronic structures are likely to be antagonistic; for example, both zinc (Zn) and Cu, which are antagonistic, are d^{10} elements. Van Campen and Scaife[36] were one of the first groups of investigators to demonstrate that high dietary Zn reduced the absorption of Cu from the gut of rats. Since then, many studies with laboratory animals have shown this to be the probable mechanism.

Although not studied as extensively as in animals, there is ample evidence of a Zn:Cu antagonism in humans as well. Patterson et al.[37] demonstrated sideroblastic anemia and low Cu status in a patient who had consumed as much as 450 mg/day of Zn for 2 years. However, one well-controlled study showed no effect of 150 mg/day of Zn for 12 weeks on plasma Cu concentrations of healthy men.[38] In addition, high oral Zn therapy has been used successfully to treat Wilson's disease patients who, because of a genetic defect, accumulate toxic amounts of Cu.[39,40]

---

* The opinions expressed in this manuscript are those of the author and not necessarily those of the U.S. Department of Agriculture, Agricultural Research Service.

Cu status also can be affected by more normal concentrations of dietary Zn, and studies suggest that a dietary Zn:Cu ratio of greater than 16:1 may have a negative effect on physiological parameters associated with Cu metabolism. Dietary intakes of Zn as low as 25 and 50 mg/day for 2 to 10 weeks have produced small changes in Cu status in both men and women.[41-45] Balance studies have shown that the amount of dietary Cu required to maintain Cu equilibrium is directly proportional to the amount of Zn in the diet.[46] Thus, it is not recommended that supplementations of Zn greater than the RDA (12 to 15 mg/day) be taken unless the intake of Cu is also relatively high.

IV. COPPER CONCENTRATIONS IN THE BODY

The human body contains about 1.1 mg of Cu per kilogram of wet weight with variable distributions in various organs and blood. The liver and brain each contain about 10% of the total body Cu, with kidney, heart, and spleen containing 1.5, 1.1, and 0.1% of the total body Cu, respectively. The Cu concentration (0.9 µg/kg) in the skeletal muscle is low when compared with other tissues, but because of the muscle mass, it contains most of the Cu in the body.

The blood contains about 6% of the total body Cu. The red cells have a Cu concentration of about 16 ± 2 µmol/l (mean $\pm$ SD) of packed cells. Plasma has an average concentration of 16.5 ± 2.5 µmol/l for men and 18.3 ± 2.5 µmol/l for women. A recent report gives the range of normal clinical values for Cu in red cells as 14.2 to 23.6 µmol/l for both men and women.[47] The normal range for Cu in plasma is 8.8 to 17.5 µmol/l for men and 10.9 to 26.6 µmol/l for women. However, plasma values consistently as low as 8.8 µmol/l might be considered a sign of low Cu status.

Most of the Cu (~93%) in plasma is firmly bound to ceruloplasmin (CP), while the remainder is lightly bound to amino acids and albumin. Ceruloplasmin is synthesized in the liver and released into the blood. The amine oxidase activity of CP in plasma is proportional to the amount of Cu present, and this activity is sometimes used as an indicator of Cu status. However, pinpointing it as a specific indicator is difficult because certain stress conditions cause the CP concentration in plasma to fluctuate, which could result in a false indication of Cu status.

Reports show that Cu concentrations and CP activity in serum, and Cu concentrations in blood and plasma change when engaging in various types of exercise and sports activities. However, the changes reported have been inconsistent. Haralambie[48] was the first to report that serum CP activity was elevated in human volunteers after they engaged in physical training. However, Dowdy and Burt[49] reported that CP activity declined after eight weeks of training and remained constant for the rest of the study. Lukaski et al.[50] found that plasma Cu concentrations were 11% higher in trained male collegiate athletes compared with non-athletes in the same age group. Studies with laboratory animals also have shown an elevation in serum or plasma Cu when the animals were exercised to exhaustion.[51,52] This led to speculation that intensive exercise or physical training might alter Cu status.

More recent studies also have shown variable results. Resina et al.[53] found that male runners trained for 6 weeks had 35% lower serum Cu concentrations than control subjects not trained. However, the change in Cu did not affect the CP activity in these subjects. On the other hand, Marrella et al.[54] found a small increase in plasma Cu of runners after a marathon when compared with values from the same subjects before the race. A total blood cell (TBC) Cu concentration, most of which was from red cells, was 30% lower in premarathon runners than in nonrunner controls. TBC Cu did not change in runners immediately after the race; however, at 24 and 72 h after the race, the Cu values were reduced even further, and significantly different from values found immediately afterwards. Anderson et al.[55] found that serum Cu concentrations were elevated in moderately trained and untrained volunteers immediately following acute exercise to exhaustion. Lukaski[56] showed that the Cu concentration and CP activity of young women swimmers were unchanged during a competitive swimming season. In addition, no differences were found between swimmers and controls who were nonswimmers.

The inconsistency among different studies is confusing, and may be caused partly by the different types of exercise or training, duration and intensity of the exercise, nutritional status of the subjects at the beginning of the program, and the age and sex of the subjects. Nonetheless, the change in serum Cu concentrations shown in some athletes does not necessarily mean that they have an altered Cu status. It could mean that the changes observed are nothing more than normal adaptive responses to strenuous exercise that result in a redistribution of Cu among various tissues, with no untoward effects on the athlete.

V. COPPER METABOLISM

A. ANTIOXIDANT FUNCTION OF COPPER

An excellent review of how free radicals and antioxidants might be involved in sports and exercise was written by Aruoma.[57] Oxygen is a toxic gas; without internal protective mechanisms all aerobic organisms, including humans, would quickly succumb to a host of reactive oxygen species (ROS) generated by the body during normal metabolic processes. When individuals engage in strenuous exercise, they increase their oxygen consumption. This makes them even more vulnerable to possible tissue damage caused by an increase in oxidative metabolites through the generation of ROS.

The oxidative metabolites produce some ROS as free radicals. A free radical is a chemical entity with one or more unpaired electrons that exists for a relatively short time. Some examples of free radicals in the living system include the hydroxyl (HO·), superoxide ($O_2\cdot^-$), peroxyl (peroxy, $RO_2\cdot$, derived from lipid oxidation), and nitric oxide (·NO). The free radicals, HO· and $RO_2\cdot$, are highly reactive species and donate an unpaired electron to other molecules. This can set up chain reactions that produce other free radicals. The free radical has an extremely short half-life and for the most part acts in the immediate area of its generation.

The body produces natural defenses against free radicals. One of these is cytosolic Cu/Zn-dependent superoxide dismutase (Cu/Zn-SOD), an enzyme that dismutates $O_2\cdot^-$ to hydrogen peroxide, which in turn is converted to water and oxygen by catalase. Hydrogen peroxide also can be acted upon by a selenium-dependent enzyme, glutathione peroxidase (GPx). Although this enzyme does not contain Cu, its activity in experimental animals is affected by low Cu status.[58,59] Some hydrogen peroxide in the presences of free iron or Cu and $O_2\cdot^-$ can be converted to OH·. This in turn may cause the generation of $RO_2\cdot$. The peroxyl radical can be scavenged by ß-carotene and α-tocopherol (vitamin E).

Therefore, keeping the concentration of $O_2\cdot^-$ in the tissues as low as possible is important. At present, only one Cu-dependent enzyme is known to attack $O_2\cdot^-$, and that is Cu/Zn-SOD. Many studies that used young growing experimental animals showed that liver Cu/Zn-SOD activity was affected by Cu deprivation.[60,61] A recent study found that liver Cu/Zn-SOD activity was proportional to the amount of Cu in the diet, ranging from <1 to about 3.5 mg/kg of dry diet. The activity was reduced by 50% when the animals were eating diets with only 1.5 mg/kg of Cu.[62] The activity of Cu/Zn-SOD may be less susceptible to low Cu in the diets of adult animals. Reeves et al.[63] found that adult mice fed diets with Cu concentrations as low as 0.8 mg/kg for 12 weeks showed no signs of low Cu/Zn-SOD activity in the liver; although they were in low Cu status as suggested by low ceruloplasmin activity (50% lower than control mice receiving 6 mg of Cu per kilogram of diet).

The human diet provides an average of about 1.5 mg/day of Cu. On a concentration basis, this is similar to animal diets. On a dry weight basis, this amounts to between 3 and 4 mg of Cu per kilogram of dry diet, or about 0.5 mg/kg fresh diet. If we can extrapolate the animal data to young growing humans, then human diets that provide less than 1.0 mg/day of Cu for an extended period could result in low Cu/Zn-SOD activity in the liver. Klevay et al.[7] found that 32% of more than 800 analyzed human diets provided less than 1.0 mg/day of Cu.

Is there real evidence that oxidative damage occurs as a result of strenuous exercise? A review of the current literature on this subject by Alessio[64] suggests that indeed the concentration of free radicals and indicators of free radical damage increase during exhaustive exercise. However, as pointed out by Alessio,[64] tissue damage of any kind is likely to produce products of lipid oxidation; thus, it becomes a question of cause and effect. It was also pointed out that other complications of exercise such as elevated catecholamine, body temperature, edema, hemoglobin autoxidation, and training status can affect lipid peroxidation in different ways. Highly trained athletes working below exhaustion level seem to be more tolerant than untrained subjects. Duthie et al.[65] could find no effect of distance running in pretrained runners on erythrocyte lipid peroxidation, and Dernbach et al.[66] found no evidence of oxidative stress during high-intensity rowing training.

Is there evidence of altered Cu/Zn-SOD activity in athletes or experimental human subjects as a result of Cu deprivation? As of this writing, no publications were found that relate Cu/Zn-SOD activity in the tissues of athletes to Cu status. However, Lukaski[56] found that erythrocyte Cu/Zn-SOD (ESOD) activity was significantly elevated at the end of a training season for female swimmers, when compared with the beginning of the season. The same was true when swimmers were compared with nonswimmer controls; the ESOD activity for swimmers was higher than the controls. Again, it was higher at the end of the training season than at the beginning for both male and female swimmers. ESOD activity was not associated with Cu status.

B. CARDIOVASCULAR AND NEUROLOGIC FUNCTIONS OF COPPER

It has been well documented in laboratory animals that Cu status is closely related to the function of the cardiovascular system.[67,68] Cu-deficient rats develop hypertrophic cardiomyopathy characterized by ventricular hypertrophy and reduced chamber volume, and they die of dissecting aneurysms. Blood pressure may be elevated or depressed, depending on the age at which the animal develops Cu deficiency.[69,70] In addition, abnormal electrocardiography is observed in Cu deficiency.[71] The latter also was observed in humans who consumed a low-Cu diet.[30,72] Some of these effects are associated with decreases in activities of Cu-dependent enzymes including lysyl oxidase necessary for collagen cross-linking, Cu/Zn-SOD for free radical scavenging, and dopamine-ß-hydroxylase for the production of norepinephrine.

Recently, Davidson et al.[61] determined the association between aerobic exercise training and Cu status in young adult male rats. They showed that although the rats had developed a mild Cu deficiency but no enlargement of the heart, anemia, or hypertension, they did develop cardiomyopathy and were unable to complete an exercise training program. The authors suggested that cardiac function during physiological stress may be compromised by developing cardiac pathology of Cu depletion. Indeed, studies by Chen et al.[73] strongly suggest that Cu deficiency in rats weakens the antioxidant defense mechanisms in the heart more so than in other tissues. This may be in part caused by inherently lower activities of Cu/Zn-SOD, catalase, and GPx in the normal heart compared with other tissues.

Cu is closely involved with the function of the nervous system.[74,75] Dopamine-ß-hydroxylase (DBH), a major enzyme in the pathway for the synthesis of the neurotransmitter norepinephrine, is Cu dependent. Studies have shown that ataxia develops in some animal species fed diets deficient in Cu, and this condition may be associated with demyelination of the nerves. Cu deficiency in animals reduces the catecholamine pool size. In severely deficient rats, brain dopamine concentrations are reduced compared with that in Cu-adequate rats.

There have been attempts to associate physical exercise with DBH activity, Cu, and plasma catecholamine concentrations in humans. Ohno et al.[76] showed that 30 min of exercise on a bicycle ergometer significantly elevated plasma Cu, DBH activity, and the concentration of dopamine, norepinephrine, and epinephrine in young sedentary men. After 30 min of rest, these parameters had returned to normal. However, no one has shown that low Cu status in athletes has an untoward effect on the values of these parameters. Neither has it been shown that low Cu status in humans is associated with neurological disorders, except in individuals with the genetic defect called Menkes' disease. This disease is characterized by low Cu absorption and results in severe Cu deficiency and progressive neurological damage in the very young.[3]

VI. DETERMINATION OF COPPER REQUIREMENTS

The Food and Nutrition Board (FNB) defined the RDAs as follows: "Recommended Dietary Allowances (RDAs) are the levels of intake of essential nutrients that, on the basis of scientific knowledge, are judged by the FNB to be adequate to meet the known nutrient needs of practically all healthy persons."[77] To arrive at a value for the RDAs, the average physiological requirement for a nutrient was estimated and then adjusted by factors to compensate for rates of absorption and utilization. As stated in the 1989 publication, there is not always agreement among the experts on the criteria for determining the physiological requirements for a nutrient. This is an understatement with regard to the determination of the RDA for Cu.

What criteria do we use to determine Cu requirements? Because of ethical reasons, there are few methods of data collection that can be used to assess Cu requirements in the human. In the past, metabolic balance studies have been used to estimate the RDA for Cu.[4] However, this method is flawed because the rate of Cu absorption varies with intake, and the values may be misinterpreted with regard to requirement. In addition, individuals may adapt to a particular intake and begin to regulate the output of Cu so that zero balance is obtained even in the face of possible long-term dietary shortages of the nutrient. Other possible criteria for determining requirement include changes in the Cu concentrations of blood or changes in the activities of Cu-dependent enzymes. However, these methods have not been very successful because the values tend to be affected by a variety of conditions not related to requirement. In addition, accurate assessment of Cu requirements may be hampered because of the limited number of noninvasive tests that are allowed in human subjects.

Of course, one of the main drawbacks to determining the requirement for any nutrient in humans, including Cu, is the enormous cost involved in conducting controlled experiments. In the past, most studies with human subjects have not been of sufficient length to overcome the adaptation responses to low intakes of Cu, or to be able to observe changes in Cu concentrations in blood or in enzyme activities. Longer experimental periods may help solve some of the problems, but present the additional problem of subject compliance. This, in turn, demands an increase in the number of subjects and the cost spirals.

Because of these difficulties, the FNB, in 1989,[6] could not amass sufficient data to establish an RDA for Cu. Instead they recommended a safe and adequate daily intake of 1.5 to 3 mg/day for both males and females over the age of 11. This was down from 2 to 3 mg/day suggested in the 1980 version.[4] In 1995, a workshop was sponsored by the FNB and the U.S. Department of Agriculture, Agricultural Research Service, to look at new approaches, endpoints, and paradigms for the assessment of mineral requirements for humans.[78] Evidence was presented to suggest that the RDA for Cu might be lower than the current ESADDI. If so, the value would be closer to the Canadian recommended requirement for Cu of 1.0 to 2.0 mg/day.[5] The current ESADDI for Cu is based on the needs of the general population. To date there is no evidence to suggest that the Cu requirements for athletes is different.

VII. CONCLUSIONS

Cu is a required nutrient. Without an adequate dietary source, health and physiological function cannot be maintained. There is a need for Cu in enzyme systems that regulate oxygen consumption, cardiovascular function, and neurological function. The safe and adequate daily dietary intake of Cu for the general adult population is 1.5 to 3.0 mg. There are indications that athletes may have a tendency to alter blood Cu concentrations and increase losses in sweat and urine during exercise. Dietary surveys of athletes also indicate that, like the general population, some may take in less than the recommended amount of Cu. However, there is no convincing evidence that low Cu status exists in athletes who consume a well-balanced diet of a variety of foods. It is highly recommended, therefore, that athletes obtain the required amount of Cu by eating a variety of foods, including those with moderate to high amounts of Cu. They should not rely upon dietary supplementations for Cu or any other nutrient unless they are found to be lacking in the nutrient by clinically recognized tests conducted under the supervision of a qualified nutritionist or physician.

REFERENCES

1. Mason, K.E., A conspectus of research on copper metabolism and requirements of man, *J. Nutr.*, 109, 1979, 1979.
2. O'Dell, B.L., *Copper, Present Knowledge in Nutrition*, Brown, M.L. Ed., International Life Sciences Institute, Nutrition Foundation, Washington, D.C., 1990, p. 261.
3. Linder, M.C., *Biochemistry of Copper*, Plenum Press, New York, 1991.
4. National Research Council, Trace elements, *Recommended Dietary Allowances*, 9th ed., National Academy Press, Washington, D.C., 1980, p. 151.
5. Health and Welfare Canada, *Recommended Nutrient Intakes for Canadians*, Department of Health and Welfare, Ottawa, ON, 1983.
6. National Research Council, Trace elements, *Recommended Dietary Allowances*, 10th ed., National Academy Press, Washington, D.C., 1989, p. 224.
7. Klevay, L.M., Buchet, J.P., Bunker, V.W., Clayton, B.E., Gibson, R.S., Medeiros, D.M., Moser-Veillon, P.B., Patterson, K.Y., Taper, L.J., and Wolf, W.R., Copper in the Western diet (Belgium, Canada, U.K. and U.S.A.), *Trace Elements in Man and Animals — TEMA 8*, Anke, M., Meissner, D., and Mills, C.F., Eds., Verlag Media Touristik, Gersdorf, Germany, 1993, p. 207.
8. Johnson, P.E., Milne, D.B., and Lykken, G.I., Effects of age and sex on copper absorption, biological half-life, and status in humans, *Am. J. Clin. Nutr.*, 56, 917, 1992.
9. Lawler, M.R. and Klevay, L.M., Copper and zinc in selected foods, *J. Am. Diet. Assoc.*, 84, 1028, 1984.
10. USDA Consumer Nutrition Data Set 456-3, U.S. Department of Agriculture, Hyattsville, MD.
11. USDA, Composition of Foods. Agriculture Handbook 8.1-12, U.S. Department of Agriculture, Hyattsville, MD.
12. Telford, R.D., Catchpole, E.A., Deakin, V., McLeay, A.C., and Plank, A.W., The effect of 7 to 8 months of vitamin/mineral supplementation on the vitamin and mineral status of athletes, *Int. J. Sport Nutr.*, 2, 123, 1992.
13. Telford, R.D., Catchpole, E.A., Deakin, V., Hahn, A.G., and Plank, A.W., The effect of 7 to 8 months of vitamin/mineral supplementation on athletic performance, *Int. J. Sport Nutr.*, 2, 135, 1992.
14. Worme, J.D., Doubt, T.J., Singh, A., Ryan, C.J., Moses, F.M., and Deuster, P.A., Dietary patterns, gastrointestinal complaints, and nutrition knowledge of recreational triathletes, *Am. J. Clin. Nutr.*, 51, 690, 1990.
15. Bazzarre, T.L., Scarpino, A., Sigmon, R., Marquart, L.F., Wu, S.M., and Izurieta, M., Vitamin-mineral supplement use and nutritional status of athletes, *J. Am. Coll. Nutr.*, 12, 162, 1993.
16. Lukaski, H.C., Hoverson, B.S., Gallagher, S.K., and Bolonchuk, W.W., Physical training and copper, iron, and zinc status of swimmers, *Am. J. Clin. Nutr.*, 51, 1093, 1990.
17. Lukaski, H.C., Siders, W.A., Hoverson, B.S., and Gallagher, S.K., Iron, copper, magnesium and zinc status as predictors of swimming performance, *Int. J. Sports Med.*, In press, 1996.
18. Milne, D.B., Klevay, L.M., and Hunt, J.R., Effects of ascorbic acid supplements and a diet marginal in copper on indices of copper nutriture in women, *Nutr. Res.*, 8, 865, 1988.
19. Klevay, L.M., Reck, S.J., Jocob, R.A., Logan, G.M., Jr., Munoz, J.M., and Sandstead, H.H., The human requirement for copper. I. Healthy men fed conventional, American diets, *Am. J. Clin. Nutr.*, 33, 45, 1980.
20. Turnlund, J.R., Keyes, W.R., Anderson, H.L., and Acord, L.L., Copper absorption and retention in young men at three levels of dietary copper by use of the stable isotope ^{65}Cu, *Am. J. Clin. Nutr.*, 49, 870, 1989.

21. Koh, E.T., Comparison of copper status in rats when dietary fructose is replaced by either cornstarch or glucose, *Proc. Soc. Exp. Biol. Med.*, 194, 108, 1990.

22. Fields, M., Ferretti, R.J., and Smith, J.C., Jr., The interactions of type of dietary carbohydrate with copper deficiency, *Am. J. Clin. Nutr.*, 39, 289, 1984.

23. Reiser, S., Ferretti, R.J., Fields, M., and Smith, J.C., Jr., Role of dietary fructose in the enhancement of mortality and biochemical changes associated with copper deficiency in rats, *Am. J. Clin. Nutr.*, 38, 214, 1983.

24. O'Dell, B.L., Fructose and mineral metabolism, *Am. J. Clin. Nutr.*, Suppl. 58, 771S, 1993.

25. Van den Berg, G.J., Yu, S., Van der Heijden, A., Lemmens, A.G., and Beynen, A.C., Dietary fructose vs. glucose lowers copper solubility in the digesta in the small intestine of rats, *Biol. Trace Elem. Res.*, 38, 107, 1993.

26. Johnson, M.A., Interaction of dietary carbohydrate, ascorbic acid and copper with the development of copper deficiency in rats, *J. Nutr.*, 116, 802, 1986.

27. Schoeneman, H.M., Failla, M.L., and Fields, M., Consequences of copper deficiency are not differentially influenced by carbohydrate source in young pigs fed a dried skim milk-based diet, *Biol. Trace Elem. Res.*, 25, 21, 1990.

28. Schoeneman, H.M., Failla, M.L., and Steele, N.C., Consequences of severe copper deficiency are independent of dietary carbohydrate in young pigs, *Am. J. Clin. Nutr.*, 52, 147, 1990.

29. Holbrook, J.T., Smith, J.C., Jr., and Reiser, S., Dietary fructose or starch: effects on copper, zinc, iron, manganese, calcium and magnesium balances in humans, *Am. J. Clin. Nutr.*, 49, 1290, 1989.

30. Reiser, S., Smith, J.C., Jr., and Mertz, W., Indices of copper status in humans consuming a typical American diet containing either fructose or starch, *Am. J. Clin. Nutr.*, 45, 245, 1989.

31. Van Campen, D. and Gross, E., Influence of ascorbic acid on the absorption of copper by rats, *J. Nutr.*, 95, 617, 1968.

32. Van den Berg, G.J., Yu, S., Lemmens, A.G., and Beynen, A.C., Dietary ascorbic acid lowers the concentration of soluble copper in the small intestinal lumen of rats, *Br. J. Nutr.*, 71, 701, 1994.

33. Van den Berg, G.J., Yu, S., Lemmens, A.G., and Beynen, A.C., Ascorbic acid feeding of rats reduces copper absorption, causing impaired copper status and depressed biliary copper excretion, *Biol. Trace Elem. Res.*, 41, 47, 1994.

34. Finley, E.B. and Cerklewski, F.L., Influence of ascorbic acid supplementation on copper status in young adult men, *Am. J. Clin. Nutr.*, 37, 553, 1983.

35. Milne, D.B., Omaye, S.T., and Amos, W.H., Jr., Effect of ascorbic acid on copper and cholesterol in adult cynomolgus monkeys fed a diet marginal in copper, *Am. J. Clin. Nutr.*, 34, 2389, 1981.

36. Van Campen, D.R. and Scaife, P.U., Zinc interference with copper absorption in rats, *J. Nutr.*, 91, 473, 1967.

37. Patterson, W.P., Winkelmann, M., and Perry, M.C., Zinc-induced copper deficiency: megamineral sideroblastic anemia, *Ann. Intern. Med.*, 103, 385, 1985.

38. Samman, S. and Roberts, D.C.K., The effect of zinc supplements on plasma zinc and copper levels and the reported symptoms in healthy volunteers, *Med. J. Aust.*, 146, 246, 1987.

39. Hill, G.M., Brewer, G.J., Prasad, A.S., Hydrick, C.R., and Hartmenn, D.E., Treatment of Wilson's disease with zinc. I. Oral zinc therapy regimens, *Hepatology*, 7, 522, 1987.

40. Brewer, G.J., Yuzbasiyan-Gurkan, V., and Lee, D.Y., Use of zinc-copper metabolic interaction in the treatment of Wilson's disease, *J. Am. Coll. Nutr.*, 9, 487, 1990.

41. Festa, M.D., Anderson, H.L., Dowdy, R.P., and Ellerseick, M.R., Effect of zinc intake on copper excretion and retention in man, *Am. J. Clin. Nutr.*, 41, 285, 1985.

42. Fischer, P.W.F., Giroux, A., and L'Abbe, M.R., Effect of zinc supplementation on copper status in adult man, *Am. J. Clin. Nutr.*, 40, 743, 1984.

43. Greger, J.L., Zaikas, S.C., Abernathy, R.P., Bennett, O.A., and Huffman, J., Zinc, nitrogen, copper, iron, and manganese balance in adolescent females fed two levels of zinc, *J. Nutr.*, 108, 1449, 1978.

44. Taper, W., Hinners, M.L., and Ritchey, S.J., Effects of zinc intake on copper balance in adult females, *Am. J. Clin. Nutr.*, 33, 1077, 1980.

45. Yadrick, M.K., Kenney, M.A., and Winterfeldt, E.A., Iron, copper and zinc status: response to supplementation with zinc or zinc and iron in adult females, *Am. J. Clin. Nutr.*, 49, 145, 1989.

46. Sandstead, H.H., Interactions that influence bioavailability of essential metals to humans, *Metal Speciation: Theory, Analysis and Application*, Kramer, J.R. and Allen, H.E., Eds., Lewis Publisher, Chelsea, MI, 1995, p. 315.

47. Tietz, N.W., *Clinical Guide to Laboratory Tests*, W.B. Saunders, Philadelphia, 1995.

48. Haralambie, G., Changes in electrolytes and trace minerals during long-lasting exercise, *Metabolic Adaptation to Prolonged Physical Exercise*, Howald, H. and Poortmans, J.R., Eds., Birkhauser Verlag, Basel, 1975, p. 340.

49. Dowdy, R.P. and Burt, J., Effect of intensive, long-term training on copper and iron nutriture in man, *Fed. Proc.*, 39, A786, 1980.

50. Lukaski, H.C., Bolonchuk, W.W., Klevay, L.M., Milne, D.B., and Sandstead, H.H., Maximal oxygen consumption as related to magnesium, copper, and zinc nutriture, *Am. J. Clin. Nutr.*, 37, 407, 1983.

51. Cordova, A., Gimenez, M., and Escanero, J.F., Changes of plasma zinc and copper at various times of swimming until exhaustion, in the rat, *J. Trace Elem. Electrolytes Health Dis.*, 4, 189, 1990.

52. Cordova, A. and Escanero, J.F., Influence of lithium and exercise on serum levels of copper and zinc in rats, *Rev. Esp. Fisiol.*, 47, 87, 1991.

53. Resina, A., Fedi, S., Gatteschi, L., Rubenni, M.G., Giamberardino, M.A., Trabassi, E., and Imreh, F., Comparison of some serum copper parameters in trained runners and control subjects, *Int. J. Sports Med.*, 11, 58, 1990.

54. Marrella, M., Guerrini, F., Solero, P.L., Tregnaghi, P.L., Schena, F., and Velo, G.P., Blood copper and zinc changes in runners after a marathon, *J. Trace Elem. Electrolytes Health Dis.*, 7, 248, 1993.

55. Anderson, R.A., Bryden, N.A., Polansky, M.M., and Deuster, P.A., Acute exercise effects on urinary losses and serum concentrations of copper and zinc of moderately trained and untrained men consuming a controlled diet, *Analyst*, 120, 867, 1995.

56. Lukaski, H.C., Effects of exercise training on human copper and zinc nutriture, *Adv. Exp. Med. Biol.*, 258, 163, 1989.

57. Aruoma, O.I., Free radicals and antioxidant strategies in sports, *J. Nutr. Biochem.*, 5, 370, 1994.

58. Olin, K.L., Walter, R.M., and Keen, C.L., Copper deficiency affects selenoglutathione peroxidase and selenodeiodinase activities and antioxidant defense in weanling rats, *Am. J. Clin. Nutr.*, 59, 654, 1994.

59. Lai, C., Huang, W., Askari, A., Klevay, L.M., and Chiu, T.H., Expression of glutathione peroxidase and catalase in copper-deficient rat liver and heart, *J. Nutr. Biochem.*, 6, 256, 1995.

60. Balevska, P.S., Russanov, E.M., and Kassabova, T.A., Studies on lipid peroxidation in rat liver by copper deficiency, *Int. J. Biochem.*, 13, 489, 1981.

61. Davidson, J., Medeiros, D.M., Hamlin, R.L., and Jenkins, J.E., Submaximal, aerobic exercise training exacerbates the cardiomyopathy of postweanling copper-depleted rats, *Biol. Trace Elem. Res.*, 38, 251, 1993.

62. Johnson, W.T., Dufault, S.N., and Thomas, A.C., Platelet cytochrome c oxidase activity is an indicator of copper status in rats, *Nutr. Res.*, 13, 1153, 1993.

63. Reeves, P.G., Rossow, K.L., and Johnson, L., Maintenance requirements for copper in adult male mice fed AIN-93M rodent diet, *Nutr. Res.*, 14, 1219, 1994.

64. Alessio, H.M., Exercise induced oxidative stress, *Med. Sci. Sports Exercise*, 25, 218, 1993.

65. Duthie, G.G., Robertsen, J.D., Maughan, R.J., and Morrice, P.C., Blood antioxidant status and erythrocyte lipid peroxidation following distance running, *Arch. Biochem. Biophys.*, 282, 78, 1990.

66. Dernbach, A.R., Sherman, W.M., Simonsen, J.C., Flowers, K.M., and Lamb, D.R., No evidence of oxidant stress during high-intensity rowing training, *J. Appl. Physiol.*, 74, 2140, 1993.

67. Schuschke, L.A., Saari, J.T., Miller, F.N., and Schuschke, D.A., Hemostatic mechanisms in marginally copper-deficient rats, *J. Lab. Clin. Med.*, 125, 748, 1995.

68. Kopp, S.J., Klevay, L.M., and Feliksik, J.M., Physiological and metabolic characterization of a cardiomy-opathy induced by chronic copper deficiency, *Am. J. Physiol.*, 245, H855, 1983.

69. Klevay, L.M., Hypertension in rats due to copper deficiency, *Nutr. Rep. Int.*, 35, 999, 1987.

70. Medeiros, D.M., Lin, K.-N., Liu, C.-C.F., and Thorne, B.M., Pre-gestation dietary copper restriction and blood pressure in the Long-Evans rat, *Nutr. Rep. Int.*, 30, 559, 1984.

71. Viestenz, K.E. and Klevay, L.M., A randomized trial of copper therapy in rats with electrocardiographic abnormalities due to copper deficiency, *Am. J. Clin. Nutr.*, 35, 258, 1982.

72. Klevay, L.M., Inman, L., Johnson, L.K., et al., Increased cholesterol in plasma in a young man during experimental copper depletion, *Metabolism*, 33, 1112, 1984.

73. Chen, Y., Saari, J.T., and Kang, Y.J., Weak antioxidant defenses make the heart a target for damage in copper-deficient rats, *Free Rad. Biol. Med.*, 17, 529, 1994.

74. O'Dell, B.L. and Prohaska, J.R., Biochemical aspects of copper deficiency in the nervous system, *Neurobiology of the Trace Elements*, Dreosti, I.E. and Smith, R.M., Eds., Humana Press, Clifton, NJ, 1983, p. 41.

75. Prohaska, J.R., Functions of trace elements in brain metabolism, *Physiol. Rev.*, 67, 858, 1987.

76. Ohno, H., Yahata, T., Hirata, F., Yamamura, K., Doi, R., Harada, M., and Taniguchi, N., Changes in dopamine-beta-hydroxylase, and copper, and catecholamine concentrations in human plasma with physical exercise, *J. Sports Med.*, 24, 315, 1984.

77. National Research Council, Definition and applications, *Recommended Dietary Allowances*, National Academy Press, Washington, D.C., 1989, p. 10.

78. Klevay, L.M. and Medeiros, D.M., *Copper, J. Nutr.*, 126, In press, 1996.

Chapter 14

CHROMIUM

Jenna D. Anding
Ira Wolinsky
Dorothy J. Klimis-Tavantzis

CONTENTS

I. PHYSIOLOGICAL ROLE

The importance of chromium (Cr) was first emphasized when Mertz and Schwartz[1] suggested that a Cr-containing agent was necessary for maintaining normal glucose tolerance in rats. This agent was later termed glucose tolerance factor (GTF) and Cr was identified as its active ingredient.[2] Although the structure has yet to be identified, GTF has been suggested to potentiate the action of insulin.[3] Other roles of Cr include nucleic acid metabolism, by which it functions in the areas of gene expression,[4] and structural integrity of nuclear strands.[5]

The use of Cr supplementation has been shown to be effective in patients with impaired glucose tolerance and elevated blood lipids.[6] For athletes Cr has become a popular nutrient of interest because of its proposed potentiating effect on insulin. Often termed the "anabolic hormone", insulin stimulates the uptakes of glucose, amino acids, and triglycerides by cells. It is suggested, then, that without Cr the action of insulin would be diminished. Because of insulin's effects on protein synthesis, Cr is often promoted as an anabolic supplement for muscle development.[7,8]

II. ESTIMATED REQUIREMENTS AND DIETARY INTAKE

Cr is an essential trace mineral. Although a recommended dietary allowance (RDA) for Cr has yet to be established, an estimated safe and adequate daily dietary intake (ESADDI) of 50 to 200 µg has been recommended by the National Research Council.[9]

Early estimated dietary Cr intake studies most likely are invalid because of laboratory difficulties in assessing the Cr content of foods.[10] More recent studies, however, using the minimum ESADDI of 50 µg, have described the dietary intake of Cr in developed countries, including the U.S., as suboptimal.[11] Anderson and Kozlovsky reported a 7-day average Cr intake of 25 and 33 µg for females and males, respectively, suggesting that the majority of Americans fail to consume the minimum ESADDI. Studies involving dietary intake of Cr among athletes are also limited. Kleiner et al.[12] assessed the dietary intake of nationally ranked elite body-builders and reported that females and males consumed diets which averaged 21 and 143 µg of Cr, respectively.

III. FACTORS AFFECTING CHROMIUM BALANCE

Because Cr intake is difficult to assess, Lefavi et al.[13] have suggested that an individual's Cr balance (Cr intake/absorption – excretion) might be an appropriate indicator of one's Cr status. Being in a prolonged state of negative Cr balance (Cr excretion > intake/absorption) could lead to a deficiency; therefore, it is important to understand the factors which may affect the absorption and excretion of this mineral.

Animal studies have suggested that the absorption of Cr occurs rapidly[14] in the duodenum[15] by nonmediated passive diffusion.[16] Normal Cr absorption ranges from 0.5 to 4%, with absorption at the upper end of the range occurring when intake is less than 40 µg per day.[16] A deficiency state of Cr, however, does not increase absorption above the upper end of the range,[17] intensifying the symptoms of a deficiency which include impaired glucose tolerance, decreased insulin receptor number, elevated serum cholesterol and triglyceride levels, decreased HDL-cholesterol, and increased incidence of aortic plaques.[18] Food sources which contain appreciable sources of chromium include brewer's yeast, mushrooms, broccoli, condiments such as barbecue sauce, and black pepper.[11,19] The manner in which foods are processed may alter the Cr content.[10]

Cr is stored in body tissues until mobilized. Because the kidneys lack the ability to reabsorb Cr, mobilization of Cr apparently commits the mineral primarily to urinary excretion[20] although a small amount of Cr is lost through hair, perspiration, and bile.[21,22]

The excretion of Cr is influenced by several types of stress including exercise[23-26] and diets high in simple carbohydrates.[27] Anderson et al.[23-26] have consistently demonstrated that exercise significantly increases Cr excretion in comparison to basal excretion levels. One might suggest that the increased energy requirement by exercising muscles would lead to an increase in glucose utilization and, hence, insulin secretion. However, Anderson et al.[26] have demonstrated that exercise will result in an insulin secretion which is unchanged or decreased, suggesting that the mineral plays a role in glucose metabolism in addition to that of insulin.

Aside from exercise, Koslovsky et al.[27] demonstrated that increasing the contribution of simple carbohydrates from 15 to 35% of total energy significantly increases basal Cr excretion. This response could be explained by the fact that an increase in the intake of simple sugars will raise the serum glucose level and trigger the pancreas to release insulin.[28] For insulin to work effectively, the GTF must be in place, in which Cr has an essential role. If the need for insulin increases to account for the increase in simple carbohydrates in the diet, the mobilization of Cr would be expected to increase as well. As previously stated, once Cr is mobilized, it cannot be reabsorbed and must be excreted.[20]

In comparison to their sedentary counterparts, athletes may be challenged to maintain a positive chromium balance for three reasons discussed by Lefavi et al.[13] First, when training for a specific event the athlete will usually increase either the intensity or duration of the exercise. Assuming Cr excretion is increased during periods of exercise in comparison to nonexercise days, there may be limited opportunities to replenish Cr stores if the athlete has more exercise than nonexercise days, although Anderson et al.[23] have reported that trained athletes have a significantly lower basal Cr excretion than men who were untrained. Second, it is not uncommon for certain athletes to alter their caloric intake when training for a specific event. If caloric intake is lowered, then there is a decreased likelihood that Cr-containing foods will be included in the diet. Third, the active lifestyle adopted by athletes along with advertisements promoting simple-sugar-containing sports drinks may encourage the athlete to adopt a diet which contains high amounts of simple sugars. For the athlete who is in a negative Cr balance, Lefavi et al.[13] have suggested that the presence of one or all of these factors might intensify or prolong that balance.

IV. EFFICACY OF CHROMIUM SUPPLEMENTATION

Research suggesting that athletes are potentially at risk for negative Cr balance, combined with slick advertisements in health and fitness magazines promoting the mineral's proposed muscle-building powers, often entice athletes to turn to supplementation to keep or gain a competitive edge. Chromium picolinate has been marketed as a safe alternative to anabolic steroids.[29] However, this and other similar supplements are marketed as nutritional supplements, not drugs. Hence, it presently escapes the Food and Drug Administration's requirement that it be proven safe and effective.[29]

The interest in Cr as an anabolic agent was probably heightened by one suggestion that chromium picolinate increased lean body mass and decreased body fat, based on two supplementation trials.[30] The first trial involved 10 male volunteers from a weight-training course who received either a daily supplement of 200 µg of Cr (in the form of chromium picolinate) or a placebo for 40 days. Percentage body fat was derived from skin folds and lean body mass was determined by subtracting body fat weight from total weight. Subjects were instructed to consume their usual diets and to maintain their normal activity with the exception of the prescribed weight-lifting program. Subjects receiving the Cr supplement increased their body weight by 2.2 kg, of which 1.6 kg was identified as lean body mass. Subjects receiving the placebo gained 1.25 kg of body weight, of which only 0.04 kg was lean body mass.

The second trial, involving 31 football players, was conducted in a similar manner. Again, subjects supplemented with Cr reported a 3.6% increase in lean body mass while subjects receiving the placebo had an increase in lean body mass which was determined to be less than 1%. A decrease in percentage body fat was noted in both groups, but was significant only among the Cr-supplemented subjects. Although dietary intake and Cr balance were not addressed, Evans concluded that Cr supplementation did result in significant increases in lean body mass.[30]

Hasten et al.[31] attempted to confirm Evans' results by supplementing 59 college students in a 12-week beginning weight-training program with either chromium picolinate or a placebo. The subjects were divided into four groups identified by gender and treatment and body weight, skinfold measurements, and the amount of weight lifted by squat and bench press were followed throughout the study. At the end of the trial the females supplemented with Cr gained significantly more body weight than the other groups. The authors suggested that this increase was in fact lean body mass based on changes in skinfolds and body density regression equations, but the supplementation did not produce an effect on muscle strength for females or males. The authors concluded that for their study chromium picolinate was beneficial for females but not males. Furthermore, the authors suggested that chromium picolinate might be more effective among trained subjects, since the initial results of weight training would appear to be dramatic whether or not Cr was supplemented. Here,[31] as with the Evans study, dietary Cr intake and Cr balance were not addressed.

Clancy et al.[32] investigated the effects of Cr supplementation on the lean body mass and strength of football players. Subjects were given either a 200-μg Cr supplement or a placebo. During the 9-week trial, Cr excretion, percentage body fat and lean body mass, strength, and dietary intake were measured. Percentage body fat and lean body mass were determined by hydrostatic weighing and 3-day food records kept prior to, during, and after the study to ensure usual dietary intake. Isometric and dynamic strength tests of the elbow and knee were identified as indicators of muscle strength. Subjects receiving the supplement demonstrated a higher urinary excretion of Cr in comparison to their counterparts, but did not demonstrate an increase in lean body mass or strength, leading the researchers to conclude that the subjects receiving the Cr supplementation failed to gain any of its proposed benefits. Although these results do not support the proposed benefits of Cr supplementation, the Clancy et al. study[32] did make an effort to account for dietary intake and Cr excretion, two important factors that were not addressed in previous studies.[30,31]

A more recent study by Lukaski et al.[34] investigated the effect of Cr supplementation in the forms of chromium picolinate and chromium chloride on 36 sedentary men with respect to body composition and strength gain. Serum and urinary chromium as well as dietary intake also were measured. Chromium supplementation in either form failed to demonstrate a significant increase in muscle mass, strength, or fat reduction, confirming those results reported by Clancy et al.[32]

V. TOXICITY OF CHROMIUM SUPPLEMENTATION

With respect to humans, the toxicity of Cr has not been shown to be a problem, most likely due to its low absorption. However, recent research by Lukaski et al.[34] suggests that Cr supplementation could interfere with the metabolism of iron. The long-term safety of Cr supplementation in humans has not been proven conclusively and remains a concern.

VI. CONCLUSIONS/RECOMMENDATIONS

Based on the available research, there is little doubt that athletes probably have an increased requirement for chromium. For the athlete with a suboptimal consumption of Cr, incorporating chromium-rich foods in the diet should be the first step in increasing intake. Although Lefavi et al.[13] have suggested that supplementation might benefit the athlete whose diet is inadequate in Cr, one must keep in mind the possibility that excessive intakes (greater than 200 μg), could interfere with the absorption of other minerals.[33,34] Chromium's proposed anabolic properties and long-term safety have not been conclusively proven and athletes who are not deficient in Cr will most likely fail to gain any physiological benefits of supplementation.[35] Until research suggests otherwise, the universal supplementation of chromium is not advised.

REFERENCES

1. Mertz, W. and Schwartz, K., Improved intravenous glucose tolerance as an early sign of dietary necrotic liver degeneration, *Arch. Biochem. Biophys.*, 58, 504, 1955.
2. Schwartz, K. and Mertz, W., Chromium III and the glucose tolerance factor, *Arch. Biochem. Biophys.*, 85, 292, 1959.

3. Mertz, W. and Roginski, E.E., The effect of trivalent chromium on galactose entry in rat epididymal fat tissue, *J. Biol. Chem.*, 238, 868, 1963.

4. Okada, S., Ohba, H., and Taniyama, M., Alterations in ribonucleic acid synthesis by chromium (III), *J. Inorg. Biochem.*, 15, 223, 1981.

5. Anderson, R.A. and Guttman, H.N., Trace minerals and exercise, in *Exercise, Nutrition and Energy Metabolism,* Hartort, E.S. and Terjung, R.L., Eds., Macmillan, New York, 1988, 180.

6. Clarkson, P.M., Nutritional ergogenic aids: chromium, exercise and muscle mass, *Int. J. Sport Nutr.*, 1, 289, 1991.

7. Evans, G.W., Chromium picolinate is an efficacious and safe supplement, *Int. J. Sport Nutr.*, 3, 117, 1993.

8. Fisher, J.A., *The Chromium Program,* Harper & Row, New York, 1990.

9. National Research Council, *Recommended Dietary Allowances*, National Academy of Sciences, Washington, D.C., 1989, 241.

10. Kumpulainen, J.T., Chromium content of foods and diets, *Biol. Trace Elem. Res.*, 32, 9, 1992.

11. Anderson, R.A., Bryden, N.A., and Polansky, M.M., Dietary chromium intake: freely chosen diets, institutional diets, and individual foods, *Biol. Trace Elem. Res.*, 32, 117, 1992.

12. Kleiner, S.M., Bazzarre, T.L., and Ainsworth, B.E., Nutritional status of nationally ranked elite bodybuilders, *Int. J. Sport Nutr.*, 4, 54, 1994.

13. Lefavi, R.G., Anderson, R.A., Keith, R.E., Wilson, G.D., McMillan, J.L., and Stone, M.H., Efficacy of chromium supplementation in athletes: emphasis on anabolism, *Int. J. Sport Nutr.*, 2, 111, 1992.

14. Polansky, M.M., and Anderson R.A., Chromium absorption and retention, *Fed. Proc.*, 42, 925, 1983.

15. Chen, N.S.C., Tsai, A., and Dyer, I.A., Effect of chelating agents on chromium absorption in rats, *J. Nutr.*, 103, 1182, 1973.

16. Dowling, H.J., Offenbacher, E.G., and Pi-Sunyer, F.X., Absorption of inorganic, trivalent chromium from the vascularly perfused rat small intestine, *J. Nutr.*, 119, 1138, 1989.

17. Mertz, W., Roginski, E.E., and Reba, R.C., Biological activity and fate of trace quantities of intravenous chromium (III) in the rat, *Am. J. Physiol.*, 209, 489, 1965.

18. Borel, J.A. and Anderson, R.A., Chromium, in *Biochemistry of the Essential Ultratrace Elements,* Frieden, E., Ed., Plenum Press, New York, 1984, 175.

19. Anderson, R.A., New insights on the trace elements, chromium, copper and zinc, and exercise, *Med. Sport Sci.*, 32, 38, 1991.

20. Stoecker, B.J., Chromium, in *Present Knowledge in Nutrition,* 6th ed., Brown, M.L., Ed., International Life Sciences Institute Nutrition Foundation, Washington, D.C., 1990, 287.

21. Hopkins, L.L., Distribution in the rat of physiological amounts of injected Cr[51] (III) with time, *Am. J. Physiol.*, 29, 155, 1965.

22. Doisy, R.D., Streeten, D.H.P., Souma, M.L., Kalafer, M.E., Rekant, S.L., and Dalakos, T.G., Metabolism of chromium[51] in human subjects, in *Newer Trace Elements in Nutrition,* Mertz, W. and Cornatzer, W.E., Eds., Marcel Dekker, New York, 1971, chap. 8.

23. Anderson, R.A., Polansky, M.M., Bryden, N.A., Roginski, E.E., Patterson, K.Y., and Reamer, D.C., Effect of exercise (running) on serum glucose, insulin, glucagon, and chromium excretion, *Diabetes*, 31, 212, 1982.

24. Anderson, R.A., Bryden, N.A., Polansky, M.M., and Deuster, P.A., Exercise effects on chromium excretion of trained and untrained men consuming a constant diet, *J. Appl. Physiol.*, 61, 249, 1988.

25. Anderson, R.A., Polansky, M.M., and Bryden, N.A., Strenuous running: acute effects on chromium, copper, zinc and selected clinical variables in urine and serum of male runners, *Biol. Trace Elem. Res.*, 6, 327, 1984.

26. Anderson, R.A., Bryden, N.A., Polansky, M.M., and Thorp, J.W., Effects of carbohydrate loading and underwater exercise on circulating cortisol, insulin and urinary losses of chromium and zinc, *Eur. J. Appl. Physiol.*, 63, 146, 1991.

27. Kozlovsky, A.S., Moser, P.B., Reiser, S., and Anderson, R.A., Effects of diets high in simple sugars on urinary chromium losses, *Metabolism*, 35, 515, 1986.

28. Granner, D.K., Hormones of the pancreas, in *Harper's Biochemistry*, Murray, R.K., Granner, D.K., Mayes, P.A., and Rodwell, V.W., Eds., Appleton & Lange, East Norwalk, CT, 1988, 547.

29. Beltz, S.D. and Doering, P.L., Efficacy of nutritional supplements used by athletes, *Clin. Pharm.*, 12, 900, 1993.

30. Evans, G.W., The effect of chromium picolinate on insulin controlled parameters in humans, *Int. J. Biosocial Res.*, 11, 163, 1989.

31. Hasten, D.L., Rome, E.P., Franks, B.D., and Hegsted, M., Effects of chromium picolinate on beginning weight training students, *Int. J. Sport Nutr.*, 2, 343, 1992.

32. Clancy, S.P., Clarkson, P.M., DeCheke, M.E., Nosaka, K., Freedson, P.S., Cunningham, J.J., and Valentine, J.J., Effects of chromium picolinate supplementation on body composition, strength, and urinary chromium loss in football players, *Int. J. Sport Nutr.*, 4, 142, 1994.

33. Clarkson, P.M. and Haymes, E.M., Trace mineral requirements for athletes, *Int. J. Sport Nutr.*, 4, 104, 1994.

34. Lukaski, H.C., Bolonchuk, W.W., Siders, W.A., and Milne, D.B., Chromium supplementation and resistance training: effects on body composition, strength and trace element status of men, in press
35. Hopkins, L.L. and Schwartz, K., Chromium (III) binding to serum proteins, specifically siderophilin, *Biochem Biophys Acta.*, 90, 484, 1964.
36. Wagner, J.L., Use of chromium and cobamamide by athletes, *Clin. Pharm.*, 8, 832, 1989.

Chapter 15

SELENIUM

Mallory Boylan
Julian E. Spallholz

CONTENTS

I. INTRODUCTION

Selenium (Se) is a trace element which is essential, yet toxic when consumed in excessive quantities. The toxicity of Se was recognized long before its essentiality, with symptoms of Se toxicity or selenosis described by Marco Polo in 1295 during his travels to China. In 1934, Franke[1] identified Se as a toxic agent found in some plant foods. About 20 years later, Schwarz and Foltz[2] became the first to demonstrate that Se was an essential dietary element which prevented liver necrosis in rats. Since that time Se deficiency syndromes have been identified in both animals and humans. Se deficiency can result in cardiomyopathy, muscle pain, and osteoarthropathy in humans.[3]

Rotruck and co-workers[4] in 1973 discovered that Se, in a selenocysteine residue, was a constituent of the enzyme glutathione peroxidase (GSHPx). Since GSHPx is the enzyme which converts hydrogen peroxide to water, most of the research in the area of Se and exercise has centered around the role of Se in this antioxidant enzyme. Strenuous exercise dramatically increases oxygen uptake and production of reactive oxygen species (ROS) including superoxide ($O_2 \cdot^-$), hydroxyl radical ($\cdot OH$), and hydrogen peroxide (H_2O_2) that may be responsible for biochemical and physiologic changes indicative of oxidative stress induced by exercise.[5,6] Peroxidative injury to tissues is also found in severe Se deficiency due to the depletion of GSHPx activity. It would also seem obvious that in the rare cases of severe Se deficiency which result in arthritis or in cardiomyopathy, or Se toxicity with nerve damage, athletic ability would be impaired.

II. SELENIUM AND ITS ROLE AS AN ANTIOXIDANT

Since the discovery of cytosolic GSHPx, other selenoproteins including additional anti-oxidant enzymes have been identified in mammals. A distinct, glycosylated GSHPx has been found in the plasma and a membrane-associated enzyme, phospholipid hydroperoxide GSHPx (PLGSHPx), is also widely distributed in tissues.[7,8] While an exact function is not totally clear, selenoprotein P is found in plasma and tissues and appears to have some antioxidant properties.[7,9] An additional enzyme which contains Se is Type I iodothyronine 5-deiodinase, which is the enzyme that catalyzes the removal of iodine from l-thyroxine (T_4) converting it to 3,3,5-triiodothyronine (T_3).[7]

The primary task of the Se-containing antioxidant enzymes is to protect cellular components from peroxidation by controlling the H_2O_2 and organic peroxide levels in aerobic cells.[7] According to Ursini and Bindoli,[10] both GSHPxs will reduce peroxidic substrates such as H_2O_2, linoleic acid hydroperoxide, *tert*-butyl hydroperoxide, and cumene hydroperoxide. Cholesteryl hydroperoxides, some prostaglandin peroxides, and peroxidized DNA are also substrates for GSHPx. Additional substrates for PLGSHPx include peroxidized phosphatidyl choline, phosphatidyl ethanolamine, and phosphatidyl serine; cardiolipin, phosphatidic acid, and peroxidized membranes. Figure 1 provides a schematic of the reactions of the GSHPxs. An adequate intercellular concentration of reduced glutathione (GSH) is needed as a substrate for both GSHPxs.[11] The riboflavin-containing enzyme glutathione reductase (GR) with flavin adenine dinucleotide (FDA) as its coenzyme and reduced nicotinamide adenine dinucleotide phosphate (NADPH) as the reducing agent converts oxidized glutathione (GSSG) back to GSH.

A. TISSUE DISTRIBUTION OF GLUTATHIONE PEROXIDASES AND EFFECT OF SELENIUM ON TISSUE ENZYME ACTIVITY LEVELS

Se and GSHPx activity are both widely distributed in animal tissues. Behne and Wolters[12] analyzed the Se content and GSHPx activity in tissues of female rats. The largest percentages of Se were found in the muscle (39.8%) and liver (31.7%) with other tissues each containing less than 10% of the remaining Se. The GSHPx activity was greatest in the liver (65.6%), followed by erythrocytes (21.2%) and muscle (6.1%), with other tissues containing 2.1% or less of the remaining GSHPx activity.

Se deficiency results in a decrease in both GSHPx and PLGSHPx activity in tissue[13] as well as an increase in tissue peroxide levels[14] and signs of peroxidative injury to tissues.[14,15] Results of a study by Weitzel et al.[13] indicated that the two GSHPxs have individual depletion kinetics, as GSHPx in liver samples from mice fed a Se-deficient diet decreased by 90% of the activity of control mice, whereas PLGSHPx was depleted by only 45% of control activity. In Se-deficient animals or humans, Se supplementation will induce production of GSHPx. In general, there is a correlation between the dietary Se intake and tissue GSHPx activity in both rats and humans.[16] Over a 20-week period, in rats fed diets ranging from a torula yeast basal diet with no added Se to a diet with 5.0 mg/kg, erythrocyte GSHPx steadily climbed as Se intake increased. However, when mice were fed a diet containing 1.0 mg Se per kilogram of diet for 6 months, liver GSHPx activity levels were lower than for mice fed an adequate 0.2 mg/kg Se diet, though still much higher than the value for mice fed a Se-deficient diet.[17]

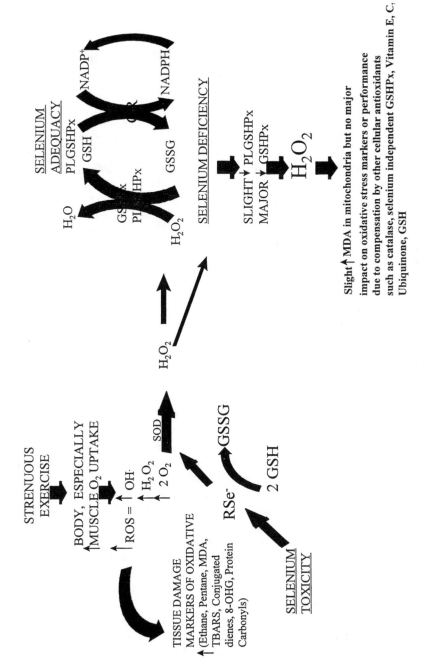

FIGURE 1 Exercise, oxidative stress, and selenium status: possible interactions. (Adapted from References 5, 6, 8, 50, 52, 55-57.)

In humans who have a hereditary lack of GSHPx in erythrocytes, ability of the erythrocytes to withstand stress induced by oxidizing agents is impaired and results in a hemolytic crisis.[18] Glutathione peroxidase and PLGSHPx are major enzyme systems responsible for detoxification of H_2O_2 and lipid hydroperoxides. Lack of sufficient quantities of these enzymes from a Se deficiency as well as genetic defects or the inability to incorporate dietary Se into GSHPx leads to signs and symptoms associated with peroxidative tissue damage.

III. SELENIUM NEEDS AND CONSEQUENCES OF SELENIUM DEFICIENCY

A. SELENIUM NEEDS

Evidence that an endemic cardiomyopathy in China called Keshan disease was linked to poor Se status and was prevented by selenium supplementation provided evidence for the nutritional essentially of Se in humans.[19] Se was recognized as an essential nutrient and was assigned a Recommended Dietary Allowance (RDA) in 1989.[20] The RDA for Se was set at 55 μg/day for women and 70 μg/day for men. Dietary Se intake in areas of China affected by Keshan disease averages about 7 to 11 μg/day of Se, with estimated minimum daily requirements of Se for adult men and women of 19 and 13 μg, respectively.[19] Using plasma GSHPx as an index of Se status, Yang et al.[19] evaluated the effect of graded doses of Se in the form of selenomethionine on Chinese men with an initial low Se status. After 5 months, plasma GSHPx levels were found to reach a stationary level in groups given 30 μg or more of the Se supplement per day in addition to the approximate 10 μg/day from their diets. As Se needs are related to body weight, and Americans tend to be taller and heavier than people from China, and using a safety factor of 1.3 (1.3 × The Chinese dietary intake), the RDA for Se is about 0.87 μg/kg body weight.[20]

B. SELENIUM DEFICIENCY-RELATED SYNDROMES

Syndromes related to selenium deficiency are often somewhat nonspecific, may be multifactorial, and are rare.[19] Se deficiency has, however, been identified as a factor in two human diseases in China, Keshan disease and Kaschin-Beck disease.[19]

Keshan disease is a cardiomyopathy, more common in women and children than in men, which is characterized by multifocal necrosis in the myocardium.[19] Signs and symptoms of Keshan disease include nausea, vomiting, chest discomfort, chills, dyspnea and palpitations on exertion, cardiogenic shock followed by congestive heart failure, and arrhythmias. Individuals with Keshan disease have been reported to have significantly lower levels of blood Se and GSHPx activity than normal subjects living in the same area in China.[21] Administration of prophylactic doses of Se to people in areas of China where Se deficiency is prevalent has been reported to result in a significant lessening in the Keshan disease incidence.[19] While Se deficiency appears to be a major factor, the etiology of Keshan disease has not been totally elucidated and other factors may be contributing to the disease.[22] Se may have a protective and stabilizing effect on membranes[23,24] due to PLGSHPx, which may lessen membrane susceptibility to environmental pathogenic agents.

Other factors associated with Keshan disease are a Coxsackie virus,[25] vitamin E deficiency,[19] pathogenic factors from endemic grains,[26] and methionine deficiency.[19] When inoculated with a Coxsackie virus CB-21 isolated from the blood of a Keshan disease patient, mice which had been fed a Se-deficient diet developed significantly more myocardial lesions than mice in normal Se status.[25] Beck et al.[27] reported that Se-deficient mice developed more severe myocardial lesions after infection with Coxsackie B3 virus than did mice with normal Se status, and Se deficiency resulted in less lymphocyte proliferation in response to mitogens and antigens. When the virus was replicated in Se-deficient mice it underwent changes associated with increased virulence.

Vitamin E and Se function as synergistic antioxidants and many of the signs and symptoms of a double deficiency of these two nutrients can be prevented or will be improved by supplementation with either nutrient.[20] Beck et al.[28] reported that vitamin E deficiency increased the cardiac pathology associated with Coxsackie B3 infection in mice, especially mice fed diets high in menhaden oil as opposed to lard for dietary fat. Work by Beck et al.[27,28] on the effects of both Se and vitamin E deficiency on myocardial injury from the Coxsackie B3 virus supports the possibility of multiple factors influencing the development of Keshan disease.

In regard to cardiovascular disease other than Keshan disease, there is some epidemiologic evidence associating low blood or dietary Se with increased risk of cardiovascular disease.[29] Pucheu and co-workers[30] reported that plasma Se values of patients with coronary artery disease and/or myocardial infarction were 80% of the values found in healthy control subjects. Other studies have found no relationship between Se and cardiovascular disease.[31,32] Possible mechanisms by which low selenium status with below normal GSHPx levels could be related to cardiovascular disease include alterations in arachidonic acid metabolites and blood-clotting mechanisms.[33-36]

Kaschin-Beck's disease is an endemic osteoarthropathy prevalent in the areas of China and Russia classified as Se-deficient zones.[19,38] It is most common in children and signs and symptoms include endochondral ossification, hyaline cartilage necrosis, joint pain and deformity, limited flexion of finger and elbows, and muscular atrophy.[19] Pain in the weight-bearing joint is described as stabbing and is intensified by exposure to cold or exercise. The principal pathological finding in Kaschin-Beck's disease is chondronecrosis.[19] While etiological factors for Kaschin-Beck's disease may be similar to those for Keshan disease, subjects with Kaschin-Beck's have been reported to have an improvement in their condition in response to Se supplementation.[39] Kaschin-Beck's patients have an increase in blood GSHPx and a decrease in lipid peroxidation products in membranes in response to Se supplements and these factors could decrease chondronecrosis. Adjuvant arthritis is more pronounced in Se-deficient rats and their macrophages have lower GSHPx activity and produce higher levels of H_2O_2 when compared to control rats.[40] These factors may lead to peroxidative cell injury and worsening of arthritis.

Se deficiency has also been noted in conjunction with protein energy malnutrition, acquired immunodeficiency syndrome, alcoholism, short bowel syndrome, long-term total parenteral nutrition without Se, and the use of formulas for inborn errors of metabolism that had no added Se.[22,41-45] In these conditions, problems related to Se deficiency may include muscle pain, nail changes, cardiomyopathy, fatty liver, poor growth, and immunosuppression. It would appear that severe Se deficiency produces signs and symptoms that would have detrimental effects on exercise performance.

IV. SELENIUM TOXICITY

Se toxicity or selenosis occurs in areas of China where dietary intake of Se is about 5 mg/day.[19] A few cases of Se toxicity have also been reported due to consumption of Se supplements such as sodium selenite, with most of the cases in individuals who were taking a supplement which, by the manufacturer's error, contained about 23 mg of Se in each tablet.[46] Some symptoms of Se toxicity were noted in a subject who consumed only 1 mg/day of Se from sodium selenite for 2 years, however.[19] Se toxicity causes dry, brittle, easily broken hair which is depigmented and lackluster; thick, brittle deformed finger and toenails; skin which is red, swollen, blistered, and itchy; nausea, vomiting, and abdominal pain; fatigue; a garlic odor; and neurological abnormalities including peripheral paresthesia, paralysis, hemiplegia, motor disturbances, extremity pain, and convulsions.[19,46]

The molecular mechanism which causes Se toxicity appears to be related to reactions between Se and GSH in which oxygen radicals are produced. Se compounds which form selenide (RSe^-) anions can oxidize GSH and other cellular thiols and produce superoxide that in turn initiates a cascade of ROS production.[47-50]

V. SELENIUM AND EXERCISE

Most research in the area of Se and exercise has focused on the role of Se in the antioxidant enzyme GSHPx which, using GSH, converts H_2O_2 to water. Whole-body and especially muscle oxygen uptake increases sharply during intense physical exercise leading to oxidative stress.[51] This oxidative stress may be related to production of ROS such as superoxide in the mitochondria during exercise. Superoxide when acted on by superoxide dismutase (SOD) produces H_2O_2 which can then be converted to water by GSHPx or catalase. In tissues which experience ischemia during exercise, reperfusion and reoxygenation contribute to a burst of ROS production. When biomembrane polyunsaturated fatty acids are acted on by ROS under aerobic conditions, a peroxidative chain reaction occurs leading to increased excretion of ethane and pentane in expired air and increased levels of malondialdehyde (MDA), conjugated dienes, and thiobarbituric acid reactive substances (TBARS) in tissues.[5,52,53] Some possible interactions among exercise, oxidative stress, and Se status are outlined in Figure 1.

Only limited animal and very limited human research has been conducted regarding Se and exercise. Types, duration, and intensity of exercise and dietary Se levels fed to animals are varied, which may account in part for the lack of continuity in results of acute exercise and training effects on activity levels of GSHPx and indicators of oxidative damage to tissues.

One consistent finding is that animals fed a Se-deficient diet have lower tissue levels of GSHPx when compared to values from animals fed adequate selenium.[54-58] Lower Se status is also associated with decreased levels of GSHPx activity in human subjects.

The only human study in which subjects were in less than optimal Se status was conducted by Edwards et al.[59] Subjects also had intermittent claudication in addition to altered Se status. Edwards and co-workers[59] evaluated the effects of treadmill exercise on patients with intermittent claudication due to peripheral vascular disease and normal controls. Subjects with intermittent claudication were found to have significantly lower plasma Se and GSHPx activity levels than in 19 control subjects. A group of 11 patients with intermittent claudication and 7 controls participated in a treadmill exercise test. Neutrophils were noted to be significantly higher in patients with claudication and were further elevated by the exercise. Plasma thromboxane, an indicator of platelet activation, and von Willebrand's factor, a marker of endothelial injury, were also higher in claudicants than in controls and both were increased 15 min after exercise in claudicants and controls ($p < .05$). Edwards and co-workers[59] speculated that reduced GSHPx activity levels in patients with claudication may contribute to unopposed action of oxygen radicals resulting in increased damage to the endothelium. No attempt was made to evaluate the effects of a Se supplement in these patients and other antioxidant enzymes were not evaluated in the study, but it does appear that in intermittent claudication patients, lower plasma GSHPx values may be one factor contributing to lack of protection from the oxidative stress of exercise.

In rats fed Se-deficient diets that are subjected to acute exercise, Brady et al.[58] found no significant effect of exercise on liver, blood, or muscle GSHPx activity levels. Lang and co-workers[57] reported decreased GSHPx, increased GSH, decreased vitamin E, and increased ubiquinone levels in tissues of Se-deficient rats. Exercise did not cause a significant rise in liver GSHPx in either control or Se-deficient animals. Plasma total GSH and oxidized glutathione were both significantly higher in animals after exercise to exhaustion, with levels in rats fed Se-deficient diets about twice the values found in control rats. While not a significant difference, the Se-deficient rats had a 16% higher mean running time to exhaustion than control rats. Adequate dietary vitamin E levels, residual GSHPx, and activation of other antioxidant pathways were suggested as mechanisms which preserved the exercise capacity in the rats fed Se-deficient diets. Ji et al.[55] did find increased levels of catalase and cytosolic SOD in livers of Se-deficient rats after acute exercise and significant increases in manganese SOD in liver, and Se-independent GSHPx in muscle after training. Manganese SOD activity was 24% higher in heart mitochondria from Se-deficient rats as compared to controls.[55]

In trained athletes participating in a half marathon, Duthie et al.[60] found no significant differences in erythrocyte GSHPx activity prerace and up to 120 h postrace. They also noted no significant change in erythrocyte catalase or SOD, but total GSH and GSH values were significantly lower than prerace values at 5 min postrace. While plasma creatinine kinase, an index of damage to muscles, was elevated in plasma postrace, conjugated dienes and thiobarbituric acid reactive substances (TBARS), indexes of oxidative damage, were not elevated by the exercise. Erythrocytes were more susceptible to hydrogen peroxide-induced peroxidation after the half marathon, however.

Acute exercise also results in an increase in pentane, which is a derivative of omega-6 fatty acid hydroperoxides, in expired air.[52] Pentane in expired air is also increased by Se deficiency.[61] Pentane excretion can be reduced in Se-deficient rats by providing them with adequate amounts of vitamin E. Muscle mitochondrial MDA levels are also elevated in untrained rats subjected to acute exercise and in rats with Se deficiency.[56] So both Se deficiency and acute exercise increase levels of substances which may be considered indicative of oxidative damage to tissues. In a double-blind, placebo-controlled study, Tessier et al.[62] evaluated the effect of Se supplementation (240 μg of an organic Se capsule containing 70% selenomethionine) or placebo on response to acute exercise and training in 24 healthy nonsmoking males. The Se-supplemented group had a significant elevation in plasma Se levels, with the supplemented group's mean values 182% of the mean value of the control group. Neither Se supplementation nor training resulted in an elevation of vastus lateralis muscle GSHPx activity levels. The intensity level of the training was higher in the animal studies which, in addition to species differences, may account for the contradictory results regarding GSHPx inducement by training in humans vs. animals. In rats, training has been reported to result in an increase in GSHPx in muscle tissue.[63-65] Before training and following a run to exhaustion, muscle GSHPx activity levels were lower than resting levels.[62] After training in the placebo group, muscle GSHPx activity declined but not to as great a degree as in the pretraining exercise test. In the Se-supplemented group, posttraining muscle GSHPx activity was increased 64 to 79% after the max aerobic capacity test. In light of the finding by Storz et al.,[66] that oxygen radicals induced transcription of messenger RNA that codes for antioxidant enzymes including peroxidases in prokaryotic cells, Tessier et al.[62] speculated that production of oxygen radicals during exercise may be a stimulus to induce higher GSHPx activity in muscle tissues after Se supplementation.

VI. CONCLUSION

Data in the area of Se status as a factor in athletic performance are scarce, and in some aspects such as the possible effect of training on elevation of muscle GSHPx, a conflict exists between results of animal and human studies. The studies have been of short duration; so while they were sufficiently long to cause a major decline in tissue activity levels of GSHPx, the activity of PLGSHPx, which depletes much more slowly than GSHPx, could have remained very well preserved. No studies reviewed evaluated the effects of any aspect of exercise on tissue activity of PLGSHPx. It does appear that in selenium deficiency, compensatory use of many of the body's other antioxidant defense mechanisms come in to play to protect the body from ROS stress induced by exercise. More research is needed before any recommendations for athletes can be made for any deviation from the RDA intake levels for Se. As Se is a toxic mineral when taken in excess, any Se supplement should be used with great caution.

REFERENCES

1. Franke, G., A new toxicant occurring naturally in certain samples of plant food-stuffs, *J. Nutr.*, 8, 597, 1934.
2. Schwarz, K. and Foltz, C., Selenium as an integral part of factor 3 against dietary necrotic liver degeneration, *J. Am. Chem. Soc.*, 79, 3292, 1957.
3. Combs, G. and Combs, S., *The Role of Selenium in Nutrition*, Academic Press, London, 1986.
4. Rotruck, J.T., Pope, A.L., Ganther, H.E., Swanson, A.B., Hafeman, D.G., and Hoekstra, W.G., Selenium: biochemical role as a component of glutathione peroxidase, *Science*, 179, 588, 1973.
5. Ji, L., Oxidative stress and antioxidant response during exercise, oxidative processes and antioxidants, *13th Ross Laboratories Conference Report*, 13,23, Ross Product Division, Abbott Laboratories, Columbus, OH, 1994.
6. Jenkins, R., Free radical chemistry: relationship to exercise, *Sports Med.*, 5, 156, 1988.
7. Zachara, B., Mammalian selenoproteins, *J. Trace Elem. Electrol. Health Dis.*, 6, 137, 1992.
8. Ursini, F., Maiorino, M., Valente, M., and Gregolin, C., Purification from pig liver of a protein which protects liposomes and biomembranes from peroxidative degradation and exhibits glutathione peroxidase activity on phosphatidylcholine hydroperoxides, *Biochem. Biophys. Acta*, 197, 710, 1982.
9. Burk, R., Molecular biology of selenium with implications for its metabolism, *FASEB, J.*, 5, 22, 1991.
10. Ursini, F. and Bindoli, A., Catalysis by selenoglutathione peroxidase, in *Biological Macromolecules and Assemblies*, Jurnak, F.A. and McPherson, A., Eds., John Wiley & Sons, New York, 1987.
11. Wendel, A., Pilz, W., Ladenstein, R., Sawatzki, G., and Weser, U., Substrate-induced redox change of selenium in glutathione peroxidase studied by X-ray photoelectron spectroscopy, *Biochem. Biophys. Acta*, 377, 211, 1975.
12. Behne, D. and Wolters, W., Distribution of selenium and glutathione peroxidase in the rat, *J. Nutr.*, 113, 456, 1983.
13. Weitzel, F., Ursini, F., and Wendel, A., Different dietary selenium requirement for the two selenoenzymes, glutathione peroxidase and phospholipid hydroperoxide glutathione peroxidase, in the mouse, Abstr., *4th Int. Symp. Selenium in Biology and Medicine*, Tubingen, West Germany, Walter de Gruyer, New York, 1989.
14. Baker, S.S. and Cohen, H.J., Increased sensitivity to H_2O_2 in glutathione peroxidase deficient rat granulocytes, *J. Nutr.*, 114, 2003, 1984.
15. Lane, H.W., Shirley, R.L., and Cerda, J.J., Glutathione peroxidase activity in intestinal and liver tissues of rats fed various levels of selenium, sulfur and α-tocopherol, *J. Nutr.*, 109, 444, 1979.
16. Hafeman, D.G., Sunde, R.A., and Hoekstra, W.G., Effect of dietary selenium on erythrocyte and liver glutathione peroxidase in the rat, *J. Nutr.*, 104, 580, 1974.
17. Boylan, M., Cogan, D., Huffman, N., and Spallholz, J., Behavioral characteristics in open field testing of mice fed selenium deficient and selenium supplemented diets, *J. Trace Elem. Exp. Med.*, 3, 157, 1990.
18. Necheles, T.F., Maldonado, N., Barquet-Chediak, A., and Allen, D.M., Homozygous erythrocyte glutathione peroxidase deficiency: clinical and biochemical studies, *Blood*, 33, 164, 1969.
19. Yang, G., Ge, K., Chan, J., and Chen, X., Selenium-related endemic diseases and the daily selenium requirement of humans, *World Rev. Nutr. Diet.*, 55, 98, 1988.
20. Food and Nutrition Board, *Recommended Dietary Allowances*, National Academy Press, Washington, D.C., 1989, chap. 10.
21. Luo, X., Wei, H., Yang, C., Xing, J., Liu, X., Qiao, C., Feng, Y., Liu, J., Liu, Y., Wu, Q., Liu, X., Guo, J., Stoecker, B.J., Spallholz, J.E., and Yang, S.P., Bioavailability of selenium to residents in a low selenium area of China, *Am. J. Clin. Nutr.*, 42, 439, 1985.
22. Zumkley, H., Clinical aspects of selenium metabolism, *Biol. Trace Elem. Res.*, 15, 139, 1988.
23. Li, G., Han, C., and Yang, J., Effect of a selenium deficient diet from a Keshan disease area on myocardial metabolism in the pig, in *Selenium in Biology and Medicine*, Part B, Combs, F.G., Spallholz, J.E., Levander, O.A., and Oldfield, J.E., Eds., AVI Book by Van Nostrand Reinhold, New York, 1987, 814.
24. Yang, F.Y. and Wo, W.H., Role of selenium in stabilization of human erythrocyte membrane skeleton, *Biochem. Int.*, 15, 475, 1987.
25. Ge, K.Y., Bai, J., Deng, X.J., Wu, S.Q., Wang, S.Q., Xue, A.N., and Su, C.Q., The protective effect of selenium against viral myocarditis in mice, in *Selenium in Biology and Medicine*, Part B, Combs, G.F., Spallholz, J.E., Levander, O.A., and Oldfield, J.E., Eds., AVI Book by Van Nostrand Reinhold, New York, 1987, 761.

26. Wang, F., Li, G., Li, C., Yang, T., and Ping, Z., Pathogenic factors of Keshan disease in the grains cultivated in endemic areas, in *Selenium in Biology and Medicine,* Part B, Combs, G.F., Spallholz, J.E., Levander, O.A., and Oldfield, J.E., Eds., AVI Book by Van Nostrand Reinhold, New York, 1987, 896.

27. Beck, M., Kolbeck, P., Shi, Q., Rohr, L., Morris, V., and Levander, O., Increased virulence of a human enterovirus (Coxsackie virus B3) in selenium deficient mice, *J. Infect. Dis.,* 170, 351, 1995.

28. Beck, M., Kolbeck, P., Rohr, L., Shi, Q., Morris. V., and Levander, O., Vitamin E deficiency intensifies the myocardial injury of Coxsackie virus B3 infection in mice, *J. Nutr.,* 124, 345, 1994.

29. Shamburger, R.J., Willis, C.E., and McCormak, L.J., Selenium and heart disease. III. Blood selenium and heart mortality in 19 states, in *Trace Substances in Environmental Health-XII,* Hemphill, D.D., Ed., University of Missouri Press, Columbia, MO, 1979, 59.

30. Pucheu, S., Coudray, C., Vanzetto, G., Favier, A., Machecourt, J., and de Leiris, J., Time course of changes in plasma levels of trace elements after thrombolysis during acute myocardial infarction in humans, *Biol. Trace Elem. Res.,* 47, 171, 1995.

31. Robinson, M.F., Clinical effects of selenium deficiency and excess, in *Clinical, Biochemical, and Nutritional Aspects of Trace Elements,* Prasad, A.S., Ed., Alan R. Liss, New York, 1982, 325.

32. Thomson, C.D., Reah, H.M., Robinson, M.F., and Simpson, F.O., Selenium concentrations and glutathione peroxidase activities in blood of hypertensive patients, *Proc. Univ. Otago Med. Sch.,* 56, 1, 1978.

33. Schoene, N.W., Morris, V.C., and Levander, O.A., Altered arachidonic acid metabolism in platelets and aortas from selenium-deficient rats, *Nutr. Res.,* 6, 75, 1986.

34. Levander, O.A., A global view of human selenium nutrition, *Annu. Rev. Nutr.,* 7, 277, 1987.

35. Bryant, R.W., Bailey, J.M., King, J.C., and Levander, O.A., Altered platelet glutathione peroxidase activity and arachidonic acid metabolism during selenium repletion in a controlled human study, in *Selenium in Biology and medicine,* Spallholz, J.E., Martin, J.L., and Ganther, H.E., Eds., AVI Publishing, Westport, CT, 1981, 395.

36. Schoene, N.W., Morris, V.C., and Levander, O.A., Altered arachidonic acid metabolism in platelets and aortas from selenium-deficient rats, *Nutr. Res.,* 6, 75, 1986.

37. Warso, M.A. and Lands, W.E.M., Presence of lipid hydroperoxides in human plasma, *J. Clin. Invest.,* 75, 667, 1985.

38. Li, J. Y., Ren, S., Cheng, D.Z., Wan, H.J., Liang, S.T., Zhang, F.J., and Gao, F.M., Distribution of selenium in the microenvironment related to Kaschin-Beck's disease, in *Selenium in Biology and Medicine,* Spallholz, J.E., Martin, J.L., and Ganther, H.E., Eds., AVI Publishing, Westport, CT, 1987, 911.

39. Liang, S., Zhang, J., Shang, X., Mu, S., and Zhang, F., Effects of selenium supplementation in prevention and treatment of Kaschin-Beck's disease, in *Selenium in Biology and Medicine,* Part B, Combs. G.F., Spallholz, J. E., Levander, O.A., and Oldfield, J.E., Eds., AVI Book by Van Nostrand Reinhold, New York, 1987, 938.

40. Parnham, M.J., Winkelmann, J., and Leyck, S., Macrophage, lymphocyte and chronic inflammatory responses in selenium deficient rodents. Association with decreased glutathione peroxidase activity, *Int. J. Immunopharmacol.,* 5, 455, 1983.

41. Kien, C.L. and Ganther, H.E., Manifestations of chronic selenium deficiency in a child receiving total parenteral nutrition, *Am. J. Clin. Nutr.,* 37, 319, 1983.

42. Lombeck, I., Kasperek, K., Feinendegen, L.E., and Bremer, H.J., Low selenium state in children, in *Selenium in Biology and Medicine,* Part B, Combs, G. F., Spallholz, J.E., Levander, O.A., and Oldfield, J.E., Eds., AVI Book by Van Nostrand Reinhold, New York, 1987, 269.

43. Dworkin, B.M., Rosenthal, W.S., Wormser, G.P., Weiss, L., Nunez, M., Joline, C., and Herp, A., Abnormalities of blood selenium and glutathione peroxidase activity in patients with acquired immunodeficiency syndrome and AIDS-related complex, *Biol. Trace Elem. Res.,* 15, 167, 1988.

44. Aaseth, J., Aadland, E., and Thomassen, Y., Serum selenium in patients with short bowel syndrome, in *Selenium in Biology and Medicine,* Part B, Combs, G.F., Spallholz, J.E., Levander, O.A., and Oldfield, J.E., Eds., AVI Book by Van Nostrand Reinhold, New York , 1987, 976.

45. Aaseth, J., Thomassen, Y., Alexander, J., and Norheim, G., Decreased serum selenium in alcoholic cirrhosis, *N. Engl. J. Med.,* 303, 944, 1989.

46. Helzlsouer, K., Jacobs, R., and Morris, S., Acute selenium intoxication in the United States, *Fed. Proc.,* 44, 1670, 1985.

47. Seko, Y., Saito, Y., and Kitahara, J., Active oxygen generation by the reaction of selenite with reduced glutathione in vitro, in *Selenium in Biology and Medicine,* Wendel, A., Ed., Springer-Verlag, Berlin, 1989, 70.

48. Xu, H., Feng. Z., and Vi, C., Free radical mechanisms of the toxicity of selenium compounds, *Huzahong Longong Daxve Xuebao,* 19, 13, 1991.

49. Yan, L. and Spallholz, J.E., Generation of reactive oxygen species from the reaction of Selenium compounds with thiols and mammary tumor cells, *Biochem. Pharmacol.,* 45, 429, 1993.

50. Spallholz, J.E., On the nature of selenium toxicity and carcinostatic activity, *Free Rad. Biol. Med.,* 17, 45, 1994.

51. Ji, L., Oxidative stress during exercise: implications of antioxidant nutrients, *Free Rad. Biol. Med.,* 18, 1079, 1995.

52. Witt, E.H., Reznick, A.Z., Viguie, C.A., Starke-Reed, P., and Packer, L., Exercise, oxidative damage and effects of antioxidant manipulation, *J. Nutr.,* 122, 766, 1992.

53. Dillard, C.J., Litov, R.E., Savin, W.M., Dumelin, E.E., and Tappel, A.L., Effect of exercise, vitamin E, and ozone on pulmonary function and lipid peroxidation, *J. Appl. Physiol.,* 45, 927, 1978.

54. Hill, K.E., Burk, R.F., and Lane, J.M., Effect of selenium depletion and repletion on plasma glutathione and glutathione-dependent enzymes, *J. Nutr.,* 117, 99, 1987.

55. Ji, L.L., Stratman, F.W., and Lardy, H.A., Antioxidant enzyme response to selenium deficiency in rat myocardium, *J. Am. Coll. Nutr.,* 11, 79, 1992.

56. Ji, L.L., Stratman, F.W., and Lardy, H.A., Antioxidant enzyme systems in rat liver and skeletal muscle: influences of selenium deficiency, chronic training, and acute exercise, *Arch. Biochem. Biophys.,* 263, 150, 1988.

57. Lang, J., Gohil, K., Packer, L., and Burk, R., Selenium deficiency, endurance exercise capacity, and antioxidant status in rats, *J. Appl. Physiol.,* 63, 2532, 1987.

58. Brady, P.S., Brady, L.J., and Ullrey, D.E., Selenium, vitamin E and the response to swimming stress in the rat, *J. Nutr.,* 109, 1103, 1979.

59. Edwards, A., Blann, A., Suarez-Mendez, V., Lardi, A., and McCollum, C., Systemic responses in patients with intermittent claudication after treadmill exercise, *Br. J. Surg.,* 81, 1738, 1994.

60. Duthie, G., Robertson, J., Maughan, R., and Morrice, P., Blood antioxidant status and erythrocyte lipid peroxidation following distance running, *Arch. Biochem. Biophys.,* 282, 78, 1990.

61. Dillard, C.J., Litor, R.E., and Tappel, A.L., Effect of dietary vitamin E, selenium, and polyunsaturated fats on in vivo lipid peroxidation in the rat as measured by pentane production, *Lipids,* 13, 396, 1978.

62. Tessier, F., Hida, H., Favier, A., and Marconnet, P., Muscle GSHPx activity after prolonged exercise, training, and selenium supplementation, *Biol. Trace Elem. Res.,* 47, 279, 1995.

63. Sen, C.K., Marin, E., Kretzschmar, J., and Hanninen, O., Skeletal muscle and liver glutathione homeostasis in response to training, exercise, and immobilization, *J. Appl. Physiol.,* 74, 1265, 1992.

64. Laughlin, M.H., Simpson, T., Sexton, W.L., Brown, O.R., Smith, J.K., and Korthuis, R.J., Skeletal muscle oxidative capacity, antioxidant enzymes, and exercise training, *J. Appl. Physiol.,* 68, 2337, 1990.

65. Schauer, J.E., Schelin, A., Hanson, P., and Stratman, F.W., Dehydroepiandrosterone and a B-agonist, energy transducers, alter antioxidant enzyme systems: influence of chronic training and acute exercise in rats, *Arch. Biochem. Biophys.,* 283, 503, 1990.

66. Storz, G., Tartaglia, L.A., and Ames, B.N., Transcriptional regulator of oxidative stress-induced genes:direct activation by oxidation, *Science,* 248, 189, 1990.

Chapter **16**

OTHER SUBSTANCES IN FOODS

———— Barbara Mc. Chrisley

CONTENTS

0-8493-8192-4/97/$0.00+$.50
© 1997 by CRC Press, Inc.

I. INTRODUCTION

Several of the elements and compounds classified as "other substances in foods" may function with regard to physical performance. Some of these include choline, carnitine, taurine, myo-inositol, and the trace element boron. Also, coenzymes, growth factors and nucleosides, amino acids, and buffers included in this classification which may function with regard to physical performance are coenzyme Q_{10}, pyrroloquinoline quinone, inosine, creatine, arginine, ornithine, aspartate, bicarbonates, and phosphate salts. Exactly which ones are "other substances in foods"? According to the 1989 edition of the *Recommended Dietary Allowances,*[1] these are substances naturally present in foods which are required by some animals or microbes but there is insufficient or no evidence of their essentiality in the diets of humans. These are further classified as nutrients not essential for humans or animals and include various growth factors, amino acids, peptides, and vitamins, frequently incorrectly referred to as being members of the B complex.

Therefore, several of these substances in the various categories will be reviewed in this chapter with respect of their current status as determined by the latest scientific reports and their implications regarding exercise performance.

II. NUTRIENTS ESSENTIAL FOR SOME HIGHER ANIMALS THAT MAY BE RELATED TO ATHLETIC PERFORMANCE IN HUMANS

Many organic and inorganic compounds are found naturally in foods and are required by humans and animals. Some of these compounds have not been proven to be required by normal humans but are nutrients essential for some higher animals. However, various compounds have been indicated to affect athletic performance in humans. Included in this group are choline, carnitine, myo-inositol, and boron.

A. CHOLINE

Choline is known to be part of the structure of acetylcholine and phosphatidylcholine. Dietary sources come from lecithin in foods such as egg yolks, liver, soybeans, and peanuts. Lecithin serves as structural component of cell membranes and plasma lipoproteins. Although choline is a dietary requirement for several animal species, it has not been shown to be essential for humans. The requirement is higher during growth and development. The average daily intake in the U.S. is about 400 to 900 mg.[2]

Essentiality of choline — Zeisel[3] has indicated recently that several lines of evidence suggest that choline is indeed an essential nutrient for humans. Human cells grown in culture require choline.[4] Healthy humans fed diets deficient in choline have decreased plasma concentrations. Humans fed intravenously with little choline develop dysfunctional liver.[5] In addition, other consequences include renal, pancreatic, memory, and growth disorders. Fatty infiltration of the liver occurs in the deficiency of choline. Phosphatidylcholine is essential in the synthesis of the very low density lipoproteins (VLDL) which transport triacyglycerol out of the liver. In the event they are not packaged and transported out of the liver, they will accumulate, thus infiltrating the liver. Choline facilitates carnitine synthesis derived from trimethyllysine. Low choline is attributed to decreased methyl groups needed for carnitine. Choline-deficient diets also contribute to carcinogenesis of the liver. Decreased methylation of DNA may contribute to excessive proliferation of fat of the liver.[6] Research reports such as these indicate the possible essentiality of choline in the diet. In fact, choline was listed as a vitamin in the Recommended Dietary Allowances publication of 1974[7] (but not in 1980 or 1989).

Choline and exercise — Because of these biological functions of choline, supplementation has been encouraged by various companies that market products as ergogenic aids. It has been indicated to "cut fat" or contribute to fat loss.[8] Choline supplementation has not been demonstrated through research to reduce adiposity in human subjects. Early research indicate conflicting reports of beneficial effects from choline supplementation on muscular power endurance and performance. Staton[9] reported no increase in grip strength after supplementation with 30 mg of lecithin for 2 weeks. Conaly et al.[10] reported decreased plasma choline concentrations in marathon runners. Studies are needed to investigate the possible decrease in performance of athletes with low choline concentrations since acetylcholine is released at neuromuscular junctions. To date, few studies have determined the increased blood levels from supplementation with the effects on methylation metabolism, creatine synthesis, or exercise performance.[6] More research is needed with regard to choline and physical performance.

B. CARNITINE

Carnitine (ß-hydroxy-[γ N-trimethylammonia] butyrate) plays an important role in energy metabolism. It is synthesized in the liver and kidney from the essential amino acids lysine and methionine.

Essentiality of carnitine — Carnitine transports long-chain fatty acids into the mitochondria, thus serving a major metabolic function. Carnitine is now viewed as a "conditionally essential nutrient".[11] Feller and Rudman[12] listed several causes for impairment of carnitine function. Some of these included limited amino acid precursors and/or cofactors for carnitine synthesis from impaired organs or malfunctioned steps in the biosynthetic pathway. Myopathies of lipid storage due to subnormal carnitine palmitoyltransferase may occur. Alterations of carnitine transport, with low levels in muscle but normal concentrations in plasma, occur due to excess loss of carnitine in hemodialysis in patients on total parenteral nutrition (TPN). In addition, infants require more carnitine when shifting from glucose to fatty acids for energy. Infants have low levels of carnitine and soy-based formulas lacking in carnitine place them at high risk.

Carnitine and exercise — Because carnitine transports long-chain fatty acids into the mitochondria, supplement advocates claim that carnitine is a "fat loss agent".[8] The average consumption of 6 g/day of carnitine over a 10-day period had little effect on resting oxygen consumption.[13] Supplementation of endurance athletes indicated an increase in $\dot{V}O_2$max [14] and reduction in respiratory quotient.[15] Other studies[16,17] do not support these findings. If increased consumption of carnitine could lead to increased use of fat, then muscle glycogen could be spared during exercise. This would be advantageous to the athlete to defer the time to exhaustion. Data have not been supportive of this suggestion, however.

Otto et al.[18] reported no effect of 500 mg carnitine supplementation of subjects daily for 4 months on free fatty acid utilization, $\dot{V}O_2$max, anaerobic threshold, exercise time to exhaustion, or work output on a cycle ergometer for 60 min. No effects were reported by other researchers[19-21] who supplemented subjects with 2 g of carnitine on fuel utilization at 50% $\dot{V}O_2$max, maximal heart rate, anaerobic threshold, $\dot{V}O_2$max, or exercise time to exhaustion. The Dal Negro et al.[13] study showed little effect on resting oxygen consumption in normal subjects when they ingested 6 g/d of carnitine over a 10-day period. Marconi et al.,[14] in a prior study, observed an increase in $\dot{V}O_2$max when subjects were supplemented with carnitine. Gorostiaga et al.[15] reported a reduction in respiratory quotient in their supplemented subjects. Cerretelli and Marconi[16] did not support these finding in a later study. Soop et al.[21] reported no muscle substrate utilization in subjects supplemented with 5 g of carnitine for 5 days before a 120-min cycle exercise session.

Wagenmaker[22] concluded that L-carnitine does not affect endurance performance or fat metabolism. Supplementation does not lead to increased levels in the muscle nor does exercise lead to a decrease in muscle carnitine content. Carnitine's usefulness as a ergogenic aid is not supported by current data. Wagenmaker[22] reported that the consequences of the D-isomer of carnitine in humans resulted in muscle weakness and myoglobinuria. Additional research is needed to answer the many questions concerning carnitine and the athlete and its use as a ergogenic aid.

C. MYO-INOSITOL

Myo-inositol is a cyclic alcohol (cyclohexanehexol). It is found in plants as phytic acid and as part of phospholipids in the membranes.[23]

Essentiality of myo-inositol — It has been found that myo-inositol serves as a messenger for mediated hormonal stimuli for mobilizing calcium intracellularly as well as a substrate for the biosynthesis of phosphatidylinositol.[24] A deficiency in rats has been reported to produce triglyceride accumulation and abnormal fatty metabolism. Abnormal levels of myo-inositol has been found in animals exhibiting diabetes mellitus, chronic renal failure, and galactosemia. Patients who experience diabetic neuropathy have demonstrated an improvement in nerve conduction when treated with additional myo-inositol. No RDA has been set for myo-inositol, although possible therapeutic roles in diabetes mellitus and chronic renal failure have been indicated. Inositol is regulated through synthesis and catabolism. The intestinal flora also synthesize myo-inositol. Serum levels reflect dietary levels under most normal conditions.

Myo-inositol and exercise — Myo-inositol is one of the substances that is often linked to a type of B vitamin. It does serve as a coenzyme like a B vitamin in some metabolic pathways. Because of this function, it may be advocated as an ergogenic aid to enhance performance and exercise. No research was found to support this possibility, however.

D. BORON

Minerals such as arsenic, nickel, silicon, and boron have been established to be essential in animals.[25] Boron, in particular, has gained attention for its essentiality and effect on exercise and performance.

Essentiality of Boron — Boron affects calcium and magnesium metabolism. Deficiencies have been reported in rats, chickens, and humans.[25,26]

Boron and exercise — Boron supplementation has been shown to affect serum phosphorus and magnesium concentration in young women and this effect was modified by exercise. Boron supplementation has been associated with balancing blood minerals, especially phosphorus, to optimize bone mineralization.[27] Another study did not verify the effects of a 3-mg boron supplement on mineral metabolism and hormone levels in postmenopausal women that had doubled serum testosterone levels.[25] But in another study in which male body builders were supplemented with 2.5 mg of boron, increased plasma testosterone, lean mass, and strength were shown.[28]

III. COENZYMES, GROWTH FACTORS, AMINO ACIDS, AND BUFFERS THAT MAY BE RELATED TO ATHLETIC PERFORMANCE IN HUMANS

Interest continues in the area of possible nutritional effects of compounds known as coenzymes, growth factors, amino acids, and buffers and their possible effects on exercise.

Celano et al.[29] investigated several polyamines, sperminic, and spermidine that were required for the normal growth of cells in the rat, and Dufour et al.[30] studied the maturation of the intestinal cells. DeLucchi et al.[31] and Kulkarni et al.[32] demonstrated immunologic suppression and the necessity of dietary nucleotides in human infants and laboratory animals. Rats and mice acquired deficiency signs when fed a diet deficient in cofactor pyrroloquinoline quinone.

Other growth factors are required in cell or tissue cultures and for bacteria and other invertebrates. Many of these are not required in human diets since they can be synthesized in the tissues of higher animals.

Many of these substances are advocated by nonscientific communities as necessary for body building and as ergogenic aids. Some of these substances are coenzyme Q_{10}, pyrroloquinoline quinone, nucleosides, inosine, creatine, arginine, ornithine, aspartates, and buffers.

A. COENZYME Q_{10}

Ubiquinone, better known as Coenzyme Q_{10} (CoQ_{10}) is a lipid which occurs naturally in the mitochondria. It is a redox carrier and is involved in the oxidative phosphorylation process.

Essentiality of CoQ_{10} — High concentrations exist in the heart and it has been used therapeutically for treatment of cardiovascular disease by utilizing its oxidative and reduction role.[33] Coenzyme Q_{10} also has been suggested to be effective for endurance athletes because of the increased oxygen uptake and exercise performance observed in cardiac patients.[34]

CoQ_{10} and exercise — Although supplementation with CoQ_{10} significantly increased serum CoQ_{10} levels of humans compared to the placebo groups, there were no significant improvements in blood lactate at submaximal or maximal workloads, heart rate, $\dot{V}O_2max$, or endurance performance.[35-37] Schardt et al.[38] compared supplemented groups (600 mg/d) with a control group of 15 patients with exercise-induced angina. The CoQ_{10} was significantly effective in reducing ischemia-related electrocardiographic segment depression as compared to the placebo group. CoQ_{10} caused only minor effects on hemodynamics. Gohil et al.[39] reported that endurance exercise training led to an adaptive increase in the CoQ_{10} content and cytochrome c reductase activity of the red quadriceps and soleus muscles in adipose tissue, but not of cardiac or white quadriceps muscles in Wister female rats. Cockerill et al.[40] reported increased girth measurements and decreased percent body fat in 13 male athletes supplemented with a combination of B vitamins, vitamin C, free-form amino acids, as well as CoQ_{10}. True effects could not be compared to controls because the study was not "blind". The effects of CoQ_{10} supplementation on athletes needs further study to determine safety, bioavailability, metabolism, if indeed it is to be used as a ergogenic aid.

B. PYRROLOQUINOLINE QUINONE

Pyrroloquinoline quinone (PQQ) is a biologically active compound with regard to growth and reproduction in mice. The structure of PQQ is that of a tricarboxylic acid-*o*-quinone. PQQ carries out redox reactions utilizing reducing equivalents from the cofactors riboflavin, ascorbic acid, niacin, and pyridoxal.[41] PQQ has been indicated as a potent growth factor, an antioxidant, and also a cofactor for various dehydrogenases in some bacteria.

Essentiality of PQQ — PQQ compounds have been isolated from human milk and blood cells. The requirement may be conditional since picomolar amounts appear sufficient in the development of the neonatal mice.[42] Various methodologies utilizing enzyme assays, as well as chemical and chromatographic separations are used for detection of PQQ. Further investigation of the biological roles of this compound will determine whether it may be considered a "conditional" vitamin.

PQQ and exercise — To date, no research has been published with respect to PQQ and physical performance. However, because of its function as a growth factor, research in the area of physical performance is warranted.

C. INOSINE

The nucleoside inosine, in increased amounts in the cells, has been advocated to force additional synthesis of adenosine and therefore provide more ATP. Inosine also may provide nucleotide precursors for DNA, RNA, and protein synthesis.[6]

Essentiality of inosine — Parenteral inosine has been shown to have therapeutic benefits in some cardiac conditions such as angina, digitalis toxicity, and senility in older patients as reported in a couple of French studies.[43,44] Excess inosine is metabolized to uric acid by the enzyme xanthine oxidase, contributing to the condition of gout. In addition, in the exercising muscle increased formation of free radicals occur from the conversion of xanthine dehydrogenase to xanthine oxidase. Thus, supplementation with inosine may contribute to toxicity and an unhealthy state.

Inosine and exercise — Inosine has been indicated as an energy enhancer and to aid in increased endurance, recuperation, and strength. Thus, supplementation of inosine has been encouraged for athletes as an ergogenic aid. However, the existing research does not support these claims.[8] Williams et al.[45] found no effect of 6 g inosine on 3-mi run time or $\dot{V}O_2$max in trained runners. Further investigation of inosine and its effect on performance is needed.

D. CREATINE

Creatine exists as free creatine as well as the high-energy bond creatine phosphate in skeletal muscle. Creatine phosphate is converted to creatine with synthesis of ATP by the enzyme creatine phosphokinase.

Essentiality of creatine — The creatine pool in the muscle represents a combination of that which has been synthesized in the muscle as well as dietary intake. This energy-rich pool delivers energy for a period of up to 15 s to the contracting muscle along with ATP before the majority of energy is generated from the energy-yielding stores of carbohydrate and fat.

Creatine and exercise — Since creatine serves as a short-term high-energy bond with phosphate, increased stores of creatine may help to prolong exercise performance. More studies are needed to investigate the effects of creatine supplementation on exercise performance. A study by Harris et al.[46] indicated an improvement in running times of men supplemented with creatine: 10 trained distance runners were given 5 g creatine or a placebo for 6 days.

E. ARGININE AND ORNITHINE

Arginine and ornithine, although individual amino acids, are mentioned here because they are particularly advocated by some of the popular media as an ergogenic aid to stimulate the release of human growth hormone which enhances muscle growth.

Essentiality of arginine and ornithine — Sufficient arginine and ornithine are acquired from protein sources. Arginine infusion has been demonstrated in several studies to release significant amounts of anabolic hormones. Doses from 15 to 30 g led to 4- to 6-fold increases in plasma arginine levels.[47] Ingestion of 6 g of oral arginine increased plasma levels by 100% without release of growth hormones.[48] However, growth hormone was elevated in plasma of subjects after the administration of 1200 g of arginine pyroglutamate combined with 1200 g of lipine hydrochloride to 15 healthy male volunteers aged 15 to 20 years.[49] Arginine supplementation also has been shown to increase the rate of creatine synthesis. The creatine pool was increased after the consumption of equimolar amounts of glycine and arginine fed to subjects at 4 g of nitrogen daily.[50] In addition, arginine supplementation has been reported to reduce ammonia toxicity in animal models. Administration of intravenous arginine of 1 to 4 g decreased elevated ammonia levels in subjects induced to high ammonia levels with intravenous amino acids.[51,52]

Arginine, ornithine and exercise — Arginine supplementation may benefit athletic performance. The stimulation of growth hormones could increase muscle growth. Increased stores of creatine may enhance creatine phosphate synthesis and the release of energy. The reduction of ammonia toxicity to the muscle may reduce fatigue. Bucci et al.[53] reported a significant rise in serum human growth hormone (HGH) of body builders 90 min after ingestion of 12 g (for 70 kg) of l-ornithine. Lower dosages of 40 and 100 mg/kg had less effect on serum HGH levels. Side effects of stomach cramping and diarrhea were reported by some of the subjects. To date, a few studies have reported conflicting results on the effects of arginine supplementation on body composition and muscular strength. Therefore, more research is needed to verify the effect of arginine and ornithine on the stimulation of growth factors and increased muscle growth.

F. ASPARTATE

Another nonessential amino acid, aspartate, with potassium and magnesium salts, has been indicated to lower the accumulation of blood ammonia occurring during exercise.[54]

Essentiality of aspartate — Aspartic acid and its amide, asparagine are completely dispensable amino acids, i.e., they are synthesized in the body and thus are not essential components of the diet. Glutamate can be transaminated with oxaloacetate to aspartate in a reaction catalyzed by aspartate aminotransferase.[54] Aspartate is one of the amino acids directly involved in urea generation by the urea cycle. It is this function of aspartate that has been suggested to lower the accumulation of blood ammonia during exercise.

Aspartate and exercise — Studies have indicated conflicting results on the effects of aspartate on blood accumulation during exercise. Maughan and Sadler[55] reported no beneficial effects of supplementation with 3 g of potassium and magnesium aspartates to 8 subjects 24 h prior to a cycle ergometer exercise to exhaustion. Wesson et al.,[56] however, supplemented their subjects with 10 g of aspartate. These subjects were exercised to exhaustion at 75% $\dot{V}O_2max$. A 15% increase in endurance performance and a significant reduction in serum ammonia levels were observed. Obviously, more research is needed to verify these conflicting reports on supplementation with aspartates.

G. BUFFERS (BICARBONATE AND PHOSPHATE SALTS)

The body has a natural buffering system controlled by bicarbonates to keep the blood pH in the range of 7.35 to 7.45, even in exercise. The production of lactic acid which is formed by anaerobic glycolysis during exercise leads to muscle fatigue. Thus, metabolic alkalosis has been an anecdote to increase the body's buffer reserve of bicarbonates for several years. Phosphate as a buffer will help keep the body's pH in the appropriate range. It, just like the bicarbonates, will increase the buffer reserves and be utilized as a metabolic alkalosis

Essentiality of bicarbonate salts — Respiratory and renal pH regulation is exerted through the bicarbonate-carbonic acid buffer system. This system is made up of the weak acid carbonic acid ($H_2CO_3^-$) and its salt, or conjugate base, bicarbonate (HCO_3). The acid dissociates reversibly into H+ and HCO_3^-. Either protons or the hydroxyl ion are added to neutralize the shifts in the equilibrium. Therefore, the hypothesis in exercise is that the increase in H+ can be neutralized by the additional bicarbonate reserve leading to less fatigue in the muscle.

Bicarbonate and exercise — Several studies[55,57,58] have reported beneficial effects on physical performance of men with sodium bicarbonate loading. Most of these studies suggest that the intensity and continuance of the activity should be longer than 60 s to derive the ergogenic benefits from bicarbonate. Diarrhea has been reported after consumption of sodium bicarbonate. Sodium citrate, when used as a buffer at 0.5 g/kg BW, appears not to cause gastrointestinal distress.

Essentiality of phosphate salts — Phosphate is an essential nutrient that serves various functions in the body. It is involved in the generation of energy sources, particularly ATP from adenosine mono- or diphosphate and creatine phosphate. Also, several of the B vitamins have to be phosphorylated in order to become activated to their coenzyme forms. In addition, phosphate participates in helping to buffer the body's pH system.

Phosphates and exercise — Conflicting results from studies indicating the effects of phosphate loading on exercise performance have been reported. Williams[59] reported no beneficial effects of phosphate supplementation on subjects involved in a 8-km (5 mi) bike race. Whereas, Cade et al.[60] reported a significant increase in preexercise serum phosphate and erythrocyte 2,3-diphosphoglycerate was found after phosphate loading of subjects. Blood lactate levels were decreased and $\dot{V}O_2$max was significantly increased. These ten subjects were trained, male distance runners. They were given 1 g of neutral-buffered phosphate 4 times per day or a crossover placebo of 0.1 g sodium citrate. More research is needed to determine the benefits of phosphate loading on aerobic capacity as well as the potential to buffer the pH.

IV. SUBSTANCES NOT DETERMINED ESSENTIAL FOR ANIMALS OR HUMANS THAT MAY BE RELATED TO ATHLETIC PERFORMANCE IN HUMANS

Vitamins are found in food and are essential nutrients in the human body. The B vitamins are particularly involved as coenzymes in the energy cycle for metabolism of protein and for many cell activities. Athletes have resorted to substances referred to as B vitamins but which do not meet the definition of "true" vitamins. Vitamin B_{15} is sometimes called pangamic acid as well as being referred to dimethylglycine. In addition, they have relied on anabolic steroids to gain the "winning edge' by increasing lean muscle mass and improving strength. Sex hormones such as testosterone are considered for their masculinizing and growth-promoting effects. Anabolic steroids, although unethical and having serious health side effects are still misused by athletes. Some of these side effects, include liver disorders, cardiovascular disease, jaundice, testicular atrophy, decreased bone growth, and increased masculinity in women.

The Anabolic Steroid Act of 1990[61] put these substances under the Controlled Substance Act's Schedule III, thus being regulated by the Drug Enforcement Administration. Many athletes have looked to alternative chemicals which are not regulated by the Drug Enforcement Administration to perform the same functions.

A. DIMETHYLGLYCINE

Dimethylglycine (DMG) originally isolated from plant seeds, grain germs, and mammalian tissues and hydrolyzed from pangamic acid, an ester compound formed between N,N-dimethylglycine and gluconic acid. DMG is often referred to as vitamin B_{15} although it is not a "true vitamin".

Essentiality of dimethylglycine — DMG is involved in transmethylation reactions through oxidation of methyl groups and transfer of one-carbon moieties to folic acid. Consequently, this function is important in biosynthesis of compounds involved in muscle metabolism.[62]

Dimethylglycine and exercise — Studies have shown that DMG lowered blood lactic acid levels in rats exposed to severe stress as well as increased oxygen utilization in human subjects. Bishop et al.[63] reported finding decreased blood lactate levels after exercise in rats as well as human subjects who were supplemented with as much as 300 mg of DMG. Pipes[64] reported that track athletes receiving 5 mg pangamic acid (form not specified) showed an increase time to exhaustion of 24% and increase on $\dot{V}O_2$max of 28%. Girondola et al.[65]

reported no effects of DMG on $\dot{V}O_2$max oxygen debt, oxygen deficit, heart rate, blood lactate, or R values during and after cycle ergometry at 76% $\dot{V}O_2$max. Other researchers[66,67] found similar results of no beneficial effects from DMG supplementation. However, equine and canine researchers[62,68] supplemented standardbreds and greyhounds with DMG and reported finding favorable results. Bishop et al.[63] in a study human study did not find positive results when trained runners were supplemented with DMG. Levine et al.[68] indicated that DMG was responsible for lower blood lactic acid levels after training 10 racing standardbreds. Gannon et al.[62] reported an increase in endurance and racing times as well as improved recovery in racing greyhounds after supplementation with DMG. In a more recent study by Bishop et al.,[63] ingestion of 135 mg DMG prior to exercise had no effects on physiological responses or performances in 16 trained runners.

An area of concern for the DMG supporter is that large doses may be hazardous to humans. DMG has been shown to be converted to nitrososarcosine, a weak carcinogen, in the stomach of mice. Nitrosatable compounds can cause cancer in humans.[69,70] Any benefit of DMG should deter its use because of the possibility of its mutagenesis effect. More research is needed with regard to DMG and physical performance.

B. ORYZANOLE AND FERULIC ACID

Oryzanole are plant sterols acquired from the processing of rice bran oil. They occur as esters of ferulic acid and function as antioxidants.[71,72]

Essentiality of oryzanole and ferulic acid — These compounds are postulated to stimulate growth and hormonal secretion in humans.

Oryzanole and ferulic acid and exercise — Gorewit[73] infused two levels of ferulic acid into cattle and the serum growth hormone was increased but affects on growth and lean body mass were not reported. Plant sterols are poorly absorbed from the digestive tract; thus ergogenic effects are not likely to be observed.

C. GLANDULARS

Glandular extracts from pituitary, thymin, adrenal, pancreas, ovary, prostate, and spleen are used to stimulate the body's own tissues and glands.

Essentiality of glandulars — No research was found to which the need of glandular extracts to stimulate the body's own tissues and glands was investigated.

Glandulars and exercise — One of the most common extracts (orchic) is from the testicles of animals. Trindell and Tannenhaus[74] has contraindicated their effectiveness to function as glands.

D. SMILAX COMPOUNDS

Smilax products are derived from the genus that contain steroids similar in structure to testosterone and estrogen. These include smilagein, sitosterol, stigmasterol, and sarsaspogenin.

Essentiality of smilax — They are indicated to boost existing levels of the hormone and a substitute for anabolic steroids.[75]

Smilax and exercise — There is no research to document their anabolic effectiveness on performance, although they are advertised as natural forms of testosterone.

E. YOHIMBINE

Yohimbine, an extract from the bark of the Yohimbe tree (*Pausinystalia yohimbe*), has also been touted as a natural source of testosterone or enhancer of testosterone.

Essentiality of yohimbine — It has been used clinically to treat impotence but its effectiveness as an ergogenic aid and anabolic steroid has not been proven.[76]

Yohimbine and exercise — Many advocates, nevertheless, market yohimbine products to promote muscular gain and increase in strength. The effectiveness of yohimbine needs to be further investigated in order to deter the market for anabolic drugs.

V. OTHER COMBINATIONS OF COMPOUNDS THAT MAY BE RELATED TO ATHLETIC PERFORMANCE IN HUMANS

Many compounds could be identified in this group and the list grows each day. In fact, this group of ergogenic aids is the subject of entire books. However, a few included here are ginseng, wheat germ oil, bee pollen, and caffeine.

A. GINSENG

Various extracts of the Panax ginseng-containing ginsenosides, steroid glycosides have been shown to spare glycogen and increase fatty acid oxidation in exercised rats.

Essentiality of ginseng — Oral or injected ginsenosides have shown similar results by increasing endurance and reduction of fatigue in exercised animals.[77,78] These effects from the use of ginseng in animals have encouraged the use of ginseng as an ergogenic aid in humans.

Ginseng and exercise — Human studies[79] have not shown positive results when subjects were given 200 or 2000 mg of ginseng root daily for 4 to 9 weeks. The results of blood lactate, glucose, growth hormone, and $\dot{V}O_2$max measurements were not different than controls. However, a very high dollar price is still put on ginseng and advocates continue to seek the beneficial effects of ginseng.

B. WHEAT GERM OIL

Octacosanol, a long-chain waxy alcohol, is the active component in wheat germ oil.

Essentiality of wheat germ oil — Wheat germ oil has been advocated for ergogenic effects. However, it has not been proven to be essential for humans.

Wheat germ oil and exercise — Cureton[80] reported improvement in endurance and reaction times from 42 studies. Improvement was contributed to increased oxygen transport. Saint-John and McNaughton[81] indicated improved conditioned reflexes but not oxygen transport or endurance. Poiletman and Miller[82] found no ergogenic benefits of wheat germ oil on the electrocardiographic T waves of the highly trained athlete. Wheat germ oil may stabilize nerve cell membranes but does not improve endurance capacity as determined from improved nervous disorders when patients were treated with wheat germ oil.

C. BEE POLLEN

Bee pollen is composed of various vitamins and minerals. These vitamins and minerals may participate in the energy cycle as cofactors.

Essentiality of bee pollen — No research was found to indicate that bee pollen is essential.

Bee pollen and exercise — There is no evidence that bee pollen induces any physiological effect in exercise performance. Several researches as cited by Brouns[34] have reported no effects of bee pollen on $\dot{V}O_2$max or endurance performance.

D. CAFFEINE

Major dietary sources of caffeine are coffee, tea, chocolate, and colas; 200 to 300 mg are easily obtained from 2 to 3 cups of coffee. Coffee, a popular beverage, was first cultivated in Arabica and introduced into Europe about 1500, where its use spread throughout countries. Brazil, Columbia, and Angola are the major suppliers of coffee to the U.S.

Essentiality of caffeine — Research has not indicated that caffeine is an essential nutrient. However, the use of caffeine may become habitual and a tolerance level developed. Some of the effects of caffeine include stimulation of CNS, diuresis, lipolysis, and gastric acid secretion. Especially because of the stimulation of lipolysis, some athletes have used caffeine as an ergogenic aid to promote better physical performances.

Caffeine and exercise — The effects of caffeine on exercise and athletic performance has been extensively studied in the last few years.[6] More accurate information has been revealed from better controlled studies and more sophisticated instrumentation for laboratory test. Most studies[83-90] cited employed cycle ergometry or treadmill running. Significant changes in performance in metabolic measurements in caffeine-treated groups were noted in exercise times of greater than 30 min.

Caffeine ingestion increased plasma FFA concentration significantly when compared to control in exercised groups in five studies utilizing trained subjects.[83-87] Two of these studies indicated increased times to exhaustion or total work, two reported nonsignificant changes (NS), and one did not report. Knapik et al.[86] indicated increases in lactate, FFA, glycerol, and glucose. One study[88] reported an increase in lactate, but another study[89] indicated NS in the lactate concentration as well as heart rate (HR), $\dot{V}O_2$max, respiratory quotient (R), and FFAs. Another study[90] utilizing marathon runners did not report performance change, but did indicate an increase in lactate but NS in heart rate, $\dot{V}O_2$max, R, FFA, glucose, or triglycerides.

Because tolerance to caffeine is developed by users, subjects are required to refrain from caffeine for a couple of days prior to the study. Fisher et al.[89] reported significant changes in metabolism and performance of subjects only after the withdrawal period of caffeine.

The general consensus of research indicates that the ingestion of caffeine increases FFA and glycerol over just exercise alone. The time to exhaustion appeared to increase in several studies as well. Athletes need to be aware that over five cups of coffee may produce urinary caffeine levels unacceptable for competition. Other side effects include diuresis, which may lead to dehydration, and stomach upset from increased gastric secretion.

VI. SUMMARY

Several elements and compounds classified as "other substances in foods" have been reviewed which may function in regard to physical performance. These compounds are identified as substances naturally present in foods which are required by some animals or microbes, but insufficient or no evidence of their essentiality in the diets of humans exists. The compounds in the group included choline, carnitine, inositol, and the trace element boron. Also included were coenzymes and growth factors such as coenzyme Q_{10}, pyrroloquinoline quinone, inosine, creatine, arginine, ornithine, aspartate, and bicarbonate and phosphate salts. As more studies are conducted, some of these may be determined to be essential vitamins or minerals for humans in the future.

"Other substances in foods" which were discussed included nutrients not determined to be essential for animals or humans included the so-called vitamin "B_{15}", glandulars, herbs, ginseng, bee pollen, and caffeine. These compounds are exploited for various healing properties or ergogenic aids, particularly for athletes.

Because of the biological function of choline, supplementation has been encouraged by various companies to market it as a "far cutting agent" or ergogenic aid for athletes. Few studies have determined the effects of increased blood levels on the effects of methylation, creatine synthesis, and exercise performance. Likewise, carnitine has been advocated as an ergogenic aid to "cut the fat" and enhance physical performance based on the role of carnitine in transporting long-chain fatty acids into the mitochondria. Carnitine is viewed as a "conditionally essential nutrient" and may prove to be essential in the future. Carnitine's usefulness as an ergogenic aid is not supported by current research. Myo-inositol, although referred to as a type of B vitamin, does not serve a coenzyme role like other B vitamins in the energy cycle. No current data implicate myo-inositol to enhance physical performance. Consistent results were not reported on effects when subjects were supplemented with boron.

Ubiquinone (CoQ_{10}) is involved in the oxidative phosphorylation process. Although CoQ_{10} has been effective in reducing ischemia in coronary patients, conflicting effects on hemodynamics of athletes have been reported. The role of pyrroloquinoline quinone (PQQ) as a growth factor has not been determined with regard to its effects on physical performance. Inosine, the nucleoside, has been indicated as an energy enhancer, but current data do not support this claim. More studies need to investigate the role of increased stores of creatine on exercise performance. Conflicting results as to the effects of arginine and ornithine supplementation on body composition and muscular strength have been reported. Aspartates have been indicated to lower ammonia accumulation during exercise. Again, conflicting results need to be resolved through additional research. Bicarbonates generally have been reported as having beneficial effects on physical performance. However, conflicting results have been reported for phosphate supplementation to relieve fatigue from lactate accumulation in the muscle.

Vitamin B_{15} (DMG) has been advocated to lower lactic acid levels and increase oxygen utilization in human subjects. Although beneficial effects have been demonstrated in stan-dardbreds and greyhounds with DMG, favorable results have not been consistent in human subjects. Other compounds such as oryzanole and ferulic acid, glandular, smilax, yohimbine, ginseng, octacosanol wheat oil, bee pollen, and caffeine have been advocated for ergogenic and anabolic benefits. Research has not been consistent; lack of well-controlled studies or lack of research at all has deterred the validity of many of these compounds. The effects of caffeine on exercise performance have been extensively reviewed. The general consensus of research indicates that the ingestion of caffeine increases FFA and glycerol over just exercise alone.

Much more research is needed on the nutrients classified as "other substances in foods" to determine their effectiveness on exercise and physical performance. In the future some of these may be classified as vitamins and trace minerals.

ACKNOWLEDGMENT

I would like to thank Jennifer S. Jones, graduate student in Communication Sciences and Disorders at Radford University for her typing skills in preparing this manuscript.

REFERENCES

1. National Research Council, *Recommended Dietary Allowances*, 10th ed., National Academy Press, Washington, D.C., 262, 1989.
2. McMahon, K.E., Choline, an essential nutrient?, *Nut. Today*, 22, 18, 1987.
3. Zeisel, S.H., "Vitamin-like" molecules: Choline, *Modern Nutrition in Health and Disease*, 7th ed., Shils, M.E. and Young, V.R., Eds., Lea and Febiger, Philadelphia, 440, 1988.
4. Eagle, H., The specific amino acid requirements of a human carcinoma cell, (strain HeLa) in tissue culture, *J. Exp. Med.*, 102, 595, 1955.
5. Sheard, N.F. Tayek, J.A., Bistrian, B.R., Blackburn, G.L., and Zeisel, S.H., Plasma choline concentration in human fed parenterally, *Am. J. Clin. Nutr.*, 43, 219, 1986.
6. Bucci, L.R., Nutritional ergogenic aids, in *Nutrition in Exercise and Sport*, Hickson, J.F. and Wolinski, I., Eds., CRC Press, Boca Raton, FL, 107, 1989.
7. National Research Council, *Recommended Dietary Allowances*, 7th ed., National Academy Press, Washington, D.C., 1989.

8. Grunewald, K.K. and Bailey, R.S., Commercially marketed supplements for body building athletes, *J. Sports Med.,* 15(2), 90, 1993.

9. Staton, W.M., The influence of soya lecithin on muscular strength, *Res. Q. Am. Health Phys. Ed.,* 22, 202, 1951.

10. Conaly, L.A., Wurtman, R.J., Blusztajn, K., Coviella, I.L.G., Maher, T.J., and Evoniuk, G.E., Decreased plasma choline concentration in marathon runners, *New Engl. J. Med.,* 315, 892, 1986.

11. Broquist, H.P., Carnitine, in *Modern Nutrition in Health and Disease,* 8th ed., Shils, M.E., Olson, J.A., and Shike, M., Eds., Lea & Febiger, Philadelphia, 459, 1994.

12. Feller, A.G. and Rudman, D., Role of carnitine in human nutrition, *J. Nutr.,* 118, 463, 1988.

13. Dal Negro, R., Pomari, C., Zoccatelli, O., and Turco, P., Changes in physical performances of untrained volunteers. Effects of L-carnitine, *Clin. Trials J.,* 23, 242, 1986.

14. Marconi, C., Sassi, G., Carpinelli, A., and Cerretelli, P., Effect of L-carnitine loading on the aerobic and anaerobic performance of endurance athletes, *Eur. J. Appl. Physiol.,* 54, 131, 1985.

15. Gorostiaga, E.M., Maurer, C.A., and Eclache, J.P., Decrease in respiratory quotient during exercise following L-carnitine supplementation, *Int. J. Sports Med.,* 10, 169, 1989.

16. Cerretelli, P. and Marconi, C., L-Carnitine supplementation in humans. The effects on physical performance, *Int. J. Sports Med.,* 11, 1, 1990.

17. Greig, C., Finch, K.M., Jones, D.A., Cooper, M., Sargeant, A.J., et al., The effects of oral supplementation with L-carnitine on maximum and submaximum exercise capacity, *Eur. J. Appl. Physiol.,* 56, 457, 1987.

18. Otto, R., Shores, K., and Perez, H., The effects of L-carnitine supplementation on endurance exercise, *J. Med. Sci. Sports Exercise,* 195, 87, 1987.

19. Oyono-Enguelle, S., Freund, H., and Ott, C., Prolonged submaximal exercise and L-carnitine in humans, *Eur. J. Appl. Physiol.,* 58, 53, 1988.

20. Wyss, V., Effects of L-Carnitine administration on $\dot{V}O_2$max and the aerobic-anaerobic threshold in normoxia and acute hypoxia, *Eur. J Appl. Physiol.,* 60, 1, 1990.

21. Soop, M., Bjorkman, O., Cederblad, G., Hagenfeldt, L., and Wahren, J., Influence of carnitine supplementation on muscle substrate and carnitine metabolism during exercise, *J. Appl. Physiol.,* 64, 2394, 1988.

22. Wagenmaker, A.J.M., L-Carnitine supplementation and performance in man, in *Advances In Nutrition and Top Sport,* Brouns, F., Ed., Karger, Basel, 1991.

23. Holub, B.J., The nutritional significance, metabolism and function of myo-inositol and phosphatidylinositol in health and disease, *Advances in Nutritional Research,* Vo. 4, Draper, H.H., Ed., Plenum Press, New York, 107, 1982.

24. Berridge, M.J. and Irvine, R.F., Inositol triphosphate, a novel second messenger in cellular signal tranduction, *Nature,* 312, 315, 1984.

25. Nielsen, F.H., Possible future implications of ultratrace elements in human health and disease, *in Current Topics in Nutrition and Disease,* Vol. 18, Prasad, A.S., Ed., Alan R. Liss, New York, 277, 1988.

26. Carlisle, E.M., Silicon: An essential element for the chick, *Science,* 178, 619, 1972.

27. Meacham, S.L. Taper, L.J., and Volpe, S.L., Effect of boron supplementation on blood and urinary calcium, magnesium, and phosphorus, and urinary boron in athletic and sedentary women, *Am. J. Clin. Nutr.,* 61, 341, 1995.

28. Ferrando, A. and Green, N.R., The effect of boron supplementation on lean body mass, plasma testosterone levels and strength in male weightlifters, *FASEB J.,* A6, 1946, 1992.

29. Celano, P., Baylin, S.B., Giardiello, F.M., Nelkin, B.D., and Casero, J.A., Jr., Effect of polyamine depletion on c-myc-expression in human colon carcinoma cells, *J. Biol. Chem.,* 263, 5491, 1988.

30. Dufour, C., Dandrufosse, G., Forget, P., Vermesse, F., Roman, N., and Lepoint, P., Spermine and spermidine induce intestinal maturation in the rat, *Gastroenterology,* 95, 12, 1988.

31. DeLucchi, C., Pita, M.L., Faus, M.J., Molina, J.A., Uauy, R., and Gil, A., Effects of dietary mucleotides on the fatty acid composition of erythrocyte membrane lipids in term infants, *J. Pediatr. Gastroenterology Nutr.,* 6, 568, 1987.

32. Kulkarni, A.D., Fanslow, W.C., Rudolph, F.B., and Van Buren, C.T., Modulation of delayed hypersensitivity in mice by dietary nucleotide restriction, *Transplantation,* 44, 847, 1987.

33. Vanfraechem, J.H.P., Picalausa, C., and Folkers, K., Effects of CoQ_{10} on physical performance and recovery in myocardial facture, *Biomed. Clin. Aspects Coenzyme Q.,* 5, 371, 1986.

34. Brouns, F., *Nutritional Needs of Athletes,* John Wiley & Sons, Chichester, 117, 1993.

35. Braun, B, Clarkson, P., and Freedson, P., The effect of coenzyme Q_{10} supplementation on exercise performance, $\dot{V}O_2$max, and lipid peroxidation in trained cyclists, *Int. J. Sports Nutr.,* 1, 1991.

36. Roberts, J., The effect of coenzyme Q_{10} on exercise performance, *Med. Sci. Sports Exercise,* 225, 87, 1990.

37. Zuliani, U., Bonetti, A., and Campana, U., The influence of ubiquinone (CoQ10) on the metabolic response to work, *J. Sports Med. Phys. Fitness,* 29, 57, 1989.

38. Schardt, F., Welzel, D., Schiess, W., and Toda, K., Effect of coenzyme Q10 on ischaemia-induced St-segment depression a double blind, placebo-controlled crossover study, *Biomed. Clin. Aspects Coenzyme Q.,* 5, 385, 1986.

39. Gohil, K., Rothfuss, L., Lang, J., and Packer, L., Effect of exercise on tissue vitamin E and ubiquinone content, *J. Appl. Physiol.,* 63, 1638, 1985.

40. Cockerill, D.L and Bucci, L.R., Increases in muscle girth and decreases in body fat associated with a nutritional supplement program, *Clin. Sports Med.,* 1, 73, 1987.

41. Steinberg, F.M. and Bucker, R.B., Pyrroloquinoline quinone, *Modern Nutrition in Health and Disease,* 8th ed., Shils, M.E., Olson, J.A., and Shike, M., Eds., Lea & Febiger, Philadelphia, 8473, 1994.

42. Paz, M.A., Fluckiger, R., Boak, A., and Kagan, H.M., Specific detection of quinoproteins by redox-cycling staining, *J. Biol. Chem.,* 266, 689, 1991.

43. Lachieze-Rey, E., Experimentation, de l' inosine en pathologie geriatrique, *Lyon Med.,* 222, 83, 1969.

44. Linquette, M., Fossati, P., Luez, G., and Lefebore, J., Experiementation clinique de l' inosine au cours des affections cardiovasculaires, et en reanimation chirurgicale, *Lille Med.,* 12, 265, 1967

45. Williams, M., Kreider, R., and Hunter, D., Effect of oral inosine supplementation on 3-mile treadmill run performance and $\dot{V}O_2$ peak, *Med. Sci. Sports Exercise,* 22, 517,, 1990.

46. Harris, R.C., Viru, M., Greenhaff, P.L., and Hultman, E., The effect of oral creatine supplementation on running performance during maximal short term exercise in man, *J. Physiol.,* 467, 74, 1993.

47. Penny, R., Blizzard, R.M., and Davis, T., Sequential arginine and insulin tolerance test on the same day, *J. Clin. Endocrinol.,* 29, 1499, 1969.

48. Braverman, E.R. and Pfeiffer, C.C., Arginine and citrulline in the healing nutrients within, *Facts, Findings and New Research on Amino Acids,* Keats Publishing, New Canaan, CT, 173, 1986.

49. Isidori, A., Lo Monaco, A., and Cappa, M., A study of growth hormone release in man after oral adminstration of amino acids, *Curr. Med. Res. Opinion,* 7, 475, 1981.

50. Crim, M.C., Calloway, D.H., and Margen, S., Creatine metabolism in men. Creatine pool size and turnover in relation to creatine intake, *J. Nutr.,* 106, 371, 1976.

51. Fahey, J.L., Toxicity and blood ammonia rise resulting from intravenous amino acid administration in man, the protective effect of L-arginine, *J. Clin. Invest.,* 36, 1647, 1957.

52. Najarian, J.S. and Harper, H.A., A clinical study of the effect of arginine on blood ammonia, *Am. J. Med.,* 25, 832, 1956.

53. Bucci, L., Hickson, J.F., Pivarnik, J.M., Wolinsky, I., and McMahon, J.C., Ornithine ingestion and growth hormone release in bodybuilders, *Nutr. Res.,* 10, 239, 1990.

54. Groff, J.L., Gropper, S.S., and Hunt, S.M., *Advanced Nutrition and Human Metabolism,* 2nd ed., West Publications, Minneapolis 172, 1995.

55. Maughan, R.J. and Sadler, D.J.M., The effects of oral administration of salts of aspartic acid on the metabolic response to prolonged exhausting exercise in man, *Int. J. Sports Med.,* 4, 119, 1983.

56. Wesson, M., McNaughton, L., and Daves, P., Effects of oral administration of aspartic acid salts on the endeurance capacity of trained athletes, *Res. Q. Exercise Sport,* 59, 234, 1988.

57. Gledhill, N., Bicarbonate ingestion and anaerobic performance, *Sports Med.,* 1, 177, 1984.

58. Heighenhauser, B. and Jones, N., Bicarbonate loading, *Ergogenics: Enhancement of Performance in Exercise and Sport,* Lamb, D. and Williams, M., Eds., Brown and Benchmark, Dubuque, IA, 1991.

59. Williams, M.H., *Nutrition for Fitness and Sport,* 3rd ed., Wm. C. Brown Publishers, Dubuque, IA, 1992.

60. Cade, R., Conte, M., Zauner, C., Mars, D., Peterson, J., Lunne, D., Hommen, N., and Packer, D., Effects of phosphate loading on 2, 3-disphosphoglycerate and maximal oxygen uptake, *Med. Sci, Sports Exerc*ise, 16, 263, 1984.

61. Title XIX, Anabolic Steroids Control Act of 1990, 101st Cong., 2nd sess., P.L. 101-647, Sec. 1902, November 29, 1990.

62. Gannon, J.R. and Kendall, R.V., A clinical evaluation of N, N_1 Dimethylglycine (DMG) and diisopropylammonium dichloroacetate (DIPA) on the performance of racing greyhounds, *Canine Pract.,* 9(6), 7, 1982.

63. Bishop, P.A., Smith, J.F., and Young, B., Effects of N, N-Dimethylglycine on physiological response and performance in trained runners, *J. Sports Med.,* 27, 53, 1987.

64. Pipes, T.V., The effects of pangamic acid on performance in trained athletes, *Med. Sci. Sports Exercise,* 12, 98, 1988.

65. Girondola, R.N., Wiswell, R.A., and Bulbulian, R., Effects of pangamic acid (B-15) ingestion on metabolic response to exercise, *Biochem. Med.,* 24, 218, 1980.

66. Black, D.G. and Suec, A.A., Effects of calcium pangamic on aerobic endurance parameter, a double blind study, *Med. Sci. Sports Exercise,* 13, 93, 1981.

67. Gray, M.E. and Titlow, L.W., Effects of pangamic acid on maximal treadmill performance, *Med. Sci. Sports Exercise,* 14, 424, 1982.

68. Levine, S.B., Grant, D., Myrhe, G.D., Smith, G.L., and Burns, J.G., Effect of a nutritional supplement containing N, N-Dimethylglycine (DMG) on the racing standard bred, *Equine Pract.,* 4, 3, 1982.

69. Friedman, M.A., Reactions of sodium nitrite with dimethylglycine produces nitrososarcosine, *Bull. Environ. Contam. Toxicol.,* 13, 226, 1975.

70. Colman, N., Herbert, V., Gardner, A., and Gerbrant, M., Mutagenicity of dimethylglycine when mixed with nitrate: possible significance in human use of pangamates, *Proc. Soc. Exp. Biol. Med.,* 164, 9, 1980.

71. Saunders, R.M., The properties of rice bran as a foodstuff, *Cereal Foods World*, 35, 632, 1990.

72. Juliano, B.O., Rice: chemistry and technology, *Am. Assoc. Cereal Chem.*, 151, 1985.

73. Gorewit, R.C., Pituitary and thyroid hormone responses of heifers after ferulic acid administration, *J. Dairy Sci.*, 66, 624, 1983.

74. Trindell, D. and Tannenhaus, N., Glandulars: the latest fad, *Am. Counc. Sci. Health News Views*, 9, 5, 1988.

75. Tyler, V.E., Bodybuilding herbs, *Nutrition Forum*, March 23, 1988.

76. Morales, A., Surridge, D.H.C., Marshall, P.G., and Fenemore, J., Nonhormonal pharmacological treatment of organic impotence, *J. Urol.*, 128, 45, 1982.

77. Avakian, E.V., Sugimoto, R.B., Taugcho, S., and Howath, S.M., Effect of panax ginseng extract on energy metabolism during exercise in rate, *Plant Med.*, 50, 151, 1984.

78. Samira, M.M.H., Attia, M.A., Allam, M., and Elwan, O., Effect of standardized ginseng extract G115 on the metabolism and electrical activity of the rabbit's brain, *J. Int. Med. Res.*, 13, 342, 1985.

79. Teves, M.A., Wright, J.E., Welch, M.J., Patton, J.F., Mello, R.P., Roch, P.B., Knapik, J.J., Vogel, J.A., and der Marderonan, A., Effects of ginseng on repeated bouts of exhaustive exercise, *Med. Sci. Sports Exerc*ise, 15, 162, 1983.

80. Cureton, T.K., The Physiological Effects of Wheat Germ Oil on Human in Exercise, Charles C Thomas, Springfield, IL, 1972.

81. Saint-John, M. and McNaughton, L., Octacosanol ingestion and its effects on metabolic responses to submaximal cycle ergometry, reaction time and chest and grip strength, Int. Clin. Nutr. Rev., 6, 81, 1986.

82. Poiletman, R. and Miller, H., The influence of wheat germ oil on the electrocardiographic T waves of the highly trained athlete, J. Sports Med., 8, 26, 1968.

83. Costill, D.L., Dalsky, G.P., and Fink, W.J., Effects of caffeine ingestion on metabolism and exercise performance, Med. Sci. Sports Exercise, 10, 155, 1978.

84. Ivy, J.L., Costill, D.L., Fink, W.J., and Lower, R.W., Influence of caffeine and carbohydrate feedings on endurance performance, *Med. Sci. Sports Exercise*, 11, 6, 1979.

85. Essig, D., Costill, D.L., and Van Handel, P.J., Effects of caffeine ingestion on utilization of muscle glycogen and lipid during leg ergometer cycling, *Int. J. Sports Med.*, 1, 86, 1980.

86. Knapik, J.J., Jones, B.J., Toner, M.M., Daniels, W.L., and Evans, W.J., Influence of caffeine on serum substrate changes during running in trained and untrained individuals, in *Biochemistry of Exercise,* Knuttgen, H.G., Vogel, J.A., and Poortmans, J., Eds., Human Kinetics, Champaign, IL, 1983, 514.

87. Powers, S., Byrd, R., Tulley, R., and Callender, T., Effects of caffeine ingestion on metabolism and performance during graded exercise, *Eur. J. Appl. Physiol.*, 40, 301, 1983.

88. Gaesser, G.A. and Rich, R.G., Influence of caffeine on blood lactate response during incremental exercise, *Int. J. Sports Med.*, 6, 207, 1985.

89. Fisher, S.M., McMurray, R.G., Berry, M., Mar, M.H., and Forsythe, W.A., Influence of caffeine on exercise performance in habitual caffeine users, *Int. J. Sports Med.*, 7, 276, 1986.

90. Casal, D.C. and Leon, A.S. Failure of caffeine to affect substrate utilization during prlonged running, *Med. Sci. Sports Exercise,* 17, 174, 1985.

Chapter 17

SUMMARY — VITAMINS AND TRACE ELEMENTS IN SPORTS NUTRITION

Judy A. Driskell
Ira Wolinsky

CONTENTS

I. INTRODUCTION

Nutrients, including vitamins and trace minerals, play many roles with regard to sports and exercise. All of the nutrients functioning in energy metabolism, either directly or indirectly, also function in exercise. Deficiencies of many of the nutrients are known to adversely affect exercise performance. In most studies initial status of subjects with regard to the nutrient under investigation was not determined prior to initiation of supplementation. The effects of supplementation in most cases are different in individuals deficient in the nutrient than in those with adequate status. Data are limited as to the effects of doses of nutrients exceeding the RDAs on exercise performance. Few well controlled studies have been published which relate vitamin or trace mineral nutriture, including supplementation, to exercise performance. Even fewer studies have related vitamin or trace mineral nutriture to sport. The presence of nutrients in optimal quantities in the body maximizes exercise performance. The overall health as well as the physical and psychological well-being of all individuals is affected by their nutrient intakes. There is not a separate set of RDAs for athletes, but some recommendations have been made specifically for athletes of different types with regard to some of the nutrients.

Supplements of vitamins and trace minerals appear to be used frequently by athletes. Studies in which data were collected from adults during the last decade[1-4] indicate that about one third to one half of adults in the U.S. use some form of vitamin/mineral supplement. Three quarters of the college athletes included in one survey[5] believed that they needed more vitamins than nonathletes. A vast majority of coaches included in another study[6] recommended that their players take vitamin supplements. Keith[7] recently reviewed the literature and found that vitamin or vitamin and mineral supplementation has been reported in college athletes, marathon runners, female body builders, dancers, and various other amateur and professional athletes. Hence, many athletes evidently believe that supplementation with some of the vitamins and minerals is beneficial to them, particularly with regard to their performance. Evidence suggests that the taking of a multivitamin/multimineral supplement makes people feel better; hence, psychologically, and perhaps physiologically, vitamin and mineral supplementation may be beneficial to athletes. This volume reviewed the various vitamins and trace minerals with regard to their roles, including the speculative ones, in physical performance.

II. WATER-SOLUBLE VITAMINS

More research has been done on ascorbic acid, vitamin C, as it relates to physical and exercise performance than any other single nutrient. Vitamin C deficiency is known to affect physical performance. Various physiological stresses (e.g., infections and tobacco usage) affect the body's need for vitamin C. Studies indicate that athletes have daily vitamin C intakes of about 100 to 500 mg, which appears to be an acceptable range of intake. Several studies indicate that vitamin C has an ergogenic effect, while just as many studies report no effect.

Thiamin is needed for optimal neuromuscular functioning. Vigorous exercise has been reported to lower blood thiamin levels, yet controlled studies indicate that comparatively low intakes of thiamin may be adequate for humans doing some aerobic exercises. Initial thiamin status was not determined in most studies prior to supplementation trials. Thiamin is needed for the metabolism of carbohydrates and certain amino acids. Currently there is more emphasis being placed on the consumption of higher percentages of calories from complex carbohydrates and lower percentages from fats. More research is needed on the thiamin needs of groups consuming high caloric amounts of carbohydrates and lower caloric amounts of fats. To date, the research findings on thiamin and exercise are equivocal.

Riboflavin functions in respiratory metabolism. Exercise in individuals who were previously sedentary or nonathletic seems to alter some of the indices of riboflavin status. It appears that athletes and physically active individuals have adequate riboflavin status, perhaps because of long-term training adaptation or the fact that they may have been consuming more riboflavin. There is no advantage of riboflavin supplementation of athletes unless these individuals are deficient in this vitamin.

Niacin, also referred to as nicotinic acid and nicotinamide, also functions in respiration. There is no evidence of inadequate niacin status in athletes or physically active individuals, and there is no need for niacin supplementation in exercise or sport.

Vitamin B_6 functions in several metabolic pathways, including several involving proteins, carbohydrates, and fats during exercise. Several studies have shown that exercise alters vitamin B_6 metabolism. Vitamin B_6 deficiency may compromise exercise performance. Conflicting reports exist as to whether sustained aerobic exercise produces short-term alterations of several of the indices of vitamin B_6 status. The current thinking is that vitamin B_6 supplementation has no beneficial effect on exercise performance; the supplementation could possibly have adverse effects such as increasing lipid peroxidation. Vitamin B_6 is involved in the protective effect of exercise on cardiovascular disease.

Folate and vitamin B_{12} are involved in several metabolic reactions in the body including those involving amino and nucleic acids. Dietary folate estimations are inexact due to problems in analytical methodologies as well as the vitamin being lost during cooking. Many individuals do not consume adequate quantities of folate and vitamin B_{12}. The use of supplements containing folate and vitamin B_{12} has decreased the prevalence of inadequate status of these two nutrients in athletes and nonathletes. The consumption of added quantities of these two B vitamins by athletes having adequate status seems to have little if any effect on endurance or athletic ability.

Pantothenic acid and biotin, both B vitamins, are involved in energy metabolism. Since pantothenic acid is found in a wide variety of foods and biotin synthesized by the intestinal microflora is available to the body, deficiencies of these two B vitamins are rare. Currently there is no clear evidence of a beneficial effect of pharmacological doses of pantothenic acid on exercise performance; however, few controlled studies have been performed. Controlled research of biotin supplementation on exercise performance is not available. Pantothenic acid and biotin are rarely taken as individual supplements.

III. FAT-SOLUBLE VITAMINS

Adult athletes reportedly are well nourished with regard to total vitamin A. Some athletes take too much vitamin A, which can be harmful and potentially toxic. A few studies indicate that vitamin A may be mobilized from the liver during exercise if the athlete remains on a diet deficient in the vitamin; however, deficiency, as assessed by plasma retinal concentrations, will not occur until the liver reserves are severely depleted and exercise may even increase these concentrations.

ß-Carotene, as an antioxidant, may affect exercise-induced lipid peroxidation and skeletal muscle damage. Equivocal results have been reported in supplementation studies of usually several antioxidants combined, not just ß-carotene, on exercise performance. ß-carotene has some promise of being beneficial with relation to protection from oxidative damage. Carotenoids, from a variety of vegetables and fruits, should be consumed for antioxidant protection, and not just as a source of vitamin A.

Individuals can obtain vitamin D from the diet or exposure to sunlight. Ingesting large doses of vitamin D can result in toxicity. A few studies have been conducted with regard to vitamin D and exercise performance. There is little evidence that vitamin D is extensively involved in physical performance.

Vitamin K may come from dietary sources and synthesis by the intestinal microflora; the body also recycles this vitamin. Low intakes along with antibiotic therapy may produce symptoms of deficiency. It may be that the functioning of the vitamin K-dependent protein osteocalcin is of importance with regard to bone formation, and hence, perhaps to exercise performance. Otherwise, no clear association appears to exist between vitamin K and exercise.

Vitamin E deficiency is rare. Exercise influences oxidative metabolism and vitamin E may lower the oxidative stress associated with exercise. Training does increase the capacity of endogenous antioxidants to neutralize reactive oxygen species; however, more antioxidants, particularly vitamin E, may be needed to maintain the oxidant:antioxidant balance. Vitamin E may be functioning along with vitamin C and the carotenoids in this regard. Several studies indicate that animals supplemented with vitamin E have a reduction in oxidative stress from physical activity. This effect has also been shown in a few controlled human studies. Most studies have shown no improvement in exercise performance of humans with vitamin E supplementation. However, individuals, including athletes, who habitually consume low levels of antioxidants may be at high risk for the harmful effects of oxygen radicals.

IV. TRACE ELEMENTS

Iron deficiency, the most prevalent single nutrient deficiency worldwide, is known to decrease physical work capacity and maximal oxygen uptake. In anemia, caused by iron deficiency among other nutrient deficiencies and pathological conditions, the amount of oxygen transported by hemoglobin in blood is low. In deficiency, a decrease in myoglobin is also observed which contributes to decreased muscle aerobic capacity. Lower concentrations of cytochromes and other iron-containing enzymes are also evident in the deficiency. Iron supplements given to individuals who are deficient or marginally deficient in iron has been shown to be beneficial with regard to aerobic work performance measurements. Thus, athletes at the greatest risk of developing altered body iron status are female athletes, distance runners, and vegetarian athletes. Iron deficiency without anemia is observed with high prevalency in female athletes. It may also be a problem in other athletic populations. Body iron may be redistributed in athletes. Improved exercise performance was not found in several studies in which athletes having adequate iron status were given iron supplements. Iron at high doses is potentially toxic.

Zinc plays many roles in carbohydrate, lipid, and protein metabolism and thus is needed for optimal performance. Exercise induces increased excretion of zinc as compared to non-exercise conditions. However, the body tends to adapt by selectively adjusting absorption and endogenous excretion of the zinc and generally the losses of zinc due to strenuous exercise are most likely compensated. Excessive intakes of zinc may induce copper deficiency. Evidence that zinc supplementation of individuals with adequate zinc status is beneficial with regard to human performance is lacking.

Copper functions as a component of the antioxidant system, yet it can be toxic by causing the generation of free radicals. Copper is involved with oxygen consumption and stress. Reports exist that various types of athletes have higher, similar, and lower blood copper levels than nonathletes. Higher than normal losses of the mineral in sweat and urine during exercise have been reported. Surveys indicate that athletes, like others, may consume less than recommended intakes of copper. There is no evidence that the copper requirement for athletes is different than that of the general population.

Chromium functions in the maintenance of blood glucose levels, perhaps by potentiating the activity of insulin. Chromium excretion is influenced by the stress of exercise as well as diets high in mono- and disaccharides and is affected by the training state of athletes. Athletes as well as the general population frequently do not consume recommended levels of this mineral. Chromium picolinate is an ergogenic product which has been suggested to increase lean body mass and decrease body fat; contradictory reports also exist. Excessive intakes of chromium may inhibit the absorption of other minerals.

Selenium, a constituent of glutathione peroxidase, functions as an antioxidant and may protect tissues from the oxidative stress induced by exercise. Selenium and vitamin E function as synergistic antioxidants. Animals fed diets deficient in selenium have lower tissue glutathione peroxidase levels but endurance was not significantly affected. No significant differences in pre- and 120-h post-race glutathione peroxidase activities were observed in trained athletes; however, erythrocytes were more susceptible to hydrogen peroxide-induced peroxidation after the race than before. When consumed in excess, selenium may be toxic.

Several of the compounds and elements classified as "Other Substances in Foods" may function in physical and exercise performance. Some of these substances also have some of the characteristics of vitamins and essential trace minerals. Those which have been implicated, generally speculatively, to function in sports nutrition are choline, carnitine, myo-inositol, boron, coenzyme Q_{10}, pyrroloquinoline quinone, inosine, creatine, arginine, ornithine, aspartates, bicarbonate and phosphate salts, dimethylglycine, organzole and ferulic acid, glandulars, smilax, yohimbine, ginseng, wheat germ oil, bee pollen, and caffeine. The little research that has been conducted indicates that these substances do not have ergogenic functions.

V. IMPLICATIONS

More research is needed on vitamins and trace minerals in relation to exercise and sport performance. Few double-blind, crossover, placebo-controlled studies have been conducted on humans. The initial vitamin or trace mineral status of the subjects should be ascertained and only subjects having adequate status should be used in supplementation studies. Individuals having higher than normal status indices of the vitamin or trace mineral also should not be used as subjects in supplementation studies, in that these individuals probably have previously taken rather large doses of the nutrient under study for several months. Exercise may affect the form of the vitamin in the plasma and in the body as a whole. Exercise may affect the distributions of the vitamins and trace minerals in the various body tissues. Vitamins and trace minerals may be effective at some dosage levels but not others. Studies should be of sufficient duration for effects, if any exist, to be observed. Some gender differences may exist. The efficacy of supplementation with the various vitamins and minerals may vary with regard to different forms of physical activity and different performance measurements. Does supplementation affect the variables on a short-term or long-term basis? How well do subjects adapt to supplementation and training? More research is needed on the interrelationships that exist between vitamins and trace minerals and exercise performance. At the present time, data are insufficient for the establishment, with any degree of certainty, of vitamin and trace mineral requirements for sports or exercise.

REFERENCES

1. Moss, A. J., Levy, A. S., Kim, I., and Park, Y. K., Use of Vitamin and Mineral Supplements in the United States: Current Users, Types of Products and Nutrients, Adv. Vital Health Stat., Department of Health and Human Services, Washington, D.C., 1989, 174.
2. Bender, M. M., Levy, A. S., Schucker, R. E., and Yetley, E. A., Trends in prevalence and magnitude of vitamin and mineral supplement usage and correlation with health status, *J. Am. Diet. Assoc.,* 92, 1096, 1992.
3. **Anon.,** Use of vitamin and mineral supplements in the United States, *Nutr. Rev.,* 48, 161, 1990.
4. Subar, A. F. and Block, G., Use of vitamin and mineral supplements: demographics and amounts of nutrients consumed — the 1987 Health Interview Survey, *Am. J. Epidemiol.,* 132, 1091, 1990.
5. Grandjean, F., Hursh, L. M., Majure, W. D., and Hanley, D. F., Nutrition knowledge and practices of college athletes, *Med. Sci. Sports Exercise,* 13, 82, 1981.
6. Bentivegna, A., Diet, fitness and athletic performance, *Phys. Sports Med.,* 7, 99, 1979.
7. Keith, R. E., Vitamins and physical activity, in *Nutrition in Exercise and Sport,* 2nd ed., Wolinsky, I. and Hickson, J. F., Eds., CRC Press, Boca Raton, FL, 1994, chap. 8.

Sports nutrition
   and immune system function, 24
   and mental fitness considerations, 22–24
   and musculoskeletal injuries, 24
   research challenges, 225
   roles of various micronutrients on
      performance, 223–225; *see also*
      specific nutrients
Steroids, plant, *see* Oryzanole
Stress, physiologic, and need for vitamin C,
   3, 32
Superoxide dismutase, and copper, 182–183

T

Thiamin, 47–53
   absorption, 50
   in brain and neural tissues, 48
   deficiency symptoms and risk, 3; animal
      exercise models, 50–51
   dietary needs and sources, 3, 50, 52
   foods with antithiamin factors, 3
   functions, 3, 48
   in sports nutrition, 222; research
      recommendations, 52–53
   status assessment, 11, 48, 50
   status and high carbohydrate/low fat diets,
      222; and exercise, 51
   toxic effects, 50
Thiamin diphosphate (TDP), *see* Thiamin
   pyrophosphate
Thiamin pyrophosphate (TPP), 48–49
Tocopherols, *see* Vitamin E
Tocopherol equivalent, of vitamin E, 120
Tocotrienols, *see* Vitamin E
Toxic minerals, 10
Trace elements, *see* Trace minerals
Trace minerals
   deficiency and exercise performance, 7,
      10, 221
   description of specific, 8–10; *see also*
      specific trace minerals
   in sports nutrition, 223–224
   status assessment methods, 12–13;
      difficulties with, 7
   supplementation by athletes, 221–222
Tricarboxylic acid (TCA) cycle
   role of flavins in, 58, 60
   role of niacin in, 67–68
Tryptophan
   conversion to niacin, 68
   sources, 68

U

Ubiquinone, *see* Coenzyme Q_{10}

V

Vegetarian diets
   carotenemia and amenorrhea in athletes
      on, 105
   and vitamin B_{12} intake, 90, 91
Vision, and vitamin A, 102
Vitamin A, *see also* Carotenoids
   deficiency symptoms and risk, 3, 102
   dietary needs, 3
   dietary sources, 3, 101
   functions, 3, 102–103
   in sports nutrition, 223
   status assessment methods, 11
   synthesis, 101–102
   toxicity and teratogenity of, 103;
      supplementation and, 107
Vitamin B_1, *see* Thiamin
Vitamin B_2, *see* Riboflavin
Vitamin B_3, *see* Niacin
Vitamin B_6, 75–81
   deficiency symptoms and risk, 4;
      ischemia/reperfusion muscle damage,
      79
   dietary intake of, 4, 76
     and exercise performance, 78
     and nutritional status in athletes,
      78–79
   dietary sources, 4
   exercise and metabolism of, 77
   functions, 4; related to exercise, 76
   group, 76
   and oxidant stress, 79
   roles, 4
     coenzyme, 76
     in homocysteinemia, 80
   in sports nutrition, 222
   status assessment methods, 11, 76
Vitamin B_{12}, *see* Cobalamins
Vitamin "B_{15}", *see* Dimethylglycine
Vitamin C, 29–41
   absorption, 30
   and copper absorption, 180
   deficiency
     and physical performance, 30, 31–32,
      40–41
     scurvy, 6, 30
     symptoms and risk, 6